Dermatology: Diagnosis and Treatment

Dermatology: Diagnosis and Treatment

Edited by Maximus Turner

hayle
medical

New York

Hayle Medical,
750 Third Avenue, 9th Floor,
New York, NY 10017, USA

Visit us on the World Wide Web at:
www.haylemedical.com

ISBN: 978-1-63241-574-5

Cataloging-in-Publication Data

Dermatology : diagnosis and treatment / edited by Maximus Turner.
    p. cm.
Includes bibliographical references and index.
ISBN 978-1-63241-574-5
1. Dermatology. 2. Dermatology--Diagnosis. 3. Dermatology--Treatment.
4. Skin--Diseases. I. Turner, Maximus.
RL72 .D47 2019
616.5--dc23

Table of Contents

Preface

Dermatology is the branch of medicine, involving the medical and surgical management of the conditions of the hair, scalp, skin and nails. Conditions of the human dermis constitute a spectrum of dermatoses as well as nonpathologic states like racquet nails and melanonychia. The diagnosis of these is made by gathering information regarding the skin lesion(s), symptoms, morphology, duration, color, etc. Nail diseases are determined by an inspection of pliability, color changes and markings, shape and texture. Some nail diseases are Onychoptosis, Paronychia, Onychia, Onychocryptosis, etc. Hair disease may usually refer to baldness or excessive shedding of hair. Balding can occur in a localized or diffused area, and can be scarring or non-scarring. Some of the dermatological therapies for the treatment of such conditions are cryosurgery, hair transplantation, tumescent liposuction, vitiligo surgery, Mohs surgery, etc. This book contains some path-breaking studies in the field of dermatology. It elucidates new techniques of diagnosis and treatment of dermatological conditions in a multidisciplinary manner. It is appropriate for students seeking detailed information in this area as well as for experts.

Various studies have approached the subject by analyzing it with a single perspective, but the present book provides diverse methodologies and techniques to address this field. This book contains theories and applications needed for understanding the subject from different perspectives. The aim is to keep the readers informed about the progresses in the field; therefore, the contributions were carefully examined to compile novel researches by specialists from across the globe.

Indeed, the job of the editor is the most crucial and challenging in compiling all chapters into a single book. In the end, I would extend my sincere thanks to the chapter authors for their profound work. I am also thankful for the support provided by my family and colleagues during the compilation of this book.

Editor

Whole Genome Sequencing in an Acrodermatitis Enteropathica Family from the Middle East

Faisel Abu-Duhier,[1] Vivetha Pooranachandran,[2] Andrew J. G. McDonagh,[3]
Andrew G. Messenger,[4] Johnathan Cooper-Knock,[2] Youssef Bakri,[5] Paul R. Heath ⓘ,[2]
and Rachid Tazi-Ahnini ⓘ[4,6]

[1]Prince Fahd Bin Sultan Research Chair, Department of Medical Lab Technology, Faculty of Applied Medical Science,
 Prince Fahd Research Chair, University of Tabuk, Tabuk, Saudi Arabia
[2]Department of Neuroscience, SITraN, The Medical School, University of Sheffield, Sheffield S10 2RX, UK
[3]Department of Dermatology, Royal Hallamshire Hospital, Sheffield S10 2JF, UK
[4]Department of Infection, Immunity and Cardiovascular Disease, The Medical School, University of Sheffield, Sheffield S10 2RX, UK
[5]Biology Department, Faculty of Science, University Mohammed V Rabat, Rabat, Morocco
[6]Laboratory of Medical Biotechnology (MedBiotech), Rabat Medical School and Pharmacy, University Mohammed V Rabat,
 Rabat, Morocco

Correspondence should be addressed to Rachid Tazi-Ahnini; r.taziahnini@sheffield.ac.uk

Academic Editor: Gavin P. Robertson

We report a family from Tabuk, Saudi Arabia, previously screened for Acrodermatitis Enteropathica (AE), in which two siblings presented with typical features of acral dermatitis and a pustular eruption but differing severity. Affected members of our family carry a rare genetic variant, p.Gly512Trp in the SLC39A4 gene which encodes a zinc transporter; disease is thought to result from zinc deficiency. Similar mutations have been reported previously; however, the variable severity within cases carrying the p.Gly512Trp variant and in AE overall led us to hypothesise that additional genetic modifiers may be contributing to the disease phenotype. Therefore whole genome sequencing was carried out in five family members, for whom material was available to search for additional modifiers of AE; this included one individual with clinically diagnosed AE. We confirmed that the p.Gly512Trp change in SLC39A4 was the only candidate homozygous change which was sufficiently rare (ExAC allele frequency 1.178e-05) and predicted deleterious (CADD score 35) to be attributable as a fully penetrant cause of AE. To identify other genes which may carry relevant genetic variation, we reviewed the relevant literature and databases including Gene Ontology Consortium, GeneMANIA, GeneCards, and MalaCards to identify zinc transporter genes and possible interacting partners. The affected individual carried variants in RECQL4 and GPAA1 genes with ExAC allele frequency <0.01 and CADD score >10. p.Gly512Trp is highly likely to be the pathogenic variant in this family. This variant was previously detected in a Tunisian proband with perfect genotype-phenotype segregation suggestive of pathogenicity. Further research is required in this area due to small sample size, but attention should be given to RECQL4 and GPAA1 to understand their role in the skin disease.

1. Introduction

Acrodermatitis Enteropathica (AE) is a rare inherited metabolic condition that affects zinc absorption and inheritance is often seen in an autosomal recessive pattern [1]. The frequency of inherited cases is estimated at 1:500,000 individuals with no obvious correlation in race or gender [2]. The manifestations of AE include alopecia, diarrhoea, dermatitis, growth retardation, and behavioural changes. Although AE has been attributed to fully penetrant homozygous mutations in the SLC39A4 gene, severity is variable even within individual families [3] suggesting that additional genetic modifiers may play a role.

Measurement of plasma zinc is the commonest method of identifying patients with AE, and reduced levels <60 ug/dL were noted in patients B03 and B06 in the original study

Family with acrodermatitis enteropathica
from Saudi Arabia

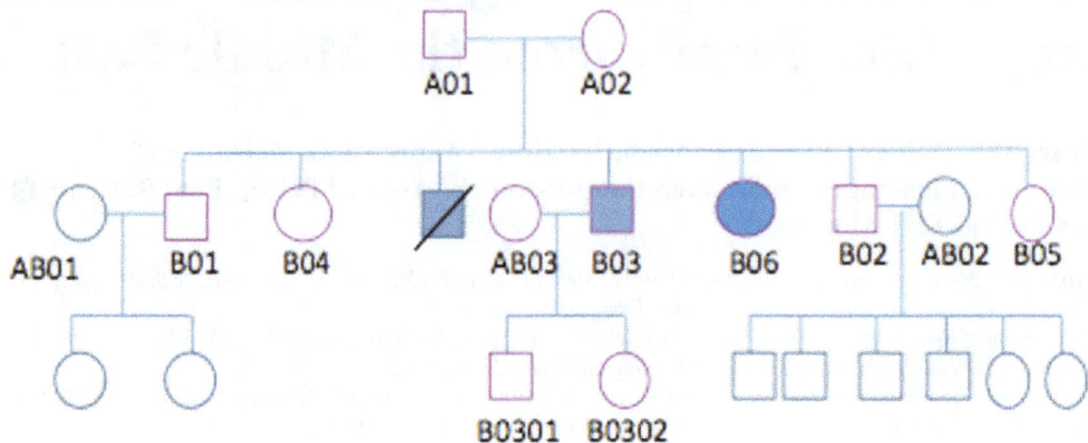

FIGURE 1: Pedigree analysis to demonstrate the family of AE and the sequenced individuals for this study. Genome sequence of the following samples: A01, A02, B03, AB01, and AB02. Only B03 and B06 are affected (one male sibling was also affected, but he died). Note. Shading in blue displays the individuals affected by the disease.

which were correlated with their typical AE symptoms. However, limitations of zinc testing have been highlighted by Garza-Rodriguez et al. (2015) [4] who reported a rare case of AE presenting with two novel missense mutations of the SLC39A4 gene associated with periorificial and acral dermatitis only and with normal plasma levels of zinc.

The family in this study was previously screened and analysed by Abu-Duhier et al. 2017 [3] to identify the pathogenic mutation. In this analysis DNA samples obtained from eleven individuals were amplified by polymerase chain reaction and Sanger sequenced. This comprised both parents and all the siblings including the affected individuals with their respective partners. A homozygous alternate allele in chromosome 8 at position 145638714 was identified in the gene SLC39A4 (solute carrier 39 member 4) which is a zinc transporter. This mutation was present only in the two affected members B03 and B06 presenting with the AE phenotype (Figure 1). The mutation gave rise to a change from the neutral aliphatic amino acid glycine to the highly hydrophobic aromatic tryptophan, with genotype c.1534G>T at position p.Gly512Trp. Although there was strong evidence that this mutation is the cause of AE in this family, severity was variable suggesting that other modifiers may be present. Moreover, because sequencing was limited to a small number of genes, it is possible that alternative homozygous pathogenic change in a zinc transporter gene may have been missed. Others have reported the p.Gly512Trp change in a patient with AE [1], but the role of genetic modifiers has not previously been examined.

To exhaustively define the genetic basis of AE in our patients, the whole genome of available family members has

now been evaluated. In this study, we aimed to identify pathogenic and relevant modifier genes associated with familial AE. On this occasion the proband B03, his parents A01 and A02, and unaffected family members AB01 and AB02 were examined by whole genome sequencing. Two additional family members were utilised as population controls in order to eliminate shared, but nonrelevant alleles.

2. Materials and Methods

Ethical approval was obtained from both University of Tabuk and University of Sheffield, and written informed consent was obtained to use genetic data for research purposes. Blood samples were available from 5 members of the family with hereditary AE and were initially sequenced (as discussed above), followed by whole genome sequencing. The individuals studied were the affected child B03, his parents A01 and A02, and two unrelated family members AB01 and AB02 who were included as individuals from the same population background (Figure 1). Both lanes of three HiSeq 2500 Rapid Run were used to multiplex and sequence the five samples. To produce fastq files, bcl2fastq version 1.8.4 was used with adapter trimming further modified to accept a single mismatch in the index sequence. BWA ALN version 0.7.5a was used to map reads by lane to the human reference genome hg19. Picard version 1.101 was used to mark duplicate reads followed by realignment around InDels using GATK version 2.6-5-gba531bd. Picard was then used to merge lane-level bam files, with additional marking of duplicates and realignment around InDels on the complete bam file. GATK HaplotypeCaller was used to call variants.

TABLE 1: "R" software was used to identify the deleterious zinc transporter gene in B03. An EXAC frequency of <0.01 and CADD score of >10 were accepted. Excluding synonymous variants, at position Chr8:145638714 of the SLC39A4 gene, c.G1534T and p.G512W, portrayed as a rare mutation in comparison to other identified genes and genetic variants. Note. Please see Sup Materials 2 for complete list of zinc transporter genes derived by "R" software for B03.

Gene	Chromosome	Start-End	Exon	Nucleotide substitution	Protein substitution	EXAC Frequency	CADD Score
SLC39A4	Chr8	145638714	10	c.G1534T	p.G512W	1.178e-05	35

The minimal calling quality was accepted at 1, allowing 10 alternative haplotypes. GATK was further used to calculate coverage statistics.

Variant calling files of the five individuals were automatically annotated using wANNOVAR to provide information including genomic annotation, frequency of variant observed in controls, and CADD scores. "R" software was used to analyse the annotated variants. Relevant literature was reviewed and GO consortium data used to identify all zinc transporter genes including SLC39A4. Variants in exonic regions of zinc transport genes were filtered by ExAC frequency and CADD score using "R" to identify rare, predicted deleterious variants present in a homozygous form (see sup materials). An ExAC frequency <0.01 and CADD score >10 were employed to suggest a deleterious variant. (ExAC allele frequency suggests the relative frequency of an allele at a genetic locus in a population [5]; CADD score helps measure the level of toxicity of a genetic variant such that a value of 10 defines the variant to be within 10% of a damaging variant in the human genome.) The analysis was repeated in the other sequenced individuals to determine whether the toxic mutation was present in relatives.

To extend the analysis beyond zinc transporter genes, GeneMANIA was used to identify genetic interactions of SLC39A4. Interacting partners were screened for potential rare deleterious variants although the requirement for homozygosity was relaxed to include heterozygous variants.

3. Results

3.1. Only the Homozygous p.Gly512Trp SLC39A4 Variant Is Sufficiently Rare and Deleterious to Cause AE in Our Pedigree. The identified deleterious SLC39A4 variant p.Gly512Trp (with ExAC frequency of 1.178e-05 and CADD score of 35) was present in homozygous form in B03 (Table 1). As would be expected the same p.Gly512Trp change was found to be present in an heterozygous form in both parents, A01 and A02, but was not found in the unaffected relatives. The remainder of identified variants in SLC39A4 and all other screened zinc transport genes demonstrated either a low CADD score or a high ExAC frequency implying a benign or uncertain significance (Sup Materials 2).

3.2. Screening SLC39A4 Interacting Partners Identified Rare Deleterious Variants in Candidate Modifier Genes. The patient B03 suffered a particularly severe form of AE and therefore is a good candidate to identify additional deleterious genetic modifiers of AE. To identify candidate

genes which are known to interact with SLC39A4, we used GeneMANIA (https://genemania.org) to identify relevant protein-protein interactions, coexpressed genes, and genes of related function based on transcription and phenotypic screening profiles. The interaction databases used by GeneMANIA included BioGRID and Pathway Commons, both including primary research studies. Databases GeneCards and MalaCards were then used to obtain information on the identified genes (Sup Materials 3). The interacting genes were screened for rare deleterious variants which may have negatively impacted upon the function of SLC39A4 and thus the AE phenotype in our patient. With specific focus on exonic regions of the genes and nonsynonymous mutations, "R" analysis demonstrated two genes that were within acceptable ExAC allele frequency and CADD score range (<0.01, >10): GPAA1 and RECQL4, suggestive of significant interaction with SLC39A4 in developing the disease phenotype in B03.

4. Discussion

AE appears to occur mainly in France and Tunisia. The p.Gly512Trp variant was previously identified in a Tunisian family [1]. All published mutations in the human SLC39A4 gene have been collated (Table 2). In the majority of cases, pathogenic variants were present in a homozygous or compound heterozygous state in AE. Families identified across a number of countries with AE have been shown to carry over 30 different mutations in SLC39A4, including deletions, nonsense, missense, and splice-site alterations [6]. Schmitt et al. [1] reported mutations including p.Gly512Trp and p.549delLeu affecting amino acids that were highly conserved between a number of species. Variants p.Gly512Trp and p.549delLeu were detected in homozygous state in Tunisian and Swedish probands, respectively, and the toxic mutation was not identified in any of 164 control chromosomes from North Africa included in their study. Moreover, there was perfect segregation between the genotype and phenotype in the pedigree suggesting a high likelihood for AE to be associated with SLC39A4 gene. As previously described by Abu-Duhier et al. [3], the mutation was located in a putative transmembrane domain and likely to alter zinc absorption by reducing transcription/ translation of SLC39A4. Heterozygous individuals tend to be asymptomatic carriers rather than manifesting the disease phenotype [7]. A significant feature of AE overall and our family in particular is variable phenotype even between individuals with the same genetic change in SLC39A4 [3]. It is anticipated the AE phenotype could be dependent on either modifier genes or an unknown putative

TABLE 2: Modified table from Schmitt et al. (2009) on genetic mutations identified up to date with AE associated SLC39A4 gene. Outlined in bold is the mutation of interest that has been identified in a Tunisian family. Note. Some reports failed to provide adequate information to complete the table.

Exon	Mutation (Nucleotide)	Influence on Amino Acid	Clinical Significance	Other findings	Study
Exon 6	c.119insC	p.Gln398fsX18	Pathogenic	(i) Homozygous (ii) Frameshift	Coromilas et al. 2011
Exon 5	c.850G>A	p.Glu284Lys	Likely/benign	(i) Missense (ii) France (iii) Homozygous	Kury et al., 2002
Exon 1	c.184T>C	p.Cys62Arg	Uncertain Significance	(i) Missense (ii) May affect protein conformation due to loss of disulfide bond (iii) Tunisia (iv) Homozygous	Kury, et al. 2003
Exon 1	c.143T>G	p.Leu48X	Likely pathogenic	(i) Nonsense (ii) Homozygous (iii) Tunisia (iv) Lacks putative zinc binding site	Kury et al. 2003 Kharfi et al. 2005 Nakano et al. 2003
Intron 1	c.192+19G>A	Donor splice site error (possibly)	Likely /Pathogenic	(i) France (ii) Compound heterozygous/homozygous (iii) Possibly altering transcripts through mis-splicing	Kury et al. 2002
Exon 2	c.283C>T	p.Arg95Cys	Pathogenic	(i) Missense (ii) Japanese (iii) Compound heterozygous (iv) Abolishes restriction enzyme site for Faul	Nakano et al. 2003
Exon 2	c.318C>A	p.Asn106Lys	Pathogenic	(i) Missense (ii) France (iii) Compound Heterozygous (iv) Deletion in one allele – failed expression of gene	Wang et al. 2002
Intron 2	c.475-2A>G	Acceptor splice site error (possibly)	Uncertain Significance	(i) Nonsense (ii) Homozygous (iii) France (iv) Appearance of premature stop codon	Kury et al. 2003
Exon 2	c.251C>T	p.Pro84Leu	Likely Benign	(i) Missense (ii) Various countries (iii) Possibly compound heterozygous (iv) Various amino acid change	Wang et al. 2002
Exon 3	c.511G>T	p.Val171Leu	Uncertain Significance	(i) Missense (ii) Heterozygous (iii) Caucasian	Schmitt et al. 2009
Exon 3	c.599C>T	p.Pro200Leu	Pathogenic	(i) Missense (ii) reduces Vmax/alter protein folding (iii) France + Austria (iv) Compound heterozygous/homozygous	Kury et al. 2002

TABLE 2: Continued.

Exon	Mutation (Nucleotide)	Influence on Amino Acid	Clinical Significance	Other findings	Study
Exon 3	c.631C>T	p.Gln211X	Likely Pathogenic	(i) Nonsense (ii) Truncated protein (iii) Tunisia (iv) Homozygous	Meftah et al. 2006
Exon 3	c.641_642ins10	p.Ser214ArgfsX30	Unknown	(i) Frameshift	Santiago et al. 2011
Exon 4	c.766delC	p.Leu256SerfsX16	Likely Pathogenic	(i) Deletion (ii) Spanish (iii) Truncated protein (iv) Heterozygous	Schmitt et al. 2009
Exon 4	c.751C>T	p.Arg251Trp	Benign	(i) Missense (ii) Homozygous (iii) France	Wang et al. 2002
Exon 5	c.850G>A	p.Glu284Lys	Likely/benign	(i) Missense (ii) Homozygous	Kury et al. 2003
Exon 5	c.909G>C	p.Gln303His	Pathogenic	(i) Missense (ii) Homozygous (iii) Substitution of highly conserved amino acid (iv) Japan	Nakano et al. 2003
Exon 5	c.926G>A	p.Cys309Tyr	Unknown	(i) Missense	Wang et al. 2002
Exon 5	c.968_971del AGTC	p.Ser324ArgfsX24	Likely/ Pathogenic	(i) Frameshift (ii) France (iii) Compound Heterozygous (iv) Alter protein function	Kury et al. 2002
Exon 6	c.989G>A	p.Gly330Asp	Likely Pathogenic	(i) Cellular mislocalization (ii) Missense (iii) Egypt (iv) Homozygous	Wang et al. 2002
Exon 6	c.1016_1017ins53	p.Thr357AlafsX10	Unknown	(i) Frameshift (ii) Premature termination codon (iii) Heterozygous (iv) Japan	Nakano et al. 2003
Exon 6	c.1115T>C	p.Leu372Pro	Likely Pathogenic	(i) Reduced protein levels (ii) Missense (iii) Egypt (iv) Homozygous	Wang et al. 2002
Exon 6	c.1120G>A	p.Gly374Arg	Pathogenic	(i) Reduced protein levels (ii) Missense (iii) France (iv) Homozygous	Kury et al. 2002
Exon 6	c.1141A>G	p.Thr381Ala	Uncertain Significance	(i) Missense (ii) Heterozygous (iii) Caucasian	Schmitt et al. 2009
Exon 6	c.1115T>G	p.Leu372Arg	Unknown	(i) Missense	Li et al. 2010
Intron 6	c.1150-2A>G	Acceptor splice site error (possibly)	Uncertain significance	(i) Homozygous (ii) France	Wang et al. 2002

TABLE 2: Continued.

Exon	Mutation (Nucleotide)	Influence on Amino Acid	Clinical Significance	Other findings	Study
Exon 7	c.1203G>A	p.Trp401X	Likely/pathogenic	(i) Nonsense (ii) Compound Heterozygote (iii) Austria (iv) Absence of zinc binding site	Kury et al. 2003
Exon 7	c.1223delC	p..Ala408fsX481	Unknown	(i) Frameshift	Vardi et al. 2009
Exon 7	c.1223_1227delCCGGG	p.Trp411ArgfsX7	Uncertain significance	(i) Frameshift (ii) Founder Effect (iii) Tunisian (iv) Homozygous	Kury et al. 2002
Exon 7	c.1229T>C	p.Leu410Pro	Uncertain Significance	(i) Missense	Wang et al. 2002
Intron 7	c.1287+2T>C	Acceptor splice site error (possibly)	Uncertain Significance		Park et al. 2010
Exon 9	c.1438G>T	p.Glu480Sto	Unknown	Stop	Nakano et al. 2009
Exon 9	c.1462_14711+delAGACTGAGCCCAGG	p.Arg488SerfsX2	Unknown	(i) Frameshift	Wang et al. 2008
Exon 10	**c.1534G>T**	**p.Gly512Trp**	**Pathogenic**	**(i) Missense (ii) Tunisia (iii) Homozygous (iv) Affect amino acids**	**Schmitt et al. 2009**
Exon 10	c.1576G>A	p.Gly526Arg	Pathogenic	(i) Reduces Vmax (ii) Missense (iii) France (iv) Homozygous	Kury et al. 2002
Exon 11	c.1784G>T	p.Gly595Val	Uncertain significance	(i) Missense (ii) Tunisia	Kharfi et al. 2010
Exon 11	c.1646_1648delTGC	p.549delLeu	Pathogenic	(i) Deletion (ii) Sweden (iii) Homozygous (iv) Affect amino acids	Schmitt et al. 2009
Exon 12	c.1888G>C	p.Gly630Arg	Pathogenic for mental retardation/X-Linked	(i) Reduced protein levels (ii) Missense (iii) Homozygous (iv) Jordan	Wang et al. 2002

TABLE 3: GeneMANIA presented the interacting partners with SLC39A4 gene. The databases GeneCards and MalaCards and the literature were reviewed to identify the function, disorder, and tissue expression. Note. The documented information only includes the main signs, symptoms, and tissue expression.

Gene	Description	Disease	Function	Signs/Symptoms	Tissue Expression
SLC39A4	Solute Carrier Family 39 Member 4	Acrodermatitis enteropathica	Encodes for a ZIP family. Required for zinc uptake in the intestine.	Growth retardation, immune-system dysfunction, alopecia, diarrhea, dermatitis.	Mostly Lungs and intestine. Overexpressed in small intestine, fetal gut and CD8 Tcells.
TSTA3	Tissue Specific Transplantation Antigen P35B	Leukocyte adhesion deficiency, type II	Catalyzes the reactions epimerase and reductase in GDP-D-mannose.	Infections, persistent leukocytosis, mental and growth retardation.	Esophagus, stomach and pancreas. Overexpressed in oral epithelium and breast
SCRIB	Scribbled Planar Cell Polarity Protein	Neural tube defects. Tick-Borne Encephalitis.	Regulates epithelial and neuronal morphogenesis.	Cleft lip, myelocystocele, urinary incontinence, hydrocephalus and lipomas.	Intestine, Ovary and Testis. Overexpressed in pancreas.
GPAA1	Glycosylphosphatidylinositol Anchor Attachment	N/A	Links proteins to cell surface membrane.	N/A	Nervous system, skin, lungs. Overexpressed in Nasal epithelium.
CYC1	Cytochrome C1	Mitochondrial complex III deficiency	Mediates the transfer of electron from Rieske iron sulphur protein to cytochrome.	Lactic acidosis, infection, insulin-responsive hyperglycemia and ketoacidosis.	Lungs, Skin, Nervous system. Overexpressed in heart.
RECQL4	RecQ Like Helicase 4	Baller-Gerold Syndrome. RAPADILINO Syndrome.	DNA helicases unwind double stranded DNAs and may modulate chromosome segregation.	Fusion of bones (neonates), slow growth, missing/malformed kneecaps.	Ubiquitously expressed. Overexpressed in Testis and Thymus.
EXOSC4	Exosome Component 4	N/A	Participates in cellular RNA processing and degradation.	N/A	Skin. Overexpressed in whole blood, testis and breast.

TABLE 4: GPAA1 and RECQL4 genes both demonstrated a likelihood of being modifier genes of SLC39A4 in developing AE in B03. Note. Please see Sup Materials 3 for "R" software version of complete list of interacting partners with SLC39A4 gene for B03.

Gene	Chromosome	Start-End	Exon	Nucleotide substitution	Protein substitution	EXAC Frequency	CADD Score
GPAA1	Chr8	145140564	11	c.G1540A	p.A514T	0.0053	15.04
RECQL4	Chr8	145740364	9	c.C1576T	p.L526F	0.0007	16.37

AE gene. Hence we have screened for additional genetic modifiers of SLC39A4 function within an individual with a particularly severe AE phenotype [3].

Our data suggests that the p.Gly512Trp change is the likely cause of disease in our family because it is the only homozygous, rare, and predicted deleterious change within a zinc transporter gene which is present within the affected patient and absent (or heterozygous) in unaffected family members. In addition we identified two rare and predicted deleterious genetic variants in SLC39A4 interacting partners which may have a role in the development of the particularly severe AE phenotype in our patient: RECQL4 and GPAA1 (Table 4). Interestingly Nistor et al. [8] reported that the complete clinical triad of features in AE was only documented in 20% of patients, questioning if only one gene is responsible and if modifier genes could be involved in the variable clinical characteristics. Patients with mutation in the RECQL4 gene have several characteristic features similar to AE; for example, Bernstein et al. [9] reported a RECQ disorder: Bloom syndrome, a rare autosomal recessive condition, which presents with mental retardation, immunodeficiency, male infertility, and increased chance of cancer. Similar features occur in some patients with AE, in the form of immunodeficiency, mental retardation, and infertility. In addition, Mann et al. [10] identified distinctive skin abnormalities in a mutant RECQL4 mouse model. Although the GPAA1 gene is known to be expressed in skin (Table 3), no disorder has been identified to date that has been directly affected by GPAA1 genetic mutation, although rare cases have been reported in which GPAA1 gene amplification and RNA and protein overexpression occurred in hepatocellular carcinoma [11]. Further research is required to explore a putative link between GPAA1 and RECQL4 mutations and AE.

Our data supports pathogenicity of the p.Gly512Trp change in SLC39A4, but in addition we have identified potentially deleterious variants in SLC39A4 interacting partners which may be important to disease pathogenesis and are potential therapeutic targets.

Consent

The participants gave their consent after they received verbal and written explanation including patient information. Individual consent has been signed by each individual.

Authors' Contributions

Rachid Tazi-Ahnini and Faisel Abu-Duhier were the principal investigators. Faisel Abu-Duhier was responsible for the acquisition of clinical materials. Faisel Abu-Duhier, Paul R. Heath, and Rachid Tazi-Ahnini were responsible for the concept and design of the study. Vivetha Pooranachandran, Rachid Tazi-Ahnini, and Paul R. Heath were responsible for the analysis and interpretation of data. Vivetha Pooranachandran and Johnathan Cooper-Knock were involved in designing software for genetic analysis. Andrew J. G. McDonagh, Andrew G. Messenger, Youssef Bakri, and Rachid Tazi-Ahnini drafted the manuscript. All authors participated in the study design, critical revision, and final approval of the manuscript. Paul R. Heath and Rachid Tazi-Ahnini contributed equally to this work.

Acknowledgments

This work was funded by University of Tabuk Prince Fahd Bin Sultan Research Chair in collaboration with University of Sheffield. Research contact grant number is R/130649-11-1. The authors are grateful to the family from Tabuk for participating in this study. The authors also thank Sheffield Diagnostic Genetics Service, Sheffield Children's NHS Trust, for genome sequencing.

Supplementary Materials

Supplementary materials include codes derived for "R" software analysis of the genome data, code used to identify the mutated zinc transporter genes in B03 sample, and code used to identify interacting partners with SLC39A4 gene in causing the disease in B03. (Supplementary Materials)

References

[1] S. Schmitt, S. Küry, M. Giraud, B. Dréno, M. Kharfi, and S. Bézieau, "An update on mutations of the SLC39A4 gene in acrodermatitis enteropathica," Human Mutation, vol. 30, no. 6, pp. 926–933, 2009.

[2] E. Maverakis, M. A. Fung, P. J. Lynch et al., "Acrodermatitis enteropathica and an overview of zinc metabolism," Journal of the American Academy of Dermatology, vol. 56, no. 1, pp. 116–124, 2007.

[3] F. Abu-Duhier, T. Lovewell, A. McDonagh, A. Messenger, A. Ibrahimi, and R. Tazi-Ahnini, "First report of SLC39A4 mutation in acrodermatitis enteropathica family from the Middle East," *International Journal of Dermatology*, vol. 56, no. 5, pp. e97–e100, 2017.

[4] V. Garza-Rodríguez, A. De La Fuente-García, C. Liy-Wong et al., "Acrodermatitis enteropathica: A novel SLC39A4 gene mutation in a patient with normal zinc levels," *Pediatric Dermatology*, vol. 32, no. 3, pp. e124–e125, 2015.

[5] Y. Kobayashi, S. Yang, K. Nykamp, J. Garcia, S. E. Lincoln, and S. E. Topper, "Pathogenic variant burden in the ExAC database: An empirical approach to evaluating population data for clinical variant interpretation," *Genome Medicine*, vol. 9, no. 1, article no. 13, 2017.

[6] S. Küry, M. Kharfi, R. Kamoun et al., "Mutation spectrum of human SLC39A4 in a panel of patients with acrodermatitis enteropathica.," *Human Mutation*, vol. 22, no. 4, pp. 337-338, 2003.

[7] A. Nakano, H. Nakano, K. Nomura, Y. Toyomaki, and K. Hanada, "Novel SLC39A4 mutations in acrodermatitis enteropathica," *Journal of Investigative Dermatology*, vol. 120, no. 6, pp. 963–966, 2003.

[8] N. Nistor, L. Ciontu, O.-E. Frasinariu, V. V. Lupu, A. Ignat, and V. Streanga, "Acrodermatitis Enteropathica," *Medicine (United States)*, vol. 95, no. 20, Article ID e3553, 2016.

[9] K. A. Bernstein, S. Gangloff, and R. Rothstein, "The RecQ DNA helicases in DNA repair," *Annual Review of Genetics*, vol. 44, pp. 393–417, 2010.

[10] M. B. Mann, C. A. Hodges, E. Barnes, H. Vogel, T. J. Hassold, and G. Luo, "Defective sister-chromatid cohesion, aneuploidy and cancer predisposition in a mouse model of type II Rothmund-Thomson syndrome," *Human Molecular Genetics*, vol. 14, no. 6, pp. 813–825, 2005.

[11] I. H. McKillop, D. M. Moran, X. Jin, and L. G. Koniaris, "Molecular pathogenesis of hepatocellular carcinoma," *Journal of Surgical Research*, vol. 136, no. 1, pp. 125–135, 2006.

2

Determination of Spearman Correlation Coefficient (r) to Evaluate the Linear Association of Dermal Collagen and Elastic Fibers in the Perspectives of Skin Injury

Naveen Kumar [ID],[1] Pramod Kumar [ID],[2] Satheesha Nayak Badagabettu [ID],[1] Melissa Glenda Lewis,[3] Murali Adiga,[4] and Ashwini Aithal Padur [ID][1]

[1]Department of Anatomy, Melaka Manipal Medical College, Manipal Academy of Higher Education, Manipal Campus, Manipal 576104, India
[2]King Fahad Central Hospital, Jazan 82666, Saudi Arabia
[3]Indian Institute of Public Health Hyderabad (IIPHH), Madhapur, Hyderabad 500033, India
[4]Department of Physiology, Kasturba Medical College, Manipal, Manipal Academy of Higher Education, Manipal 576104, India

Correspondence should be addressed to Pramod Kumar; pkumar86@hotmail.com

Academic Editor: Bruno A. Bernard

Background. Difference in scar formation at different sites, in different directions at the same site, but with changes in the elasticity of skin with age, sex, and race or in some pathological conditions, is well known to clinicians. The inappropriate collagen syntheses and delayed or lack of epithelialization are known to induce scar formation with negligible elasticity at the site of damage. Changes in the elasticity of scars may be due to an unequal distribution of dermal collagen (C) and elastic (E) fibers. *Materials and Methods.* Spearman correlation coefficients (r) of collagen and elastic fibers in horizontal (H) and in vertical (V) directions (variables CV, CH, EV, and EH) were measured from the respective quantitative fraction data in 320 skin samples from 32 human cadavers collected at five selected sites over extremities. *Results.* Spearman's correlation analysis revealed the statistically significant ($p < 0.01$) strong positive correlation between C_H and C_V in all the areas, that is, shoulder joint area ($r = 0.66$), wrist ($r = 0.75$), forearm ($r = 0.75$), and thigh ($r = 0.80$), except at the ankle ($r = 0.26$, $p = 0.14$) region. Similarly, positive correlation between E_H and E_V has been observed at the forearm ($r = 0.65$, moderate) and thigh ($r = 0.42$, low) regions. However, a significant moderate negative correlation was observed between C_V and E_V at the forearm ($r = -0.51$) and between C_H and E_H at the thigh region ($r = -0.65$). *Conclusion.* Significant differences of correlations of collagen and elastic fibers in different directions from different areas of extremities were noted. This may be one of the possible anatomical reasons of scar behavior in different areas and different directions of the same area.

1. Introduction

Collagen and elastic fiber contents of the dermis perform a complimentary role in maintaining skin shape and firmness. While rigidity of the skin is provided by the collagen content, the elastic fiber content maintains the skin elasticity by forming a three-dimensional network between the collagen fibers. Injury to the skin that results in damage to the collagen network will often have an adverse effect on wound healing. Therefore, the mechanical quality of the skin is mostly achieved by collagen fibers with their strong tensile strength

and cross-link appearance [1]. Elastin, though remarkably less than collagen, plays a critical role in wound healing mechanism as evidenced by the following observations by clinicians:

(i) Transplantation of the epidermis and superficial portion of the dermis from healthy skin (split skin graft) is the most successful and standard treatment in the case of full-thickness loss of the skin. The major drawback of this approach is that the healed split skin graft usually lacks elasticity and increased fragility associated with sensory disturbances. These changes in the transplanted split skin graft may be attributed to changes in the arrangement and content (ratio) of collagen and elastic fibers together with the extracellular matrix proteins [2].

(ii) Langer's line or skin cleavage line has been a well-known direction for making incisions to obtain an esthetic result for many years. Besides, there are many other concepts of lines on the skin that have been demonstrated and made the idea of Langer's line debatable. According to Albert Borges, this is the single best choice of line; however, it is still questionable to fulfil complete satisfaction of wound healing [3]. Nevertheless, the concept of Langer's line over the pattern of arrangement of dermal collagen in a particular direction cannot be ruled out.

(iii) The varied quantity and asymmetric distribution of collagen and elastic fibers in different orientations of the skin plane are known to manipulate the scar appearance [4–6].

In addition to the above observations, it is presumed that relative correlations between these two predominant connective tissue fibers could also be equally responsible for the unpredictable behavior of a scar, despite the incisions made in accordance with the standard lines of choice. Hence, the present work has been undertaken to determine the role of dermal collagen-elastic correlation in the region of upper and lower extremities of the human body. The descriptions presented herewith serve as an essential tool in the esthetic therapy as well as in scar management.

2. Materials and Methods

Skin excision tissues were collected from five different areas involving both extremities from formalin embalmed adult male human cadavers with the age range between 55 and 70 years. The samples from each region were obtained in two directions, namely, horizontal and vertical. Institutional human ethical clearance was obtained through the proper standard protocol before the study.

2.1. Topographic Sites of Sample Collection

Shoulder Area. At the region just lateral to the surface projection overlying the acromion process of the scapula, skin tissue that was taken along the circumferential line of joint was considered as "horizontal," while that perpendicular to it was considered as "vertical."

Wrist. Over the wrist area, skin samples in two directions were taken at the site of proximal crease line of the flexor surface.

Ankle. Skin tissues were obtained at the site about one centimeter above the insertion of the tendo calcaneus.

Forearm. This is located along the midline on the flexor compartment of the forearm between the midpoints of the elbow joint and the wrist joint.

Thigh. This is collected at the midpoint of the thigh between the pubic tubercle and the medial tibial condyle.

2.2. Histopathological Processing. The skin samples were processed for the special Verhoeff–van Gieson (VVG) stain. VVG is employed for the selective demonstration of elastic fibers that appear black in the background of the pink collagen fiber content.

2.3. Image Analysis Details. The digital images of VVG stained sections were acquired at 20x magnification using ProgRes CapturePro 2.1 Jenoptik microscopic camera with the resolution of 694×516 VGA. The collagen fiber tissue which is expressed in pink shades in the image was segmented out by appropriately adjusting the color settings in the software. A similar configuration was employed for the study of all the photos. The area occupied is calculated by the software regarding the number of pixels. In the same way, the elastic fibers which take up black shades upon staining were also selectively segmented, and the area occupied by them was also calculated in terms of the number of pixels. These values were further calculated based on the percentage area occupied by these fibers that is referred to as quantitative fraction.

The images were analyzed using the software named "TissueQuant," which is designed for color quantification in the image [7, 8]. This software provides the facility to choose a color for selectively measuring the areas in the image.

2.4. Spearman Correlation Analysis. Spearman correlation coefficient (r) was estimated to determine the linear association between the following variables:

(i) C_H and C_V (collagen content between horizontal and vertical directions).

(ii) C_H and E_H (between collagen and elastic fiber contents in the horizontal direction).

(iii) C_V and E_V (between collagen and elastic fiber contents in the vertical direction).

(iv) E_H and E_V (elastic fiber content between horizontal and vertical directions).

The outcome results were interpreted according to the degree of association as strong ($r = 0.7$–1), moderate ($r = 0.5$–0.7), or low ($r = 0.3$–0.5) after taking significant correlation ($p < 0.01$ or $p < 0.05$) values into consideration.

3. Results

Descriptive statistics of Spearman's correlation coefficient (r) and the level of significance (p) as tested at the extremity region were tabulated (Table 1) and the comprehended correlation data between the significant variables were depicted (Table 2). Significant correlations were represented as scatter plots (Figures 1–3).

Spearman's correlation analysis revealed the statistically significant strong positive correlation between C_H and C_V in all the areas under study [shoulder joint ($r = 0.66$, $p < 0.01$), wrist ($r = 0.75$, $p < 0.01$), forearm ($r = 0.75$, $p < 0.01$),

TABLE 1: Spearman's correlation coefficient (r) and its level of significance (p) for pattern at extremities.

Variables between	Shoulder joint		Wrist		Ankle		Forearm		Thigh	
	r	p	r	p	r	p	R	p	r	p
C_H & C_V	0.66	**0.000[#]**	0.75	**0.000[#]**	0.26	**0.14**	0.75	**0.000[#]**	0.80	**0.000[#]**
C_H & E_H	−0.15	**0.39**	0.01	**0.9**	0.11	**0.54**	−0.14	**0.41**	−0.65	**0.000[#]**
C_V & E_V	−0.30	**0.94**	−0.01	**0.92**	0.23	**0.20**	−0.51	**0.003[#]**	−0.25	**0.15**
E_H & E_V	−0.34	**0.05**	0.20	**0.26**	0.19	**0.28**	0.65	**0.000[#]**	0.42	**0.01[*]**

[#]Correlation is significant at 0.01 level ($p < 0.01$). [*]Correlation is significant at 0.05 level ($p < 0.05$) (C_H: collagen in horizontal direction; C_V: collagen in vertical direction; E_H: elastic in horizontal direction; E_V: elastic in vertical direction).

TABLE 2: Comprehensive correlation pattern of dermal collagen and elastic fibers between horizontal and vertical directions at extremities.

	Between C_H and C_V	Between C_H and E_H	Between C_V and E_V	Between E_H and E_V
Shoulder joint	Moderate positive ($r = 0.66$)	-	-	-
Wrist	Strong positive ($r = 0.75$)	-	-	-
Ankle	-	-	-	-
Forearm	Strong positive ($r = 0.75$)	-	Moderate negative ($r = −0.51$)	Moderate positive ($r = 0.65$)
Thigh	Strong positive ($r = 0.80$)	Moderate negative ($r = −0.65$)	-	Low positive ($r = 0.42$)

r: Spearman's correlation coefficient (C_H: collagen in horizontal direction; C_V: collagen in vertical direction; E_H: elastic fibers in horizontal direction; E_V: elastic fibers in vertical direction).

and thigh ($r = 0.80$, $p < 0.01$)] except at the ankle ($r = 0.26$, $p = 0.14$).

Moderate negative correlation between C_H and E_H was at the thigh area ($r = −0.65$, $p < 0.01$) and between C_V and E_V at the forearm ($r = −0.51$, $p < 0.05$) areas, which were found to be significant.

Significant positive correlation was also observed between E_H and E_V at forearm ($r = 0.65$, $p < 0.01$, with moderate correlation) and thigh ($r = 0.42$, $p < 0.05$, with low correlation) areas of extremities.

4. Discussion

A study has shown that, in the process of skin graft, an imbalance between collagen synthesis and its cross-linkage and/or the lack of dermal appendages make it relatively less elastic and vulnerable to immobility (contracture) [2]. The progression of healing following skin grafting/skin injury is similar [9].

Among the joint areas, positive correlations between C_H and C_V were observed at shoulder joint (moderate) and wrist areas (strong). No other significant correlation pattern was found. The ankle did not show any significant correlations among the variables tested. On the other hand, both the forearm and thigh areas did show a strong positive correlation between C_H and C_V and positive correlations (medium positive for forearm and low positive for thigh) between E_H and E_V. This observation could be due to strain and frequency of movement of joint.

Further, forearm exhibited a moderate negative correlation between C_V and E_V whereas thigh area showed a moderate negative correlation between C_H and E_H. Thus, collagen and elastic fiber content will have a negative correlation with each other in the horizontal direction of thigh area, whereas a similar relation between them could be seen in the vertical direction at forearm. This difference of trend could be due to the difference of direction of strain due to supination and pronation specific to the forearm and flexion and extension at the knee.

The results of quantitative fraction analysis in these sites exhibited significantly higher content of elastic fibers in the vertical direction (E_V) at shoulder and wrist areas. But for the collagen content, there was a higher proportion in horizontal (C_H) direction at shoulder joint area and in vertical (C_V) direction for wrist area (Table 3). The maximum effect of burst force and minimum effect of stretch force at the shoulder joint and vice versa at the wrist are said to be responsible for the alternative dominance of collagen content, but the uniform predominance of elastic fiber content was ruled out.

The elastic fiber content of the thigh is higher in horizontal (E_H) direction, and it is higher in the vertical direction (E_V) at the ankle area. Both areas, however, have shown no difference or a negligible difference for collagen content in either of the courses (C_H and C_V) specified. The stretch force exerted by slow circumferential expansion of the thigh due to changes in the bulk of thigh muscles during knee movements and compensatory effect of elastic fiber on excess stretching and laxity at ankle area during plantar flexion/dorsiflexion

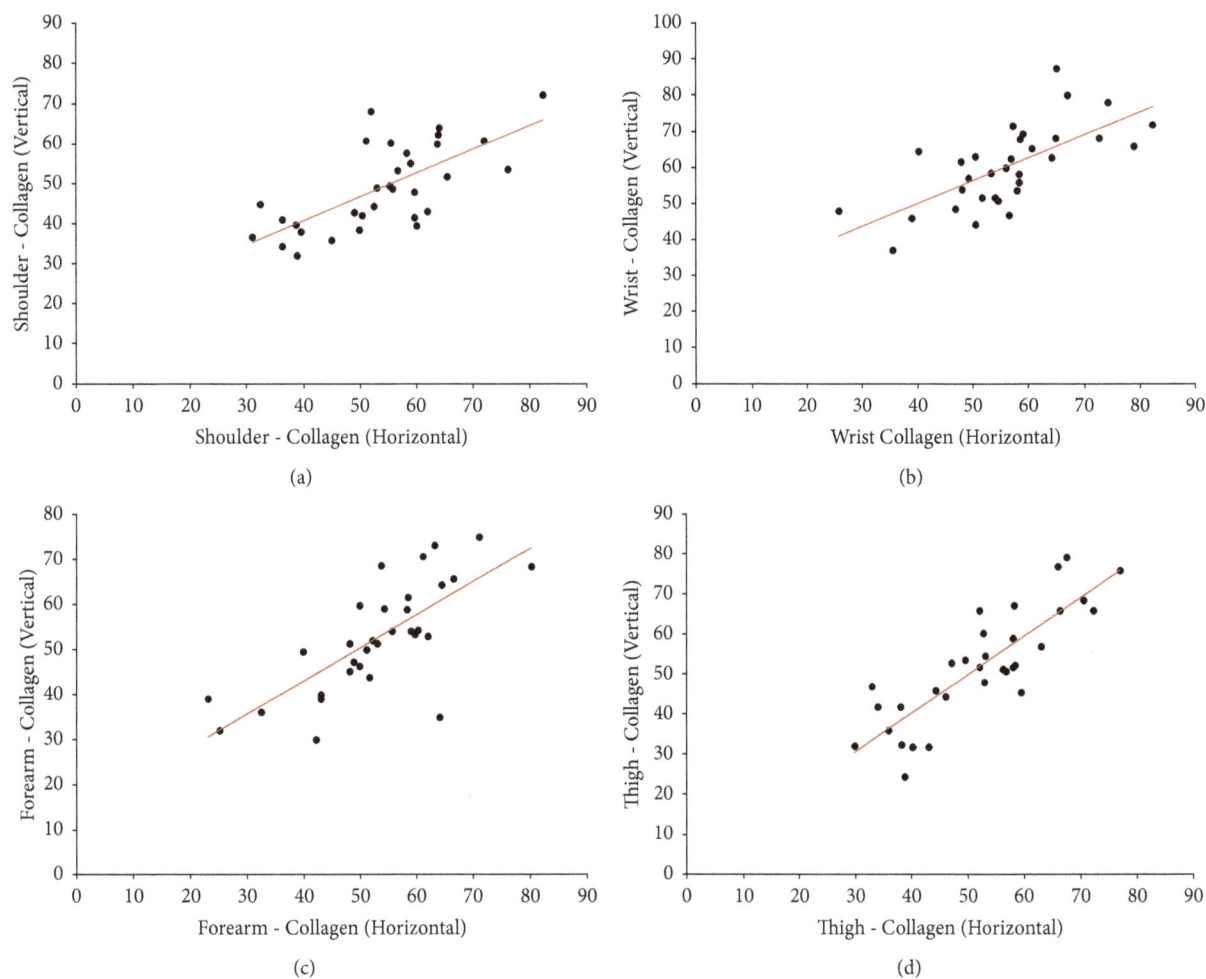

FIGURE 1: Scatter plot showing significant (two-tailed) Spearman positive correlation of collagen in horizontal versus vertical directions at (a) shoulder joint area (moderate; $r = 0.66$), (b) wrist (strong; $r = 0.75$), (c) forearm (strong; $r = 0.75$), and (d) thigh (strong; $r = 0.80$) areas.

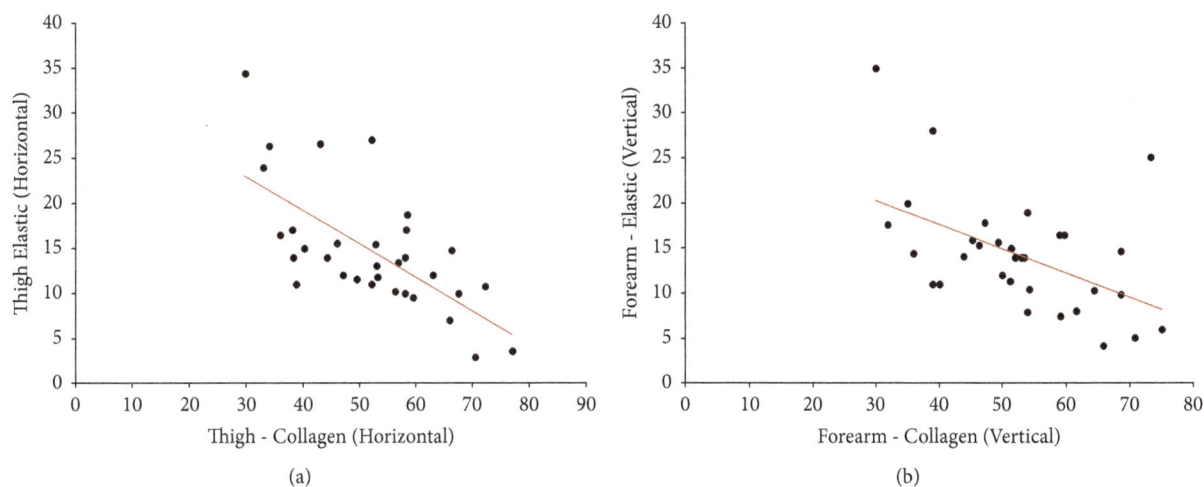

FIGURE 2: Scatter plot showing significant (two-tailed) Spearman negative correlation between collagen and elastic fibers in horizontal direction in the (a) thigh (moderate; $r = -0.65$) and negative correlation between collagen and elastic fibers in the vertical direction at the (b) forearm (moderate; $r = -0.51$).

TABLE 3: Summary of dominance pattern of dermal collagen and elastic fiber content at extremity region. C_H: Collagen in horizontal direction; C_V: collagen in vertical direction; E_H: elastic in horizontal direction; E_V: elastic in vertical direction.

	C_H	C_V	E_H	E_V
Shoulder joint	↑			↑
Wrist		↑		↑
Thigh	-	-	↑	
Ankle	-	-		↑
Forearm	-	-	-	-

↑: *significantly increased content between horizontal and vertical directions.*

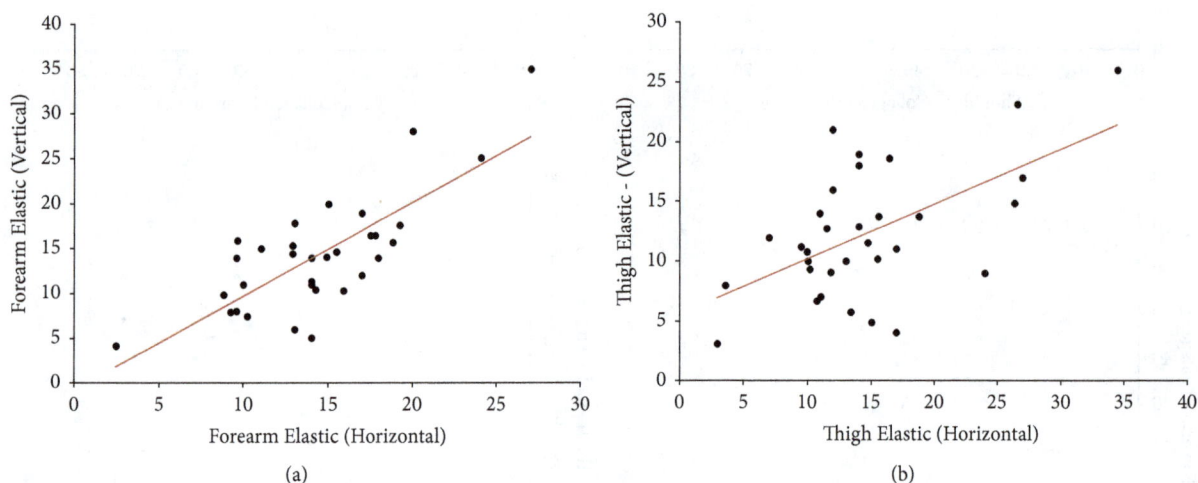

FIGURE 3: Scatter plot showing significant (two-tailed) Spearman positive correlation of elastic fibers between horizontal and vertical directions at (a) forearm (moderate; $r = 0.65$) and (b) thigh (low; $r = 0.42$) areas.

indicated the alternative predominant pattern of elastic fiber content [6].

Various clinical studies also support our assumption that relative correlation between the connective tissue fibers, apart from other reasons, could also be responsible for the unpredictable behavior of a scar.

An interventional study performed on excision wounds of the trunk and extremities when treated with bilayered closure procedure involving the deep dermis (that avoids stretching of scar) revealed an overall better appearance of the scar than subcuticular epidermal closure procedure of the same [10].

A hypertrophic scar is familiar in knees and ankles due to the constant tension (stretching during more frequent movements during locomotion) [11, 12], whereas the shoulder is said to be a common site for keloid [13]. It could be attributed to the dominance of both Cv and Ev at the shoulder but for Ev at the ankle only (Table 3). A study on evaluating the pattern of skin cleavage lines of cadaveric feet suggested that incision should be along or parallel to skin cleavage lines. If this is not entirely possible due to operative requirements, to get an optimal result as far as the scar is concerned, at least a large part of the incision should follow these lines [14].

Research studies performed on animal models reported an incremental mean area per unit of collagen fibers in their posterior limb compared with the abdominal area. That is because the limb is exposed to continuous tensions during movements compared to other parts of animals [15].

Changes in the pattern of arrangement of collagen fibers were also observed in the animal models with the inference of direction of extracellular matrix changes according to the type of stress and their movements [16, 17]. This supports the anatomical arrangement of the collagen fibers that lie more or less parallel to the epidermis in abdomen area when compared to perpendicular arrangement to the epidermis in posterior limb of animals [15].

These results probably uphold the fact that scar behavior will be different at different age due to the difference in production of collagen and elastic proteins in the human body as the age advances. In addition to age factor, chronic exposure of the skin to UV rays [18] or treatment with laser light [19] also affect the collagen content of scar. Therefore, the wounds would heal more slowly and the skin will be more vulnerable to environmental stressors [2].

In conclusion, the significant differences in correlations among the collagen and elastic fiber content of the skin in different areas of extremities are dependent on the effect of localized forces. Hence, the linear association of dermal collagen and elastic fibers in the different region and different directions, apart from tension lines, could be one of the possible anatomical reasons of unpredictable scar behavior in different areas and different orientations of the same area.

Additional Points

Limitations of the Study. In the present study, we have analyzed the data of samples obtained from the male human cadavers with the age ranging from 55 to 70 years. Due to nonavailability of female cadavers and the other age ranges, the comparison of the effect of age and sex on the correlation coefficient could not be performed.

References

[1] E. E. Peacock, *Structure synthesis and interaction of fibrous protein and matrix in wound repair*, WB Saunders Company, Philadelphia, Pa, USA, 3rd edition, 1984, Pp 56-101.

[2] N. L. Rosin, N. Agabalyan, K. Olsen et al., "Collagen structural alterations contribute to stiffening of tissue after split-thickness skin grafting," *Wound Repair and Regeneration*, vol. 24, no. 2, pp. 263–274, 2016.

[3] A. F. Borges, "Relaxed skin tension lines (RSTL) versus other skin lines," *Plastic and Reconstructive Surgery*, vol. 73, no. 1, pp. 144–150, 1984.

[4] K. Naveen, K. Pramod, N. B. Satheesha, P. Keerthana, K. Ranjini, and C. V. Raghuveer, "Histomorphometric analysis of dermal collagen and elastic fibers in skin tissues taken perpendicular to each other from Head and Neck region," *Journal of Surgical Academia*, vol. 4, no. 1, pp. 30–36, 2014.

[5] N. Kumar, P. Kumar, S. N. Badagabettu, K. Prasad, R. Kudva, and C. V. Raghuveer, "Quantitative fraction evaluation of dermal collagen and elastic fibres in the skin samples obtained in two orientations from the trunk region," *Dermatology Research and Practice*, vol. 2014, Article ID 251254, 7 pages, 2014.

[6] K. Naveen, N. B. Pramod, P. Satheesha, K. Keerthana, and R. C. Vasudevarao, "Surgical implications of asymmetric distribution of dermal collagen and elastic fibres in two orientations of skin samples from extremities," *Plastic Surgery International*, vol. 2014, Article ID 364573, 7 pages, 2014.

[7] K. Prasad, P. B. Kumar, M. Chakravarthy, and G. Prabhu, "Applications of "TissueQuant"—a color intensity quantification tool for medical research," *Computer Methods and Programs in Biomedicine*, vol. 106, no. 1, pp. 27–36, 2012.

[8] K. Naveen, K. Pramod, P. Keerthana, and N. B. Satheesha, "A histological study on the distribution of dermal collagen and elastic fibers in different regions of the body," *International Journal of Medicine and Medical Sciences*, vol. 4, no. 8, pp. 171–176, 2012.

[9] G. C. Gurtner, S. Werner, Y. Barrandon, and M. T. Longaker, "Wound repair and regeneration," *Nature*, vol. 453, no. 7193, pp. 314–321, 2008.

[10] M. Alam, W. Posten, M. C. Martini, D. A. Wrone, and A. W. Rademaker, "Aesthetic and functional efficacy of subcuticular running epidermal closures of the trunk and extremity: rater – blinded randomized control trial," *Archives of Dermatology*, vol. 142, no. 10, pp. 1272–1278, 2006.

[11] H. K. Hawkins and C. T. Pereira, "Pathophysiology of the burn scar," *Total Burn Care*, pp. 608–619, 2007.

[12] S. W. Norman, J. K. Christopher, and P. R. O'Connell, "Abnormal scars Inflammation and abnormal wounds after healing," in *Bailey and Love's Short Practice of Surgery*, pp. 598-599, Hodder Arnold, 25th edition, 2008.

[13] F. B. Niessen, P. H. M. Spauwen, J. Schalkwijk, and M. Kon, "On the nature of hypertrophic scars and keloids: a review," *Plastic and Reconstructive Surgery*, vol. 104, no. 5, pp. 1435–1458, 1999.

[14] J. Andermahr, A. Jubel, A. Elsner, P. R. Schulz-Algie, G. Schiffer, and J. Koebke, "Cleavage lines and incisions in foot surgery," *Der Orthopäde*, vol. 36, no. 3, pp. 265–272, 2007.

[15] A. A. Sawsan, "Morphometric and distribution of collagen fibers in the dermis of local canine skin in Basrah province," *Basrah Journal of Veterinary Research*, vol. 12, no. 1, pp. 127–134, 2013.

[16] K. A. Holbrook, P. H. Byers, and S. R. Pinnell, "The structure and function of the dermal connective tissue in normal individuals and patients with inherited connective tissue disorders," *Scan Electron Microscopy*, vol. 4, pp. 1731–1744, 1982.

[17] G. Zanna, D. Fondevila, L. Ferrer, and Y. Espada, "Evaluation of ultrasonography for measurement of skin thickness in Shar-Peis," *American Journal of Veterinary Research*, vol. 73, no. 2, pp. 220–226, 2012.

[18] Y. Nishimori, C. Edwards, A. Pearse, K. Matsumoto, M. Kawai, and R. Marks, "Degenerative alterations of dermal collagen fiber bundles in photodamaged human skin and UV-irradiated hairless mouse skin: Possible effect on decreasing skin mechanical properties and appearance of wrinkles," *Journal of Investigative Dermatology*, vol. 117, no. 6, pp. 1458–1463, 2001.

[19] B. D. A. U. Lins, K. C. R. Lucena, A. V. Granville-Garcia, E. M. Dantas, M. H. C. V. Catao, and L. G. V. Neto, "Biostimulation effects of low-power laser in the repair process (Review)," *An Bras Dermatol*, vol. 85, pp. 849–855, 2010.

3

Comparing the Efficacy of Triamcinolone Acetonide Iontophoresis versus Topical Calcipotriol/Betamethasone Dipropionate in Treating Nail Psoriasis: A Bilateral Controlled Clinical Trial

Nasrin Saki ⓘ,[1,2] Shahla Hosseinpoor,[1,2] Alireza Heiran ⓘ,[3]
Ali Mohammadi,[3] and Mehdi Zeraatpishe[3]

[1]Molecular Dermatology Research Center, Shiraz University of Medical Sciences, Shiraz, Iran
[2]Dermatology Department, Shiraz University of Medical Sciences, Shiraz, Iran
[3]Student Research Committee, Shiraz University of Medical Sciences, Shiraz, Iran

Correspondence should be addressed to Alireza Heiran; heiran.alireza@gmail.com

Academic Editor: Giuseppe Stinco

Background and Objective. Psoriasis is a common chronic inflammatory skin disorder affecting any age and gender. The clinical presentation of the nail disease depends on the location of the pathology: nail bed or nail matrix. We aimed to compare the therapeutic effects of triamcinolone acetonide iontophoresis (TI) and topical calcipotriol/betamethasone dipropionate in the nail bed and nail matrix involvements of psoriasis using Nail Psoriasis Severity Index (NAPSI). *Materials and Methods.* In the present bilateral comparison clinical trial, sixteen patients with clinical diagnosis of nail psoriasis were enrolled and randomized to receive six monthly TI treatment sessions either on their right or on the left hand target nails and daily application of topical calcipotriol/betamethasone dipropionate for six months on their other hand. Clinical efficacy was evaluated according to target nails NAPSI before and after the treatment. Wilcoxon sign-rank test and repeated measures ANOVA were used to compare the efficacy of the treatments. *Results.* The results did not show any difference between the therapeutic effects of TI and topical calcipotriol/betamethasone dipropionate regarding the nail bed score (P value = .356), matrix score (P value = .137), and total NAPSI (P-value = .098). *Conclusion.* Monthly TI has an equal efficacy compared to daily topical calcipotriol/betamethasone dipropionate. It can be used as a safe, easy, and compliant treatment for nail psoriasis. This study is registered under IRCT2017050233778N1.

1. Introduction

Psoriasis is a common chronic inflammatory skin disorder affecting any age or gender [1]. It may involve the extensor surfaces, scalp, joints, creases, or nails. Nail disease can occur even in patients without skin involvements [2]. Although nails account for a small proportion of the body surface area, psoriasis on such visible parts of the body, such as the face and hands, has a major negative impact on physical, psychological, and social aspects of the patient's quality of life [3]. As a result, treatment of nail psoriasis, whether skin is involved or not, is a topic of concern.

Regarding the location of the nail pathology, the clinical presentation is different; pitting, leukonychia, red spots in the lunula, nail plate crumbling, beaus lines, and trachyonychia are signs of nail matrix involvement and onycholysis, oil drop discoloration or salmon patch, subungual hyperkeratosis, and splinter hemorrhage indicate nail bed disease. Matrix involvement is more recalcitrant to the therapeutic options compared to nail bed disease [4]. Due to the significant impact of nail involvement diagnosis on the outlook and severity of psoriasis, dermatologists put Nail Psoriasis Severity Index (NAPSI) in their toolbox to score the disease severity and evaluate the treatment response. NAPSI is a numeric, reproducible, objective, and simple tool for evaluation of the severity of nail bed and nail matrix psoriasis based on the area of involvement in the nail unit [5–7].

Treatment options for nail psoriasis depend on various factors including clinical presentations and patient-related factors [8] and are aimed to inhibit epidermal proliferation, inflammation, or both [4]. They include topical and systemic agents, biologic drugs, phototherapy, intralesional corticosteroid injection, or pulse dye laser [9, 10]. Iontophoresis is a delivery system which enhances the absorption and movement of different metal ions or drugs across biological tissues, such as the skin, muscles, tendons, and joints via a low power electrical current [11].

Triamcinolone acetonide (TI) is a synthetic corticosteroid used by several routes; topical, intramuscular, or intravenous injections, for different therapeutic aims in dermatology [12].

Topical calcipotriol/betamethasone dipropionate is a yellow-to-white substance including 50 $\mu g/g$ calcipotriol and 500 $\mu g/g$ betamethasone dipropionate. Calcipotriol is a vitamin D derivative and acts similar to vitamin D, making a reversible temperature-dependent equilibrium between calcipotriol and precalcipotriol. This drug is recommended for once daily application in treating plaque-type psoriasis [13].

With regard to anatomical structure of the nail, achieving sufficient concentrations of topical antipsoriatic drugs in the nail plate, nail bed, or nail matrix is an issue; therefore, innovative methods providing adequate penetration of the agents are desirable. In this study, we aimed to compare the therapeutic efficacy between TI iontophoresis and topical calcipotriol/betamethasone dipropionate regarding nail bed score, matrix score, and total NAPSI.

2. Materials and Methods

2.1. Participants. This bilateral comparison clinical trial was conducted on sixteen patients with bilateral nail psoriasis referred to the Faghihi Hospital Dermatology Clinic, Shiraz, Iran, affiliated to University of Medical Science from March 2015 to March 2016. Patients with mild-to-moderate nail psoriasis were enrolled in the study after dermatologist clinical diagnosis confirmation and tissue biopsy. Patients who were on systemic medications did not stop their drugs considering the fact that the bilateral design resolves the demographic and baseline matching problems.

Exclusion criteria were having pacemakers, pregnancy, metal orthopedic implant, intrauterine device (IUD), and cardiac arrhythmia, hypersensitivity to any assigned medication and patients' dissatisfaction.

This study was approved by the local Ethics Committee of Shiraz University of Medical Sciences (code: IR.SUMS.MED.REC.1396.37) and registered by the Iranian Registry of Clinical Trials (code: IRCT2017050233778N1). All the patients signed the written informed consent form prior to initiation of the trial.

2.2. Materials and Procedures. Hand randomization for each patient was carried out through flipping a coin to receive six monthly scheduled triamcinolone acetonide (Sina Darou, Iran) iontophoresis treatment sessions either on the right or on the left hand target nails and daily application of calcipotriol/betamethasone dipropionate ointment (Leo Pharma, Ltd) for six months on the other hand.

The investigator dermatologist conducted the iontophoresis procedure in Faghihi Hospital Dermatology Clinic. To perform Iontophoresis (Irantronics Co., Iran), a low power electrical current was exploited to deliver triamcinolone into the skin. Fifty *ml* distilled water combined with 5 *ml* triamcinolone (40 *mg/ml*) as a homogenous mixture (final concentration of 4 *mg/ml*) was prepared and put in a shallow plastic container in which all fingernails of a hand were dipped. The current of 4 *mA* (pulse duration of 0.2 second) was passed through the solution for 20 minutes.

2.3. Clinical Assessments. At baseline a questionnaire was filled for each patient including demographic data, degree of skin involvement, and systemic medication consumption.

NAPSI of both hands' fingers was calculated at baseline and six monthly follow-ups by a well-trained dermatologist in line with six monthly triamcinolone acetonide iontophoresis sessions and daily application of calcipotriol/betamethasone dipropionate ointment for six months. To calculate NAPSI of a hand, nail plates were divided into four quadrants by imaginary longitudinal and horizontal lines. Each nail plate/bed was scored through 0-4; 0 if a nail plate/bed was intact and 4 if nail plate/bed involvement was present in all 4 quadrants; thus each nail has a matrix score (0-4) and a nail bed score (0-4), and the total nail score is 0-8. NAPSI of a hand was the sum of the total score of all fingernails (0-40).

2.4. Statistical Analysis. We used SPSS statistical package (IBM Corp. Released 2012. IBM SPSS Statistics for Windows, Version 21.0. Armonk, NY: IBM Corp.). The Wilcoxon sign-rank test was used to compare the efficacy of TI and topical calcipotriol/betamethasone dipropionate. Repeated measures ANOVA were applied to analyze the pattern of expected reduction in each treatments, separately. *P value* ≤ 0.05 was considered as statistically significantly different.

3. Results

The baseline features and nail findings are depicted in Figures 1 and 2. Sixteen patients completed the study: eleven females (68.8%) and five males (31.2%). No patient discontinued the study. The mean age was 34.31 ± 17.3 (ranged between 6 and 70 years of age). Three of them (18.8%) had skin involvement and two patients (12.5%) had positive history of systemic medication consumption.

Four patients (25%) showed only bed involvement, two patients (12.5%) had only matrix involvement, and ten patients had both bed and matrix involvements. The minimum and the maximum number of nail involvements were four and ten, and the mean number of nail involvement in hands treated with TI and topical calcipotriol/betamethasone dipropionate were 4 ± 1.15 and 4.07 ± 1.

TABLE 1: Mean severity score reduction during the course of study.

Treatment	Anatomical site	Mean severity score ± SD Measurement number							P-value
		0	1	2	3	4	5	6	
TI	Nail bed score	5.63 ± 3.59	5.63 ± 3.59	5.63 ± 3.59	5.06 ± 3.49	3.44 ± 2.68	1.94 ± 2.02	0.44 ± .89	< .001
	Matrix score	6.88 ± 8.16	6.88 ± 8.16	6.81 ± 8.1	6.13 ± 7.77	4.88 ± 7.06	4.31 ± 6.77	3.38 ± 5.91	.011
	NAPSI	12.5 ± 6.31	12.5 ± 6.31	12.44 ± 6.3	11.19 ± 6.07	8.31 ± 5.9	6.25 ± 6.44	3.81 ± 5.86	< .001
CB	Nail bed score	5.5 ± 3.5	5.5 ± 3.5	5.5 ± 3.5	5.38 ± 3.42	4.5 ± 3.37	2.5 ± 2.48	1 ± 1.71	< .001
	Matrix score	6.44 ± 8.49	6.44 ± 8.49	6.44 ± 8.49	6.38 ± 8.38	5.63 ± 7.56	4.88 ± 7.22	4.31 ± 6.81	.104
	NAPSI	11.94 ± 6.42	11.94 ± 6.42	11.94 ± 6.42	11.75 ± 6.42	10.13 ± 5.84	7.38 ± 6.65	5.31 ± 6.68	< .001

TI: triamcinolone acetonide iontophoresis, CB: calcipotriol/betamethasone dipropionate, and SD: standard deviation.

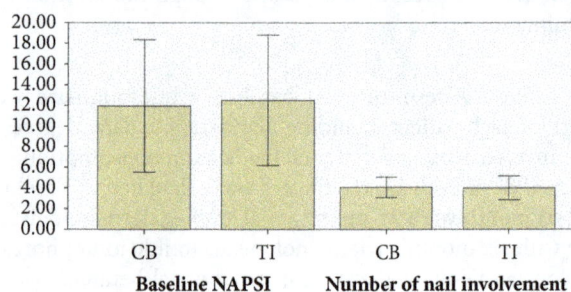

FIGURE 1: Baseline characteristics; TI: triamcinolone acetonide iontophoresis; CB: calcipotriol/betamethasone dipropionate.

At baseline, there was not difference between TI or calcipotriol/betamethasone dipropionate groups, regarding nail bed score (TI: 5.63 ± 3.59 versus calcipotriol/betamethasone dipropionate: 5.5 ± 3.5; P value = .836), matrix score (TI: 6.88 ± 8.16 versus calcipotriol/betamethasone dipropionate: 6.44 ± 8.49; P value = .672), and NAPSI (TI: 12.5 ± 6.31 versus calcipotriol/betamethasone dipropionate: 11.94 ± 6.42; P value = .472).

Initial NAPSI reduction by TI after third and fourth follow-up was recorded for 7 (43.75%) and 13 (81.25%) patients, while it was achieved by topical calcipotriol/betamethasone dipropionate in 3 (18.75%) and 10 (62.5%) patients. Failure to both treatments (constant NAPSI) was observed in a patient with twenty-nail dystrophy. Bilateral complete response (NAPSI of zero) was observed in three patients.

When comparing TI and calcipotriol/betamethasone dipropionate for the overall decrease (∆) in severity score, no difference between the therapeutic effect of TI and topical calcipotriol/betamethasone dipropionate was observed, regarding the nail bed score (TI (∆): −5.19 ± 3.25 versus calcipotriol/betamethasone dipropionate (∆): −4.5 ± 3.46, P value = .356), matrix score (TI (∆): −3.5 ± 4.83 versus calcipotriol/betamethasone dipropionate (∆): −2.13 ± 4.70, P value = .137), and NAPSI (TI (∆): −8.69 ± 4.05 versus calcipotriol/betamethasone dipropionate (∆): −6.63 ± 4.26, P value = .098) (Figure 3, Table 1).

The mean ± SD of nail bed score, matrix score, and NAPSI at the baseline and six monthly follow-up visits for both treatments were shown at Table 1 and Figure 3.

Considering the interventions separately, in the hands treated with TI a diminution pattern was observed for nail bed score (P value < .001), matrix score (P value = .011), and NAPSI (P value < .001), and in the hands treated with topical calcipotriol/betamethasone dipropionate the same trend was observed for nail bed score (P value < .001) and NAPSI (P value < .001) but not for matrix score (P value = .104).

Patients' satisfaction was evaluated by a visual analog scale (VAS) and no difference between the two therapies was observed (P value = .42). Figure 4 depicts the improvement of matrix lesion (pitting) and nail bed lesion (onycholysis) over the study.

4. Discussion and Conclusion

The puzzling treatment of nail psoriasis still remains unanswered, since topical treatments minimally influence nail involvements and systemic therapies are accompanied with several side effects such as hepatotoxicity, hypertension, renal dysfunction, immunosuppression, and severe infections, and hence they are not suitable for those with mild nail psoriasis without severe skin involvements [10, 14–16].

In a recently published review study on treatment strategies, all biologic agents including antitumor necrosis factor-a, anti-interleukin (IL) 17, and anti-IL-12/23 antibodies were introduced as the highly effective available therapies, followed by systemic therapies comprising methotrexate, cyclosporine, acitretin, and apremilast, as well as intralesional corticosteroids. In mild cases, topical treatments, including corticosteroids, calcipotriol, tacrolimus, and tazarotene could be applied. Finally, Pasch discussed the present heterogeneity of outcome measures and scarcity in trials and addressed the demand on more studies [2].

The key factor in treating nail psoriasis is to accumulate the therapeutic concentration of pharmacological agent into the site of psoriatic inflammation, the nail bed, or the nail matrix. Due to the low permeability of most drugs across the nail plate and challenging structural issues in the nail diseases, many efforts have been made to invent creative methods to set up the efficient concentration of so-called safe topical therapies with marginal side effects.

The iontophoresis, a physical method to enhance nail penetration, perhaps decreases the treatment time and enhances the efficacy by increasing drug molecules transport

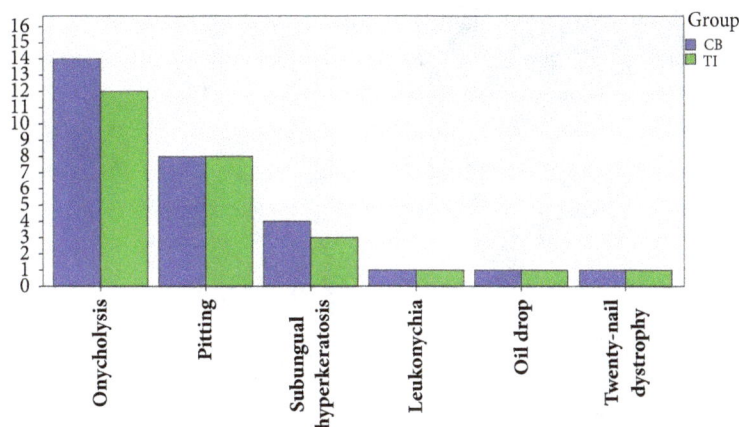

FIGURE 2: Patient's nail findings; TI: triamcinolone acetonide iontophoresis; CB: calcipotriol/betamethasone dipropionate.

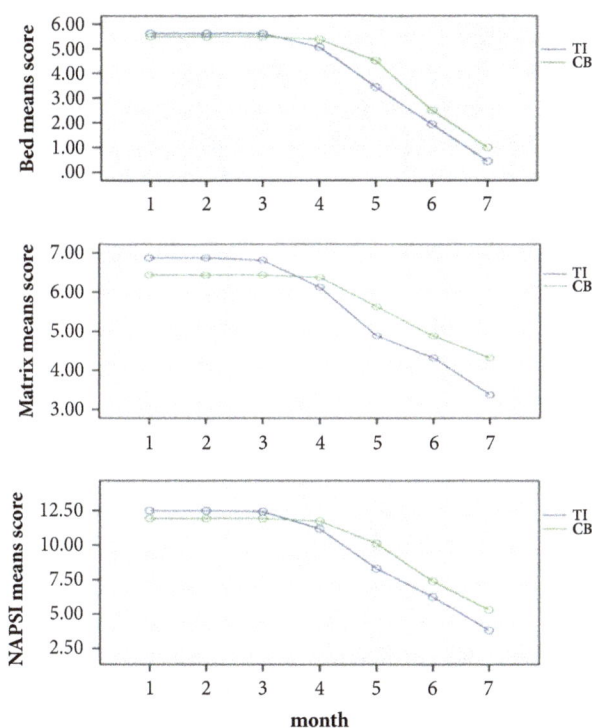

FIGURE 3: Mean nail bed, matrix, and NAPSI score reduction over the study; TI: triamcinolone acetonide iontophoresis; CB: calcipotriol/betamethasone dipropionate. Numbers 1 and 7 are indicator of baseline and 6 months.

across and into the nail plate and the consequent higher concentration of drugs. Additionally, this technique might be a more rapid-more concentrated alternative delivery system to oral route in drugs which are poorly soluble in water through lipophilicity augmentation of many molecules, as it is applied after ablative laser procedures or variety of other cosmetic procedures [17].

Studies investigating iontophoresis efficacy on nail diseases are scarce. In a study published in 2012, Van Le and Howard [18] investigated dexamethasone iontophoresis efficacy on twenty-seven patients with nail psoriasis. After all, twenty-two (81%) patients showed clinical improvement and NAPSI reduction with mean improvement score and mean duration for initial response (month) of eight and four, respectively. Terbinafine, conventionally orally taken, is regarded as a main therapy for onychomycosis, but side effects and poor solubility in water make iontophoresis a rational alternative modality to deliver terbinafine to the nails. Indeed consecutive studies showed promising findings in treating onychomycosis [19, 20]. However, more studies on different drugs are required to get conclusive results regarding the clinical efficacy of iontophoresis in treating nail diseases and this field is an untraveled road.

To the best of our knowledge, the present research is first study comparing iontophoresis with another modality, and first triamcinolone acetonide iontophoresis evaluation as well. Additionally, as an advantage each patient served as her/his own control to reduce confounding factors and personal differences. The present study showed that both treatments improved the overall and Patients did not develop any side effects.

TI was effective in treating nail bed and matrix lesions during the 6-month course of treatment with superior impact on nail bed lesions and more rapid onset of improvement compared to topical calcipotriol/betamethasone dipropionate. Studies on intralesional injection of triamcinolone acetonide [9, 21–26] showed that this modality is particularly effective for improving nail matrix lesions and moderately effective for nail bed lesions [2]. But intralesional injection is a painful procedure and accompanied with numerous reported adverse effects such as subungual hematomas, short-term paresthesia, loss of nail plate, atrophy at the injection sites, epidermal inclusion cysts, tattooing with minute rubber particles, rupture of extensor tendon, and blood splash-back on the instrument and the physician [2, 9, 21, 25–28]; hence, this procedure cannot be a preferred choice of treatment. In addition, our findings were obtained from more severe cases, higher mean baseline NAPSI, compared with milder nail psoriasis patients enrolled in most of the aforementioned studies on intralesional steroid injections.

Combination therapy with corticosteroids, particularly the combination of topical betamethasone with calcipotriol,

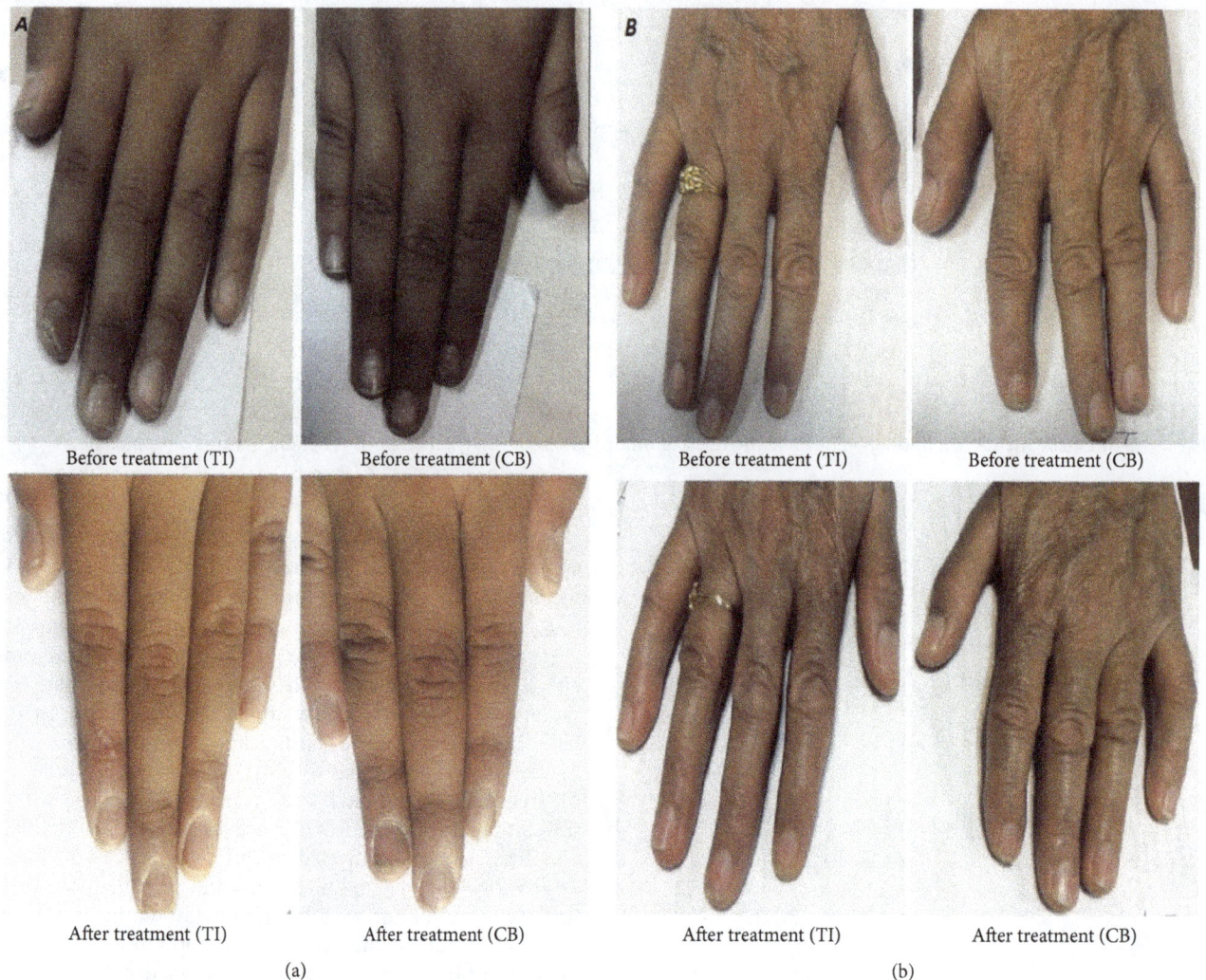

FIGURE 4: (a) A patient with nail matrix involvement (pitting); (b) patient with nail bed involvement (onycholysis); TI: triamcinolone iontophoresis; CB: calcipotriol/betamethasone dipropionate.

has been investigated in several studies [16, 18, 29, 30] and currently is used as a first line treatment for nail psoriasis, especially bed involvements. In a recent research performed by Rigopoulos et al. [29], twenty-five psoriatic patients with nail and mild skin involvements were instructed to apply daily combined calcipotriol-betamethasone ointment for 12-weeks on affected nails. Outcome measures were assessed by NAPSI at baseline and 4th, 8th, and 12th weeks. Overall improvement was 72% reduction in NAPSI (Δ: -4.2). Significant improvement for hyperkeratosis and onycholysis, moderate improvement for oil drops, and slight improvement for pitting were observed. However, such results were obtained from mild nail psoriasis cases since baseline mean NAPSI was 5.8. This result was almost in line with our study that topical calcipotriol/betamethasone dipropionate had a significant effect on nail bed lesions, but such trait was not found for the matrix lesions. The overall reduction obtained with topical calcipotriol/betamethasone dipropionate was greater with regard to the more treatment sessions in our study.

Patients did not develop any side effects in our study. Besides the bilateral comparison design and side effect free treatments, one of the TI advantages was monthly sessions; hence patients' time was saved, the procedure was cheaper, and they had a better compliance.

We found that monthly TI has equal efficacy compared to daily topical calcipotriol/betamethasone dipropionate in improving the nail bed score, matrix score, and NAPSI. It can be used as a safe and easy treatment for nail psoriasis. However, knowledge on iontophoresis in treating nail psoriasis is scarce and more studies in this field are needed. We recommend conducting studies focusing on the other aspects of nail psoriasis iontophoresis including use of other drugs to find an optimum iontophoresis protocol for nail psoriasis [31, 32].

Acknowledgments

The present article was extracted from the thesis written by Dr. Shahla Hosseinpoor, which was financially supported by the Shiraz University of Medical Sciences [Grant no. 8747] [33].

References

[1] A. Yorulmaz and F. Artuz, "A study of dermoscopic features of nail psoriasis," *Advances in Dermatology and Allergology*, vol. 1, pp. 28–35, 2017.

[2] M. C. Pasch, "Nail Psoriasis: A Review of Treatment Options," *Drugs*, vol. 76, no. 6, pp. 675–705, 2016.

[3] V. M. R. Heydendael, C. A. J. M. De Borgie, P. I. Spuls, P. M. M. Bossuyt, J. D. Bos, and M. A. De Rie, "The burden of psoriasis is not determined by disease severity only," *Journal of Investigative Dermatology Symposium Proceedings*, vol. 9, no. 2, pp. 131–135, 2004.

[4] L. I. Arango-Duque, M. Roncero-Riesco, T. Usero Bárcena, I. Palacios Álvarez, and E. Fernández López, "Treatment of nail psoriasis with Pulse Dye Laser plus calcipotriol betametasona gel vs. Nd:YAG plus calcipotriol betamethasone gel: An intrapatient left-to-right controlled study," *Actas Dermo-Sifiliográficas*, vol. 108, no. 2, pp. 140–144, 2017.

[5] Y. Hashimoto, M. Uyama, Y. Takada, K. Yoshida, and A. Ishiko, "Dermoscopic features of nail psoriasis treated with biologics," *The Journal of Dermatology*, vol. 44, no. 5, pp. 538–541, 2017.

[6] P. Rich and R. K. Scher, "Nail psoriasis severity index: a useful tool for evaluation of nail psoriasis," *Journal of the American Academy of Dermatology*, vol. 49, no. 2, pp. 206–212, 2003.

[7] K. Reich, "Approach to managing patients with nail psoriasis," *Journal of the European Academy of Dermatology and Venereology*, vol. 23, supplement 1, pp. 15–21, 2009.

[8] M. A. Radtke, F. C. Beikert, and M. Augustin, "Nail psoriasis - a treatment challenge," *JDDG: Journal der Deutschen Dermatologischen Gesellschaft*, vol. 11, no. 3, pp. 203–220, 2013.

[9] M. Nantel-Battista, V. Richer, I. Marcil, and A. Benohanian, "Treatment of nail psoriasis with intralesional triamcinolone acetonide using a needle-free jet injector: A prospective trial," *Journal of Cutaneous Medicine and Surgery*, vol. 18, no. 1, pp. 38–42, 2014.

[10] F. Ricceri, L. Pescitelli, L. Tripo, A. Bassi, and F. Prignano, "Treatment of severe nail psoriasis with acitretin: An impressive therapeutic result," *Dermatologic Therapy*, vol. 26, no. 1, pp. 77–78, 2013.

[11] B. Gazelius, "Iontophoresis-theory," in *Innovations in Microvascular Diagnosis*, PERIMED, Sweden, 1999.

[12] Wikipedia, "Triamcinolone acetonide," https://en.wikipedia.org/wiki/Triamcinolone_acetonide.

[13] NEW ZEALAND DATA SHEET, "Name of Medicine [Internet]. New Zealand Datasheet," https://medsafe.govt.nz.profs.Datasheet.d.Daivobetgel.pd.

[14] R. G. Langley, J. H. Saurat, and K. Reich, "Recommendations for the treatment of nail psoriasis in patients with moderate to severe psoriasis: a dermatology expert group consensus," *Journal of the European Academy of Dermatology and Venereology*, vol. 26, no. 3, pp. 373–381, 2012.

[15] S. M. Jones, J. B. Armas, M. G. Cohen, C. R. Lovell, G. Evison, and N. J. Mchugh, "Psoriatic arthritis: Outcome of disease subsets and relationship of joint disease to nail and skin disease," *Rheumatology*, vol. 33, no. 9, pp. 834–839, 1994.

[16] D. Rigopoulos, D. Ioannides, N. Prastitis, and A. Katsambas, "Nail psoriasis: A combined treatment using calcipotriol cream and clobetasol propionate cream [3]," *Acta Dermato-Venereologica*, vol. 82, no. 2, p. 140, 2002.

[17] M. Elman, "A new lightening approach to acne treatment-combining therapy modalities for maximizing acne treatment: phototherapy (lhe), drugs, skin rejuvenation and skin tightening," *Laser Therapy*, vol. 20, no. 1, pp. 35–37, 2011.

[18] T. Y. Tzung, C. Y. Chen, C. Y. Yang, L. PY, and Y. H. Chen, "Calcipotriol used as monotherapy or combination therapy with betamethasone dipropionate in the treatment of nail psoriasis," *Acta Dermato-Venereologica*, vol. 88, no. 3, pp. 279-280, 2008.

[19] V. B. Rajendra, A. Baro, A. Kumari, D. L. Dhamecha, S. R. Lahoti, and S. D. Shelke, "Transungual drug delivery: an overview," *Journal of Applied Pharmaceutical Science*, vol. 2, no. 1, pp. 203–209, 2012.

[20] M. B. Delgado-Charro, "Iontophoretic drug delivery across the nail," *Expert Opinion on Drug Delivery*, vol. 9, no. 1, pp. 91–103, 2012.

[21] W. Gerstein, "Psoriasis and lichen planus of nails. Treatment with triamcinolone," *JAMA Dermatology*, vol. 86, no. 4, p. 419, 1962.

[22] E. ABELL and P. D. SAMMAN, "Intradermal triamcinolone treatment of nail dystrophies," *British Journal of Dermatology*, vol. 89, no. 2, pp. 191–197, 1973.

[23] J. J. Bleeker, "Intralesional triamcinolone acetonide using the Port-O-Jet and needle injections in localized dermatoses," *British Journal of Dermatology*, vol. 91, no. 1, pp. 97–101, 1974.

[24] R. D. G. Peachey, R. J. Pye, and R. R. M. Harman, "The treatment of psoriatic nail dystrophy with intradermal steroid injections," *British Journal of Dermatology*, vol. 95, no. 1, pp. 75–78, 1976.

[25] D. A. de Berker and C. M. Lawrence, "A simplified protocol of steroid injection for psoriatic nail dystrophy," *British Journal of Dermatology*, vol. 138, no. 1, pp. 90–95, 1998.

[26] K. Saleem and W. Azim, "Treatment of nail psoriasis with a modified regimen of steroid injections," *JCPSP — Journal of College of Physicians and Surgeons Pakistan*, vol. 18, no. 2, pp. 78–81, 02.2008/JCPSP.7881.

[27] A. Björkman and P. Jörgsholm, "Rupture of the extensor pollicis longus tendon: A study of aetiological factors," *Journal of Plastic Surgery and Hand Surgery*, vol. 38, no. 1, pp. 32–35, 2004.

[28] J. Jakubik, "Finger tendon rupture following local application of triamcinolone-acetonide (Kenalog A-40)," *Acta chirurgiae plasticae*, vol. 23, no. 3, Article ID 6169243, pp. 180–188, 1981.

[29] D. Rigopoulos, S. Gregoriou, C. R. Daniel III et al., "Treatment of nail psoriasis with a two-compound formulation of calcipotriol plus betamethasone dipropionate ointment," *Dermatology*, vol. 218, no. 4, pp. 338–341, 2009.

[30] E. Tan and H. Oon, "Effective treatment of severe nail psoriasis using topical calcipotriol with betamethasone dipropionate gel," *Indian Journal of Dermatology, Venereology and Leprology*, vol. 82, no. 3, p. 345, 2016.

[31] H. N. Shivakumar, A. Juluri, B. G. Desai, and S. N. Murthy, "Ungual and transungual drug delivery," *Drug Development and Industrial Pharmacy*, vol. 38, no. 8, pp. 901–911, 2012.

4

Effectiveness of Traditional Healers in Program to Control Leprosy in Nagan Raya District in Aceh

Teuku Alamsyah,[1] **Said Usman** (ID),[2] **Mutia Yusuf,**[1] **and Said Devi Elvin**[1]

[1]*Health Polytech Facility of Health Minister, Department of Nursing, Banda Aceh 23245, Indonesia*
[2]*Medicine Faculty, Syiah Kuala University, Banda Aceh 23245, Indonesia*

Correspondence should be addressed to Said Usman; saidusmanmkes@yahoo.co.id

Academic Editor: Giuseppe Stinco

Aceh Province had the highest rate of leprosy in Indonesia; in 2014, 436 new Multibacillary cases were reported. Nagan Raya was the District in Aceh with the highest number of cases; new cases in 2015 comprised 26 with Paucibacillary (PB) and 21 with Multibacillary (MB) with a total of 4.26% with Grade II disability. The phenomena of handling and treatment by the people in Nagan Raya involve treatment by traditional healers, *"Tabib"*, to treat the leprosy, with treatments known as *Peundang* locally. The purpose of this study was to find out and to take steps to improve the effectiveness of the Tabib in controlling leprosy in Nagan Raya. The main object of this study, which used a quasi-experimental design, was to find out and to improve the treatment of leprosy patients by the Tabib who treat them there. Data was gathered using a questionnaire with an interview and the intervention was to provide training and a pocket book about leprosy and how to detect, control, and manage it there and the role that the Tabib can play in controlling leprosy in the future. The results of the study showed that there was a significant difference in knowledge about leprosy between the EG (Experimental Group) Tabib after they got the training including the pocket book and the Tabib in the Control Group (CG); i.e., that did not get any training nor the pocket book. Furthermore, after the training, there was also a significant difference in the attitude towards leprosy between the EG and the CG of Tabib. There was also a significant difference in the future role of the Tabibs to control the spread of leprosy between the EG and the CG. Based on these results, it is hoped that the District Health Department can implement a partnership model with the Tabib in Nagan Raya (and elsewhere) to use the pocket book with training to implement a program to control the spread of leprosy and also to always support the Tabib to improve their role in controlling and eliminating leprosy amongst the village people.

1. Introduction

Leprosy is a chronic, infectious disease caused by a rod shaped, acid-fast bacteria called *Mycobacterium leprae* (*M. leprae*). This disease primarily affects the skin, the peripheral nerves, the mucosa in the upper respiratory tract, and also the eyes [1].

The World Health Organization [2] reports that in 2014 there were 180,618 official cases in 103 countries and in the same year there were 215,656 new cases. At present Indonesia is one of the countries with a high rate of leprosy. In 2013 Indonesia was number 3 in the world after India and Brazil with 16,856 cases and a total of 9.86% of new cases with Grade II disability [3]. Leprosy is one of eight Neglected Tropical Diseases (NTD) that still plague Indonesia including Filaria, Frambusia, Dengue, Helminthiasis, Schistosomiasis, Rabies, and Taeniasis.

The Province of Aceh is one of the areas with the highest levels of leprosy in Indonesia. In 2014, the number of new Multibacillary leprosy cases was 436 or 75% of new cases in Aceh and there were 145 cases of Paucibacillary leprosy or 25% of the total of 581 new cases. In 2014, the prevalence of leprosy in Aceh was 1.29 per 10.000 and the number with Grade II disability was 1.4 per 100.000 population. The district with the highest number of Grade II disabled persons was Aceh Barat Daya with 3 per 100.000 [4]. In 2015 in neighboring Nagan Raya District there were 26 new cases of Paucibacillary (PB) type and 21 of Multibacillary (MB) type and the total of Grade II disabled persons was 4.26%. There were 25 Tabibs actively treating lepers [5].

Until now, leprosy still carries a stigma, so that it is difficult to find the leprosy cases and to manage appropriate treatment for them. The disfigurement from leprosy is often hideous to look at which can result in great fear of the sufferers which is called lepraphobia. Even after leprosy patients have finished their therapy and have obtained Release from Treatment (RFT), the stigma of leprosy stays with them for life. This stigma then becomes a psychological problem for the former sufferers. They feel disappointed, afraid, and deeply sad inside; they lack self-confidence and feel ashamed and worthless and of no use with their self-stigma. Furthermore, the public stigma also causes the leprosy patients and their families to distance themselves from other families as they are ostracized by other people [6]. Sufferers and People Who Have Had Leprosy (PWHHL) suffer stigma and discrimination in the form of rejection at schools and work places and in getting opportunities for work. PWHHL especially those who are severely crippled depend both physically and financially on others and end up in poverty. The problems that come from leprosy are not just medical but also social, economic, and educational problems. Most people in Nagan Raya District still have a negative stigma of leprosy patients and PWHHL; they still assume that leprosy is the result of a curse or a spell, of great sin, or of eating wrong foods or even is inherited. The result of the stigma is that the PWHHL are ostracized by people who think that they look disgusting and must be kept at a distance so sufferers try to find alternative treatments. This has resulted in the culture of handling and treating leprosy sufferers in Nagan Raya by traditional healers or Tabib as a form of local wisdom from the people there.

Tabibs are traditional healers who live in Nagan Raya. Leprosy sufferers, who do not know that leprosy can be treated at the local Health Department clinics or Puskesmas, will usually try to get treatment for their leprosy from a Tabib. The treatment method for leprosy from the Tabib usually uses special prayers "rajah" and water that has been blessed plus ointment made from plants which are rubbed onto the diseased skin and other concoctions made from plants which are given through inhaling smoke made from smouldering them. These treatments are known as "Peundang" in Acehnese. Cures using Tabib treatments are doubtful and not yet proven scientifically [7]. According to several PWHHL who have previously been treated with "Peundang", this type of treatment is very hard to follow [8].

The role of the Tabib in handling and treating cases of leprosy in Nagan Raya is very significant. The villagers very much respect and value the Tabib so they believe what they say and will follow it. The phenomenon of the Tabib and their handling of sufferers and PWHHL has become a problem for the program to control leprosy being implemented by the government Health Service in Nagan Raya District.

The role of the Tabib from one side is positive as they are capable of empowering the sufferers and the PWHHL who are put into isolation by their families and other villagers. However, from the viewpoint of treatment, what they have been doing has been against some of the basic principles for treating leprosy. This was influencing the results of the program to control leprosy being implemented by the Nagan Raya Health Service. The Tabib as a local wise man can be involved in 4 of the 8 stages of the strategy to control leprosy, namely, in early identification of cases, spreading information (about treatment), elimination of stigma, and empowerment of leprosy patients and PWHHL.

Based on data and the phenomena which have been described above, the researchers wanted to try to find out how effective the role of the Tabib could be in the Program to Manage Leprosy in Nagan Raya. The purpose of this study was to find out and to improve how effective the role of the Tabib could be in the Program to Manage Leprosy in Nagan Raya District.

2. Literature Review

Leprosy is a chronic skin disease caused by acid-fast bacteria, *Mycobacterium leprae*, which initially attacks the outer nerves and then, if not treated appropriately, spreads to other organs like the skin, the mucous glands, the kidneys, the testes, and the eyes: it can cause great physical disfigurement and distress to sufferers and their families. Leprosy can start as a result of specific causes *[9]. Specifically, the cause of leprosy is the bacteria, *Mycobacterium leprae*, getting into the human body through flesh wounds in the skin or through droplets inhaled when breathing and surviving and multiplying [10]. The WHO [11] has said that leprosy can be confirmed from the cardinal signs or primary symptoms of leprosy, namely, (a) spots on the skin where there is no feeling; the spots can be white (hypopigmentation) or reddish (erythematous) with thickening of the skin (plaque infiltrate) or in the form of lumps; the loss of feeling can happen when rubbed or cut or when heated or cooled, e.g., by ice, and the symptoms can be total or only in some places; and (b) thickening of the outer nerves accompanied by pain and interference with the functioning of the nerves concerned; sensory nerves lose their feeling, and motoric nerves experience loss of muscular strength (paralyse) and even paralysis and disturbance of the autonomic nervous system accompanied by dry and cracked skin. Symptoms usually suffered by lepers include fever while feeling cold and shivering, loss of appetite, and/or feeling sick inside and occasionally vomiting: lepers also suffer from headaches, inflammation of the testes, inflammation of the pleura (the chest), inflammation of the kidneys and sometimes malfunctioning of them too, enlargement of the liver and also of the gall bladder, and inflammation of the nerve fibres [12]

The psychological effects of leprosy on its sufferers include the stigma held by the villagers, namely, that leprosy is an incurable, inherited disease which can be spread in many ways. This stigma, held by fellow villagers, can cause leprosy patients to suffer terrible depression and even want to commit suicide [13]. Stigmas like these, which are deeply held by the villagers, cannot be easily overcome; legislation and successful rehabilitation of sufferers and elimination of recurrence of new cases of leprosy over time are needed to kill the stigma of leprosy. Also, in programs to handle leprosy, the spiritual factor, which is so important, is often overlooked and the focus is only on detection and treatment so that the programs for handling leprosy do not run well. The care of leprosy

TABLE 1: Tabibs' knowledge, attitude, and effectiveness prior to and after treatment.

Factor	EG	CG	Diff	P Values
Prior Knowledge of Leprosy	32	29	3	0.442
Knowledge After Treatment	36	26	19	0.010
Prior Attitude to Leprosy	33	28	5	0.194
Attitude After Treatment	35	27	8	0.040
Prior Effectiveness of Tabibs	31	30	1	0.795
Effectiveness After Treatment	40	22	18	0.001

patients involves various aspects: after the person is physically healthy again, treatment must be continued, sometimes for a long time, to treat the person psychologically and emotionally [14]. According to Hatzenbuehler et al. [15], a stigma is any kind of physical and social attribute which lowers the self-esteem and social acceptance of a person in some way including physically, socially, sexually, and/or ethnically [16] (Kumar, 2001). The process of stigmatization occurs, according to ILEP [17] when someone is seen as different, in a negative way, and is labeled accordingly, e.g., as a "leper" (note: this term is now taboo as it labels the sufferer forever; it is now appropriate to talk of "people with leprosy" for current sufferers and "PWHHL" for ex-sufferers). Villagers then tend to prejudge, from a traditional viewpoint saying that it is infectious, a curse, due to sins, and dangerous and cannot be controlled and the person concerned cannot make decisions. The leprosy patient gets two stigmas, namely, the social or public stigma from the villagers, which is the reaction of the villagers to the leprosy, and the self-stigma which is the personal reaction of the person when (s)he finds out that (s)he has leprosy and these stigmas are connected with stereotypes, prejudice, and discrimination [18]. Leprosy patients get stigmatized very easily due to uncivilized and primitive behaviour (by other people). Negative stigma from the villagers affects social interactions with leprosy patients so that, frequently, they do not get opportunities to work and so they remain unemployed. Discrimination at work also occurs when a person is denied work because of some physical factor (e.g., physical impairment due to leprosy) without looking at their qualifications or ability [19]. Furthermore, unemployment causes people to lose self-confidence, to isolate themselves, and eventually to give up, i.e., self-stigma. Unemployment and lack of opportunities to get a career are key factors in mental health which can cause psychological pressures from slight to serious depression and even for some lepers to want to and sometimes to succeed at committing suicide [20].

3. Method

A quasi-experimental design, with a training program and a pocket book for the Experimental Group (EG), was used for this research: this study was done to find out and to improve the effectiveness of the role of the Tabib, the traditional healers, in the Program to Manage Leprosy in Nagan Raya District. Data was obtained from a questionnaire

(See Appendix 1) plus interviews and document study. Before the field work for this study began the District Health Service (DHS) prepared a pocket book for identification, management, treatment, and cure of leprosy, based on current knowledge, best practices, and a literature survey [6, 21]. The Health Service in Nagan Raya has a list of all the Tabib practicing traditional medicine there: from this list, 120 Tabibs were selected by random sampling and these were randomly divided into two groups, 60 in the EG to get training and 60 in a Control Group (CG). On 25 July 2016, each group was invited to separate meetings at the DHS offices in Suka Makmur, Nagan Raya, where they were given the pretest questionnaire (Supplementary Section). Then after their pretest the EG were trained on identifying and managing leprosy and were given a copy of the pocket book that had been prepared [6]. During the next two weeks, DHS Officers made in situ visits to the EG Tabibs in their villages to observe their management of leprosy. Then, on 12 August, both groups, EG and CG, were again invited to separate meetings in Suka Makmur where they were again given the same questionnaire (Supplementary Section), this time as a posttest. The results obtained were later analysed statistically and are summarized in this paper.

4. Results

Based on Table 1, in the pretest no significant difference was found between prior knowledge about leprosy of the EG compared with that of the CG but there was a significant difference in the knowledge about leprosy in the posttest results from the EG Tabibs with the results from the CG Tabibs.

Based on Table 1 we find that for the pretest of the attitudes to leprosy there was no significant difference between the mean values of the EG and those of the CG in the pretest of their attitudes to leprosy but there was a significant difference in the attitudes to leprosy in the posttest results from the EG Tabibs compared with that from the CG Tabibs. Based on Table 1, we find that for the pretest of the effectiveness of their role in controlling leprosy there was no significant difference between the mean values of the EG and those of the CG in the pretest for effectiveness of role in controlling leprosy but there was a very significant difference in the effectiveness of their roles for controlling leprosy in the posttest results from the EG Tabibs compared with the results from the CG Tabibs.

5. Discussion

5.1. Knowledge about Leprosy. The results from Table 1 show that in the first pretests there was no significant difference in knowledge about leprosy between the Tabibs in the Experimental Group (EG) and those in the Control Group (CG). However, the results of the posttest, after the treatment, show that there was now a significant difference in knowledge about leprosy of the EG with that of the CG Tabibs showing that the training plus the pocket books about leprosy had been effective in increasing the knowledge about leprosy of the Tabibs.

This result of the study concerning knowledge about leprosy of the Tabib is in accordance with the theories of Notoadmodjo [22], who has said that health education is an activity to create behaviour amongst people which will be conducive to better health outcomes. Meaning that health education is an effort made to raise the awareness and knowledge (about health) amongst people so that they will maintain their health and avoid or prevent things that will damage their health and that of other people and they will know where to find treatment if they become sick and so on.

The purpose of health education is to develop and increase 3 behavioural domains, namely: the cognitive, affective, and psychomotor domains.

Based on the explanations above, in summary it can be said that because the Experimental Group of Tabibs had been given some training and had absorbed the contents of the pocket book their knowledge about leprosy and how to control it had increased significantly.

5.2. Attitudes to Leprosy. The results in Table 1 show that in the pretests there was no significant difference in attitude towards leprosy between the Tabibs in the EG and those in the CG. However, the results of the posttest, after the treatment with the pocket books show that there was now a significant difference in attitudes to leprosy of the EG with that of the CG Tabibs showing that the training with the pocket books about leprosy had been effective in improving the attitudes of the EG Tabibs to leprosy.

The results above from this study concerning the attitudes of the Tabib to leprosy are parallel with those found by Azwar [23]; in particular, factors which affect the attitudes of a person include experience, i.e., events and happenings which occur repeatedly and continuously and which are absorbed by the individual will affect their attitudes [16]. In this study, the EG Tabibs were given continuous explanations about how to control leprosy from the pocket book so that step-by-step the attitudes of the EG Tabibs to leprosy and how to manage it changed.

Azwar [23] has said that another factor which affects attitudes is the environment (including the local culture) which helps form the personality of a person.

Personality is a consistent pattern of behaviour which results from reinforcement. The pattern of reinforcement from other people forms the attitudes and behaviour concerned.

The connection between this with the present study concerning the attitudes of the Tabibs was the creation of an environment where the EG Tabibs could learn about controlling leprosy through interventions resulting from changes in the role of the Tabibs including early identification of new cases, spreading information (about management of leprosy), removing the stigma of leprosy, and empowering their leprosy patients, so strengthening the role of the Tabibs through the pocket book affects the attitude of the Tabibs to their leprosy patients. To summarize, the use of the pocket book to improve the role of the Tabibs in controlling leprosy effectively improved the attitudes of the EG Tabibs to be significantly more positive when treating leprosy patients in Nagan Raya.

5.3. Role in Handling Leprosy. The results from Table 1 show that in the pretests there was no significant difference between the two groups of Tabibs concerning the role of the Tabibs in the management of leprosy. However, the results from the posttests after the EG had had the treatment with the pocket book show that there was now a significant difference between the role of the EG Tabibs in the management of leprosy with that of the CG Tabibs showing that the training with the pocket books about leprosy had been effective in changing the EG Tabibs views of their role in managing leprosy, whilst the views of the CG Tabibs concerning their role had not changed.

The increase in the self-image of the EG Tabibs in their role in managing leprosy was because of the motivation given to them by the researchers through the pocket book that they had prepared and distributed to the EG Tabibs.

These results are similar to those found by Notoatmodjo [22], which showed that motivation is a requirement of people to participate, without motivation it is difficult to get people to participate in any program.

The growth of self-motivation must come from the people themselves whilst outsiders can only provide support and external motivation. As a result, health education is very much needed to provide the framework for motivation to grow amongst people.

Another factor which helped increase the role the Tabibs could play in managing leprosy was the involvement and partnership with the leprosy specialist workers from the Nagan Raya Health Division in managing leprosy in the district.

This is in accordance with the concepts for empowering people in health management; i.e., the involvement of people in health management depends very much on the needs of the people, the level of involvement, and the program of partnership between the people and the government (Kemenkes RI, 2012).

Furthermore, the National Health Department (Kemenkes RI, 2012) says that the role of people in health management is very much influenced by directly feeling the (health) benefits of the activities and the opportunities for the people to participate in the maintenance of health as well as the role of the local leaders (in the activities). In this study, the EG Tabibs were given information about the benefits to all villagers from taking steps to manage, control, and eliminate leprosy.

The Tabibs were also given the opportunity to be directly involved with the leprosy health workers from the Nagan Raya Health Division in activities with the villagers to promote health measures to avoid leprosy, to stop its spread, to permanently cure lepers, and to empower the PWHHL or ex-leprosy sufferers.

Based on the above, it can be seen that after the EG Tabib learnt the true facts about leprosy from the pocket book and training provided by the researchers working with the Nagan Raya Health Service, the role of these Tabibs in controlling leprosy in Nagan Raya increased greatly.

6. Conclusions

The results from this study can be summarized as follows.

No difference was found in the prior knowledge about leprosy between the training group (EG) of Tabibs and the control group (CG) in the pretest. Then after training and studying the pocket book, the results from the posttest showed that knowledge about leprosy amongst the EG of Tabibs who got the training was then significantly greater than that of the CG of Tabibs.

There was no difference in the initial attitude to leprosy amongst the EG of Tabibs and the CG which was shown by the pretests. Then after the training with the pocket book the posttest results showed that the EG Tabibs had a much better attitude to leprosy than the CG Tabibs.

There was no difference in the initial role for controlling and management of leprosy between the EG of Tabibs and the CG as shown by the pretests. Then after the training and studying the pocket books the posttest results showed that the EG Tabibs had a significantly better attitude to their role in controlling and managing leprosy than the CG Tabibs.

To summarize, the training of the Tabibs and supplying them with a pocketbook about the identification, management, treatment, and curing of leprosy increased the Tabibs' knowledge about leprosy, improved their attitude towards leprosy, and empowered the traditional Tabib to play a much better role in the identification, management, and curing of villagers with leprosy in partnership with the treatment provided by the local District Health Service and it is to be hoped that this successful intervention for the identification, treatment, management, and curing of leprosy can be replicated in all areas of Aceh and expanded to all areas of Indonesia until leprosy is eliminated from Indonesia and indeed from Asia and even the world, so it becomes a legend in the future.

Acknowledgments

The authors thank the Head of the Health Service in Nagan Raya District, Mr. T. Jamalul Alamuddin, for giving them permission to do this research study and for permission to publish the results. They also thank all the Tabibs for agreeing to participate in this research study and for giving permission to use the data and information they gave to the study anonymously. The authors thank the Aceh Health Polytechnic for funds provided to do this research amounting to Rp.30,482,000 {about US$ 2,000}.

Supplementary Materials

The Supplementary Materials comprise the Supplementary File which is a translated copy of the questionnaire used to survey the sample of Tabibs both before treatment and after treatment and after the EG Tabib had been given the pocket book. The questionnaire has four sections: namely, personal data, knowledge about leprosy, attitude to leprosy, and role of the traditional healer (Tabib). *(Supplementary Materials)*

References

[1] M. D. Amiruddin, *Penyakit kusta sebuah pendekatan klinis*, Brilian Internasional, Surabaya, Indonesia, 2012.

[2] WHO, *Leprosy*, 2015, http://www.who.in/.

[3] WHO, *Enhanced Global Strategy for Further Reducing the Disease Burden due to Leprosy*, Regional Office for South-East Asia, Indraprastha Estate, Mahatma Gandhi Marg, New Delhi, India, 2011.

[4] Dinkes Aceh, *Profil Kesehatan Provinsi Aceh Tahun*, 2015, Profil Kesehatan Provinsi Aceh Tahun.

[5] Dinkes Nagan Raya, "Data Kusta Kab. Nagan Raya, 2015. Not published".

[6] R. I. Kemenkes, *Buku Pedoman Nasional Pemberantasan Penyakit Kusta*, Depkes RI, Jakarta, Indonesia, 2013.

[7] S. I. Shadiqin, "Di Bawah Payung Tabib: Sejarah, Ritual, Dan Politik Tarekat Syattariyah Di Pantai Barat Aceh," *Substantia*, vol. 19, no. 1, pp. 75–98, 2015.

[8] T. S. Daud, *Tabib Seunagan dan Thariqat Syattariyah*, Karya Sukses, Jakarta, Indonesia, 2009.

[9] C. Dessinioti and A. D. Katsambas, "Leprosy (Hansens disease)," in *European Handbook of Dermatological Treatments*, pp. 513–519, Springer, 2015.

[10] R. M. Bhat and C. Prakash, "Leprosy, an overview of pathophysiology," *Interdisciplinary perspectives on infectious diseases*, 2012.

[11] WHO, *WHO Expert Committee on Leprosy: eighth report*, WHO, Geneva. Switzerland, 2012.

[12] J. Farrar, P. J. Hotez, T. Junghanss et al., *Manson's Tropical Diseases E-Book*, Elsevier Health Sciences, 2013.

[13] S. Sermrittirong and W. H. Van Brakel, "Stigma in leprosy: concepts, causes and determinants." *Leprosy Review*, vol. 85, no. 1, pp. 36–47, 2014.

[14] A. Grzybowski, J. Sak, J. Pawlikowski, and M. Nita, "Leprosy: Social implications from antiquity to the present," *Clinics in Dermatology*, vol. 34, no. 1, pp. 8–10, 2016.

[15] M. L. Hatzenbuehler, J. C. Phelan, and B. G. Link, "Stigma as a fundamental cause of population health inequalities," *American Journal of Public Health*, vol. 103, no. 5, pp. 813–821, 2013.

[16] Goffman, "Stigma of mental illness: changing minds, changing behaviour," *The British Journal of Psychiatry*, 2002.

[17] ILEP, *The Guidelines To Reduce Stigma: Holland*, The International Federation of Anti-Leprosy Associations (ILEP) and the Netherlands Leprosy Relief (NLR), 2011.

[18] S. Sermrittirong and W. Van, "How to reduce stigma in leprosya systematic," *Leprosy Review*, vol. 85, pp. 149–157, 2014.

[19] C. A. S. Garbin, A. J. Í. Garbin, M. E. O. G. Carloni, T. A. S. Rovida, and R. J. Martins, "The stigma and prejudice of leprosy: Influence on the human condition," *Journal of the Brazilian Society of Tropical Medicine*, vol. 48, no. 2, pp. 194–201, 2015.

[20] C. White and C. Franco-Paredes, "Leprosy in the 21st century," *Clinical Microbiology Reviews*, vol. 28, no. 1, pp. 80–94, 2015.

[21] R. I. Depkes, *Buku Pedoman Nasional Pemberantasan Penyakit Kusta*, Depkes RI, Jakarta, Indonesia, 2006.

[22] S. Notoatmodjo, *Promosi Kesehatan dan Ilmu Perilaku*, Rineka Cipta, Jakarta, Indonesia, 2007.

[23] Azwar, *Sikapmanusia teori dan pengukurannya*, Pustaka Pelajar, Yogyakarta, Indonesia, 2009.

5

Efficacy and Safety of the Traditional Japanese Medicine Keigairengyoto in the Treatment of Acne Vulgaris

Kotaro Ito,[1,2] **Saori Masaki,**[1] **Manabu Hamada,**[3] **Tetsuo Tokunaga,**[4] **Hisashi Kokuba,**[5] **Kenji Tashiro,**[6] **Ichiro Yano,**[7] **Shinichiro Yasumoto,**[8] **and Shinichi Imafuku** ⓘ[1]

[1]*Department of Dermatology, Fukuoka University School of Medicine, Fukuoka, Japan*
[2]*Ito Dermatology Clinic, Oita, Japan*
[3]*Hamada Dermatology Clinic, Fukuoka, Japan*
[4]*Tokunaga Dermatology Clinic, Fukuoka, Japan*
[5]*Sakurazaka Dermatology Clinic, Fukuoka, Japan*
[6]*Tashiro Dermatology Clinic, Fukuoka, Japan*
[7]*Yano Dermatology and Urinary Clinic, Fukuoka, Japan*
[8]*Yasumoto Dermatology Clinic, Fukuoka, Japan*

Correspondence should be addressed to Shinichi Imafuku; tsujita@fukuoka-u.ac.jp

Academic Editor: Luigi Naldi

Several traditional Japanese medicines including Keigairengyoto (KRT) are used to treat acne vulgaris, but there is no robust evidence of their effectiveness. In this study, we examined the effectiveness and safety of KRT in treating acne vulgaris. An open-label, randomized, parallel control group comparison was conducted with a conventional treatment group (adapalene and topical antibiotics; control group) and a KRT group (control treatment plus KRT). The test drugs were administered for 12 weeks to patients (15 to 64 years, outpatient) with inflammatory acne on their face, and the amount of acne at 2, 4, 8, and 12 weeks was measured. Sixty-four patients were enrolled; 29 patients in each group were included in the analysis. Twenty-eight patients in the control group and 24 patients in the KRT group were included in the efficacy analysis. The number of inflammatory skin rashes at 4 and 8 weeks in the KRT group was significantly decreased compared with the control group. There was no significant difference between the two groups in noninflammatory eruptions and general rashes. There were no serious adverse events in both groups. KRT may be a useful agent in patients with inflammatory acne in combination with conventional treatments. This trial is registered with UMIN 000014831.

1. Introduction

Acne vulgaris is a chronic skin disorder in which a complex combination of abnormal lipid metabolism, abnormal keratosis, and proliferation of bacteria is involved in the pilosebaceous gland system. Acne starts with comedones (noninflammatory rash) with sebaceous secretion port obstruction resulting from abnormal proliferation and activation of keratinocytes and swelling of hair follicles. The disease progresses to pimples or pustules (inflammatory skin rashes) where acne bacteria and oxidized metabolites in the skin induce inflammation, accompanied by migration and infiltration of inflammatory cells. Exacerbation of inflammatory rash causes intractable conditions such as cysts and nodules, and the resulting scarring reduces the patient's quality of life. Therefore, it is important to prevent acne from progressing into inflammation. To achieve this, a quicker treatment response is required to improve patient compliance.

The main conventional treatment for acne consists of topical application of retinoid, benzoyl peroxide, and antibacterial agents [1]. The retinoid selectively binds to the retinoic acid receptor and suppresses keratinocyte proliferation and activation. A representative retinoid agent, adapalene, is used as a key drug during all stages of acne vulgaris. Benzoyl peroxide has a bactericidal action against *Propionibacterium acnes* and an anti-inflammatory action, and it produces few resistant bacteria. Recently, combination therapy using these drugs or a prescription drug combination was recommended [1]. Various antibiotics are positively prescribed when bacterial infection is the leading factor. However, adverse events such as skin irritation and resistant bacteria require a new treatment strategy [2–7].

In Japan, the traditional medication Keigairengyoto (KRT) in the form of extracted granules for ethical use (product number TJ-50; Tsumura & Co., Tokyo, Japan) has been approved for medicinal use by the Japanese Ministry of Health and Welfare and is widely prescribed for patients with inflammatory diseases including acne vulgaris, empyema, and rhinitis. The base powder of KRT was obtained by spray-drying a hot water extract mixture of the following 17 crude drugs: Scutellariae radix, Phellodendri cortex, Coptidis rhizoma, Platycodi radix, Aurantii fructus immaturus, Schizonepetae spica, Bupleuri radix, Gardeniae fructus, Rehmanniae radix, Paeoniae radix, Cnidii rhizoma, Angelicae radix, Menthae herba, Angelicae dahuricae radix, Saposhnikoviae radix, Forsythiae fructus, and Glycyrrhizae radix. KRT includes large amounts of various types of medicinal ingredients such as alkaloids, flavonoids, and triterpenoids, which exhibit antimicrobial, anti-inflammatory, antilipogenesis, and antioxidant effects [8–14]. It was recently reported that KRT suppressed development of bacteria-induced dermatitis in an experimental model, through enhancing bacterial clearance in innate immune cells [15]. However, no published clinical study has shown the efficacy of KRT. Our aim was to evaluate the efficacy and safety of KRT in a comparative study between the conventional treatment using adapalene and local antibiotics and this treatment combined with KRT therapy.

2. Methods

This study was a multicenter, open-label, randomized parallel group comparison study conducted at eight dermatologic medical facilities in Japan (UMIN000014831). This study was approved by the Ethics Review Committee of Fukuoka University Hospital.

2.1. Patients. Patients (15 to 64 years, male or female unconscious) with inflammatory acne who visited one of the eight facilities between August 2014 and January 2016 and agreed to participate in this research were enrolled. For patients under 18 years of age, consent was obtained from their parent or guardian. Exclusion criteria were as follows: (1) severe complications such as liver disease, renal disease, heart disease, blood disease, or metabolic disease; (2) being pregnant, lactating, or planning to become pregnant during the study observation period; (3) taking concomitant medications and research medicines within 1 week before the start of the study; (4) participation in another trial within one month before the initiation of this study; (5) scheduling to undergo a chemical peel or laser therapy during the study observation period; (6) a history of allergies to traditional Japanese medicine; and/or (7) patients for whom, in the opinion of the study scientist or collaborating research doctor, it is not in their best interest to be enrolled into the study.

2.2. Study Design. Patients were randomized into two groups: a conventional treatment group (control group) and a KRT plus conventional treatment group (KRT group). Patients in the control group received treatment with one of the antimicrobial agents (clindamycin gel or nadifloxacin cream) in addition to 0.1% adapalene gel. Vitamins (vitamin A, B2, B6, C, and E) were allowed in combination with the research medications. Antimicrobial oral medicine, herbal medicine, and hormonal drugs were prohibited as concomitant medications, and physical treatments such as a chemical peel and laser therapy were also prohibited. Patients in the KRT group received the conventional treatment mentioned above and Tsumura Keigairengyoto extract granules (Tsumura & Co.) divided into 7.5 g oral doses to be taken 2 to 3 times per day, before or between meals. Patients were treated for 12 weeks.

2.3. Assessments of Efficacy and Safety. The amount of inflammatory and noninflammatory acne on the face was counted at baseline (study entry) and at weeks 2, 4, 8, and 12. The reduction in this number was calculated for inflammatory, noninflammatory, and total acne. Adverse events including local and systemic symptoms were collected throughout the study period. Laboratory testing was performed before treatment and at 12 weeks (or at the time of discontinuation), and abnormal fluctuation was judged. The severity of adverse events was judged to be either "serious" or "not serious".

2.4. Statistical Analysis. Evaluation of the effectiveness was performed by group and compared using the Wilcoxon rank-sum test, with the change from premedication to posttreatment as an index. Significance was set to 5% on both sides. Wilcoxon's signed-rank test was also used for intragroup analysis of longitudinal change.

3. Results

3.1. Patient Background. The patient background information for both groups is shown in Table 1. A total of 64 patients were enrolled: 31 in the control group and 33 in the KRT group. There were no differences between groups for age, sex, duration of disease, and severity of acne before treatment. There were a total of 58 patients in the full analysis set (FAS) and in the safety evaluation set (SES) (29 patients in the control group and 29 patients in the KRT group) and 52 patients in the efficacy analysis group (28 patients in the control and 24 patients in KRT group).

3.2. Reduction in the Amount of Acne. In the control and KRT groups, the amount of acne decreased throughout the course of treatment (Figures 1(a), 1(b), and 1(c)). The amount of inflammatory acne in the KRT group declined significantly faster at 4 and 8 weeks compared with the control group. A significant difference was not observed in the amount of noninflammatory acne. There was no significant difference between the two groups in the total (inflammatory and noninflammatory) acne.

3.3. Representative Images. The treatment course of a representative patient with inflammatory acne in the KRT group is presented in Figures 2(a) and 2(b).

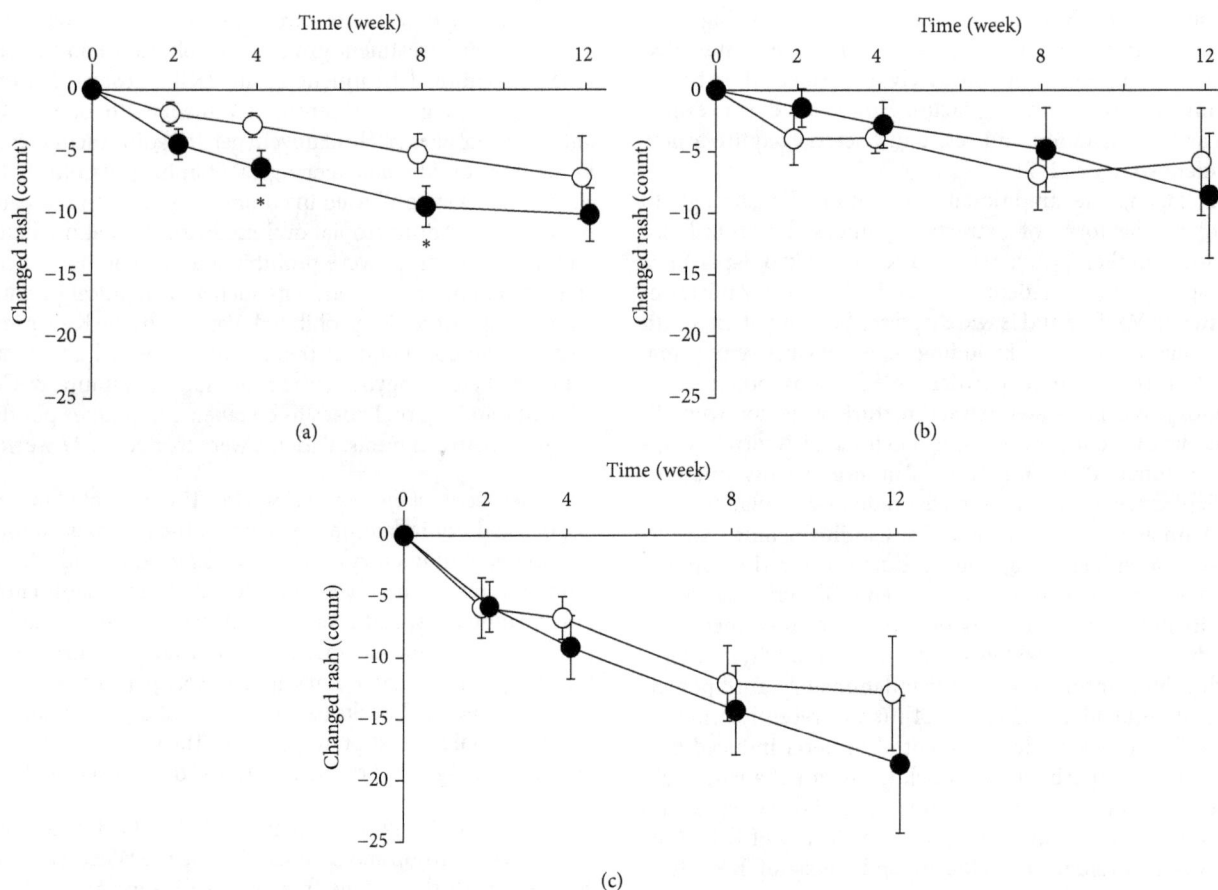

FIGURE 1: *Effect of Keigairengyoto on the number of acne rashes.* Patients were randomized into a conventional treatment group (control group, white circles) and a group with conventional treatment and Keigairengyoto (KRT group, filled circles), and they were treated for 12 weeks. The amount of inflammatory and noninflammatory acne on the face was counted at baseline (study entry) and at weeks 2, 4, 8, and 12. Time-dependent changes of inflammatory (a), noninflammatory (b), and total (c) acne are shown as a reduction in the number of the respective rashes. Data are presented as the mean ± standard error. The number of patients at the time of each control and KRT group evaluation is as follows: pretreatment: control 28 and KRT 24; week 2: 24 and 23; week 4: 20 and 22; week 8: 21 and 19; and week 12: 16 and 14. ∗P<0.05, Wilcoxon rank-sum test.

3.4. Stratified Analyses by Median Acne Duration. The median acne duration in all patients in this study was 2.6 years. The total amount of noninflammatory and inflammatory acne in patients with a disease duration of 2.6 years or more was examined. Although there was a difference in the number of patients among the groups, the KRT group showed a significantly greater reduction in the amount of acne at week 12 (Figure 3).

3.5. Safety. Adverse events and adverse reactions from the 58 patients in the SES population were collected, and these are summarized in Table 2. In the control group, four adverse events in three patients were observed throughout the study period, three of which were local skin irritants, which seemed to be related to adapalene. In the KRT group, erosion of the lesion was seen in one of the 29 patients in the SES population. No event was serious.

4. Discussion

Although there have been clinical reports that traditional Japanese medicines are effective for treating acne [16], most of the research was not of high quality. In our multicenter, open-label, randomized controlled trial, KRT objectively showed the potential to reduce inflammatory acne at an early stage.

This study also suggests that KRT is not effective for non-inflammatory acne and selectively suppresses inflammatory rashes. This selectivity suggests that KRT's point of action is different from that of adapalene or antibiotics. Because the amount of noninflammatory acne was not different at any time between the two groups, KRT may not affect keratinization abnormalities and sebaceous activity that subsequently cause comedones.

The significant point of this study is that adding KRT reduced the amount of inflammatory acne more than conventional therapy at 4 and 8 weeks. In treating acne, a rapid

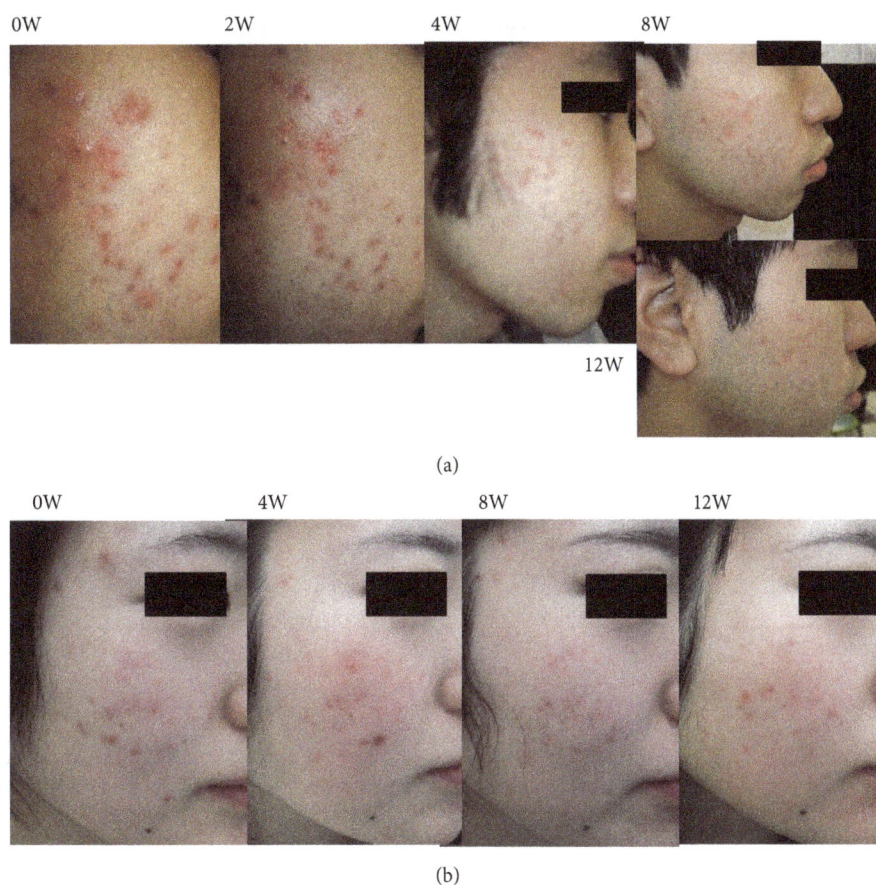

FIGURE 2: *Representative images of patients treated with Keigairengyoto.* Acne in two representative patients ((a) and (b)) treated with Keigairengyoto (KRT) at study entry and at weeks 2, 4, 8, and 12.

onset of the treatment effect is desirable to motivate patients to continue the therapy for this chronic condition.

Further stratification analyses were performed by duration of the acne. The total amount of noninflammatory and inflammatory acne in patients with a median disease duration (2.6 years or more) was examined. The KRT group showed a significantly greater reduction in the amount of acne at week 12 although there was a difference in the number of patients among the groups. For the change in inflammatory acne in patients with a disease duration of 2.6 years or more, the amount of acne at 2, 4, and 8 weeks was lower in the KRT group compared with the control group, with a significant difference at 2 and 8 weeks (data not shown). KRT may help patients more with longer history of inflammatory acne.

KRT is composed of the 17 crude drugs as described in the Introduction. Each component is identified by its external morphology and authenticated by marker compounds of plant specimens according to the methods of the Japanese Pharmacopoeia and quality standards defined at Tsumura Co. In the manufacturing process, KRT has been standardized with quantification of marker compounds including glycyrrhizin, berberine, and paeoniflorin and with specification levels for impurities such as heavy metal, pesticides, phytotoxins, and bacterial contamination under modern quality control. KRT has a large amount of various types of medicinal

ingredients such as alkaloids (e.g., berberine), flavonoids (e.g., genistein, liquiritigenin, and baicalin), and triterpenoids (e.g., glycyrrhizin, saikosaponin) [8, 17–21]. Alkaloids and flavonoids are known to possess antimicrobial activity against a wide variety of microorganisms [8–10]. KRT exhibited the strongest effect in an antimicrobial assay using *P. acnes* among 10 kinds of kampo drugs that were evaluated [22]. According to a recent report, KRT drastically reduced the number of inoculated bacteria in a mouse cutaneous infection model using live *Staphylococcus aureus* [15]. It is unclear whether the antibacterial effect of KRT could be involved in clinical effects to ameliorate acne, but KRT may have the potential to affect an antibacterial spectrum in a manner that is different from the antibiotics used in the present study and/or to enhance the effects of the other drugs combined with KRT therapy.

A recent report showed that KRT's flavonoids, genistein and liquiritigenin, function as agonists for the nuclear estrogen receptor in macrophages, leading to enhancement of bacterial clearance by macrophages in both *in vivo* and *in vitro* assays [13]. KRT is reported to suppress bacteria-induced skin edema and enhanced bacteria phagocytosis by resident macrophages in a model of abscess-forming dermatitis induced by heat-killed *Staphylococcus aureus* [15]. Some flavonoids such as genistein and liquiritigenin were thought to contribute to the adjuvant effects of KRT. In acne

TABLE 1: Background and number of acne patients.

	Control group	KRT group	Sum of the groups
Assigned number	31	33	64
FAS/SES number	29	29	58
PPS number			
Entry	28	24	52
2nd week	24	23	47
4th week	20	22	42
8th week	21	19	40
12th week	16	14	30
Age (year)	24.0±9.0	24.3±5.9	24.1±7.7
Gender M/F	12 / 16	9 / 15	21 / 31
Disease duration (year)	5.2±7.9	3.2±2.9	4.3±6.2
Severity poluration at entry (%)			
Mild	6 (21.4%)	3 (12.5%)	9 (17.3%)
Moderate	19 (67.9%)	18 (75.0%)	37 (71.2%)
Severe	2 (7.1%)	3 (12.5%)	5 (9.6%)
Very severe	1 (3.6%)	0	1 (1.9%)
Number of rash at entry			
Total rash	33.7±28.8	26.2±19.9	30.2±25.1
Inflammatory rash	14.6±22.3	12.5±9.9	13.7±17.6
Non-inflammatory rash	19.0±21.1	13.7±16.5	16.6±19.1

Patients were randomized into the conventional treatment group (control group) or the conventional treatment and Keigairengyoto group (KRT group), and they were treated for 12 weeks. Data on age, disease duration, and amount of acne at entry are shown as the mean ± standard deviation.
FAS, full analysis set; SES, safety evaluation set; PPS, per protocol set.

TABLE 2: Safety assessment.

	Control group				KRT group
	Patient #1	Patient #1	Patient #2	Patient #3	Patient #4
Adverse event	Dry skin	Erythema on right cheek	Cold	Xerotic eczema	Exacerbated rash
Severity	Not serious	Not serious	Not serious	Not serious	Not serious
Speculated drug	Adapalene	Adapalene	-	Adapalene	Keigairengyoto
Outcome	Improved	Improved	Recovered	Recovered	Recovered
Observation time[†]	1 week	1 week	3 weeks + 5 days	3 weeks + 1 day	4 days
Belonging to PPS	Yes	Yes	Yes	Yes	No

Patients were randomized into the conventional treatment group (control group) or the conventional treatment group with Keigairengyoto (KRT group), and they were treated for 12 weeks. Adverse events of local and systemic symptoms were collected throughout the study period.
[†]Observation time shows the duration from the start of treatment in the present study to finding an adverse event. PPS, per protocol set.

patients' skin, resident macrophages play a host-defensive role to exclude *P. acnes* that is secreted via the pilosebaceous apparatus, dead cells, and debris generated by inflammation. If KRT can improve acne via upregulating macrophage functions, KRT is a unique drug that is different from the existing antiacne drugs.

Previous studies showed that flavonoids reduce development of contact or allergic dermatitis in experimental models [23, 24] and that tea flavonoids improve acne symptoms in humans [25]. Moreover, KRT is reported to show a radical scavenging effect in an assay using human peripheral white blood cells [26]. Blood pharmacokinetic and antioxidant studies focusing on KRT-related flavonoids [27] showed that flavonoids are important ingredients that contribute to the antiacne effect of KRT.

The limitations of this study are as follows: (1) there were a small number of patients; (2) the study was not double-blind, and thus conclusions based on these exploratory results should be made with caution. Larger studies that address these limitations are necessary in the future.

In summary, adding oral KRT onto conventional therapy significantly increased the reduction of inflammatory acne in

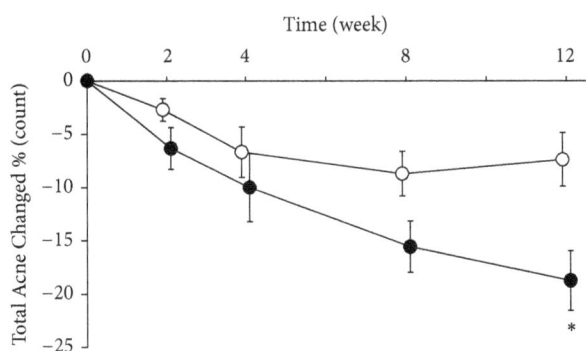

FIGURE 3: *Effect of Keigairengyoto in a stratified analysis focusing on patients with disease duration of 2.6 years or more.* Patients were randomized into a conventional treatment group (control group, white circle) and a group with conventional treatment and Keigairengyoto (KRT group, filled circle), and they were treated for 12 weeks. The median acne duration for all patients in this study was 2.6 years. The total sum of noninflammatory and inflammatory acne in patients with an acne duration of 2.6 years or more was examined. Although there was a difference in the number of patients among the groups, the KRT group showed significantly greater reduction in the amount of acne at week 12. For the change in inflammatory skin rash in patients with an acne duration of 2.6 years or more, the amount of inflammatory acne at 2, 4, and 8 weeks was lower in the KRT group compared with the control group, with a significant difference at 2 and 8 weeks. Data are shown as the mean ± standard error. The number of patients at each evaluation time point for the control and KRT groups is as follows: pretreatment: control 15 and KRT 9; week 2: 14 and 9; week 4: 9 and 9; week 8: 10 and 7; and week 12: 8 and 4. ∗P<0.05, Wilcoxon rank-sum test.

the early stage of acne compared with conventional therapy alone. There was only one side effect in the KRT group during this study. KRT may be an option as a useful agent to treat inflammatory acne.

References

[1] A. L. Zaenglein, A. L. Pathy, and B. J. Schlosser, "Guidelines of care for the management of acne vulgaris," *Journal of the American Academy of Dermatology*, vol. 74, no. 5, pp. 945–973e933, 2016.

[2] B. Bergler-Czop, M. Bilewicz-Stebel, A. Stańkowska, and T. Bilewicz-Wyrozumska, "Side effects of retinoid therapy on the quality of vision," *Acta Pharmaceutica*, vol. 66, no. 4, pp. 471–478, 2016.

[3] M. Kawashima, S. Harada, C. Loesche, and Y. Miyachi, "Adapalene gel 0.1% is effective and safe for Japanese patients with acne vulgaris: A randomized, multicenter, investigator-blinded, controlled study," *Journal of Dermatological Science*, vol. 49, no. 3, pp. 241–248, 2008.

[4] S. Sawleshwarkar, V. Salgaonkar, and C. Oberai, "Multicenter study to evaluate efficacy and irritation potential of benzoyl peroxide 4% cream in hydrophase base (Brevoxyl) in acne vulgaris," *Indian Journal of Dermatology, Venereology and Leprology*, vol. 69, no. 1, pp. 19–22, 2003.

[5] C. Foti, P. Romita, A. Borghi, G. Angelini, D. Bonamonte, and M. Corazza, "Contact dermatitis to topical acne drugs: A review of the literature," *Dermatologic Therapy*, vol. 28, no. 5, pp. 323–329, 2015.

[6] G. G. Aubin, M. E. Portillo, A. Trampuz, and S. Corvec, "Propionibacterium acnes, an emerging pathogen: From acne to implant-infections, from phylotype to resistance," *Médecine et Maladies Infectieuses*, vol. 44, no. 6, pp. 241–250, 2014.

[7] S. Humphrey, "Antibiotic resistance in acne treatment," *Skin Therapy Letter*, vol. 17, no. 9, pp. 1–3, 2012.

[8] Z.-J. Huang, Y. Zeng, P. Lan, P.-H. Sun, and W.-M. Chen, "Advances in structural modifications and biological activities of berberine: An active compound in traditional Chinese medicine," *Mini-Reviews in Medicinal Chemistry*, vol. 11, no. 13, pp. 1122–1129, 2011.

[9] C. Caliceti, P. Franco, S. Spinozzi, A. Roda, and A. F. G. Cicero, "Berberine: New insights from pharmacological aspects to clinical evidences in the management of metabolic disorders," *Current Medicinal Chemistry*, vol. 23, no. 14, pp. 1460–1476, 2016.

[10] J. Luo, B. Dong, K. Wang et al., "Baicalin inhibits biofilm formation, attenuates the quorum sensing-controlled virulence and enhances Pseudomonas aeruginosa clearance in a mouse peritoneal implant infection model," *PLoS ONE*, vol. 12, no. 4, Article ID 0176883, 2017.

[11] K. B. Pandey and S. I. Rizvi, "Plant polyphenols as dietary antioxidants in human health and disease," *Oxidative Medicine and Cellular Longevity*, vol. 2, no. 5, pp. 270–278, 2009.

[12] B. Dinda, S. Dinda, S. DasSharma, R. Banik, A. Chakraborty, and M. Dinda, "Therapeutic potentials of baicalin and its aglycone, baicalein against inflammatory disorders," *European Journal of Medicinal Chemistry*, vol. 131, pp. 68–80, 2017.

[13] A. Kaneko, T. Matsumoto, Y. Matsubara et al., "Glucuronides of phytoestrogen flavonoid enhance macrophage function via conversion to aglycones by β-glucuronidase in macrophages," *Immunity, Inflammation and Disease*, vol. 5, no. 3, pp. 265–279, 2017.

[14] L. J. Ming and A. C. Yin, "Therapeutic effects of glycyrrhizic acid," *Natural Product Communications*, vol. 8, pp. 415–418, 2013.

[15] J. Koseki, A. Kaneko, Y. Matsubara et al., "Keigairengyoto, a traditional Japanese medicine, promotes bacterial clearance by activating innate immune cells in mouse cutaneous infection models," *Trends in Immunotherapy*, vol. 1, no. 1, pp. 35–49, 2017.

[16] S. Higaki, T. Toyomoto, and M. Morohashi, "Seijo-bofu-to, Jumi-haidoku-to and Toki-shakuyaku-san suppress rashes and incidental symptoms in acne patients," *Drugs under Experimental and Clinical Research*, vol. 28, no. 5, pp. 193–196, 2002.

[17] H. Sun, H. Wang, A. Zhang et al., "Chemical discrimination of cortex Phellodendri amurensis and cortex Phellodendri chinensis by multivariate analysis approach," *Pharmacognosy Magazine*, vol. 12, no. 45, pp. 41–49, 2016.

[18] R.-X. Liu, G.-H. Song, P.-G. Wu et al., "Distribution patterns of the contents of five biologically activate ingredients in the root of Scutellaria baicalensis," *Chinese Journal of Natural Medicines*, vol. 15, no. 2, pp. 152–160, 2017.

[19] H.-F. Chen, W.-G. Zhang, J.-B. Yuan, Y.-G. Li, S.-L. Yang, and W.-L. Yang, "Simultaneous quantification of polymethoxylated flavones and coumarins in *Fructus aurantii* and *Fructus aurantii immaturus* using HPLC-ESI-MS/MS," *Journal of Pharmaceutical and Biomedical Analysis*, vol. 59, no. 1, pp. 90–95, 2012.

[20] S. Zhou, J. Cao, F. Qiu, W. Kong, S. Yang, and M. Yang, "Simultaneous determination of five bioactive components in radix glycyrrhizae by pressurised liquid extraction combined with UPLC-PDA and UPLC/ESI-QTOF-MS confirmation," *Phytochemical Analysis*, vol. 24, no. 6, pp. 527–533, 2013.

[21] B. Yuan, R. Yang, Y. Ma, S. Zhou, X. Zhang, and Y. Liu, "A systematic review of the active saikosaponins and extracts isolated from radix bupleuri and their applications," *Pharmaceutical Biology*, vol. 55, no. 1, pp. 620–635, 2017.

[22] S. Higaki, S. Morimatsu, M. Morohashi, T. Yamagishi, and Y. Hasegawa, "Susceptibility of Propionibacterium acnes, Staphylococcus aureus and Staphylococcus epidermidis to 10 Kampo formulations," *Journal of International Medical Research*, vol. 25, no. 6, pp. 318–324, 1997.

[23] Y. W. Kim, R. J. Zhao, S. J. Park et al., "Anti-inflammatory effects of liquiritigenin as a consequence of the inhibition of NF-κB-dependent iNOS and proinflammatory cytokines production," *British Journal of Pharmacology*, vol. 154, no. 1, pp. 165–173, 2008.

[24] M. Y. Yun, J. H. Yang, D. K. Kim et al., "Therapeutic effects of Baicalein on atopic dermatitis-like skin lesions of NC/Nga mice induced by dermatophagoides pteronyssinus," *International Immunopharmacology*, vol. 10, no. 9, pp. 1142–1148, 2010.

[25] J. Y. Yoon, H. H. Kwon, S. U. Min, D. M. Thiboutot, and D. H. Suh, "Epigallocatechin-3-gallate improves acne in humans by modulating intracellular molecular targets and inhibiting *P. acnes*," *Journal of Investigative Dermatology*, vol. 133, no. 2, pp. 429–440, 2013.

[26] H. Akamatsu, Y. Asada, and T. Horio, "Effect of keigai-rengyo-to, a Japanese kampo medicine, on neutrophil functions: A possible mechanism of action of keigai-rengyo-to in acne," *Journal of International Medical Research*, vol. 25, no. 5, pp. 255–265, 1997.

[27] T. Matsumoto, Y. Matsubara, Y. Mizuhara et al., "Plasma pharmacokinetics of polyphenols in a traditional Japanese medicine, jumihaidokuto, which suppresses propionibacterium acnes-induced dermatitis in rats," *Molecules*, vol. 20, no. 10, pp. 18031–18046, 2015.

Skin Cancer Knowledge, Attitudes, and Practices among Chinese Population: A Narrative Review

Philip M. Stephens [iD],[1] Brian Martin,[1] Ghazal Ghafari,[1]
James Luong,[1] Vinayak K. Nahar [iD],[2] Linda Pham,[1] Jiangxia Luo,[3,4]
Marcelle Savoy,[5] and Manoj Sharma [iD][6]

[1]DeBusk College of Osteopathic Medicine, Lincoln Memorial University, Harrogate, TN, USA
[2]Center for Animal and Human Health in Appalachia, College of Veterinary Medicine, DeBusk College of Osteopathic Medicine, and School of Mathematics and Sciences, Lincoln Memorial University, Harrogate, TN, USA
[3]Department of English, Gannan Medical University, Ganzhou, Jiangxi, China
[4]Carter and Moyers School of Education, Lincoln Memorial University, Harrogate, TN, USA
[5]Lon and Elizabeth Parr Reed Health Sciences Library, DeBusk College of Osteopathic Medicine, Lincoln Memorial University, Harrogate, TN, USA
[6]Department of Behavioral & Environmental Health, School of Public Health, Jackson State University, Jackson, MS, USA

Correspondence should be addressed to Vinayak K. Nahar; naharvinayak@gmail.com

Academic Editor: Gavin P. Robertson

Skin cancers are becoming a substantial public health problem in China. Fair skin and increased exposure to ultraviolet B (UVB) rays from the sun are among the most substantial risk factors for skin cancer development, thus making the Chinese people vulnerable to this group of diseases. The purpose of this article is to present a narrative review of the knowledge, attitudes, and practices (KAP) related to skin cancers within the Chinese population. A systematic electronic search of MEDLINE (PubMed), CINAHL, ScienceDirect, and Google Scholar databases yielded nine articles that met the inclusion criteria. The review found that although sunscreen application was a commonly used method of skin protection among the general Chinese population, educational interventions enhancing current knowledge and attitudes about the effects of UVB rays on skin from undue sun exposure were limited in many smaller communities of the country. Hence, there is an essential need to design effective, evidence-based educational programs promoting sun protection behaviors in both congregated and sparsely populated areas of China.

1. Introduction

Skin cancers, the most commonly diagnosed of all cancers, are typically viewed as ailments affecting primarily Caucasian populations in countries such as Australia, New Zealand, Slovenia, and Norway [1–3]. However, worldwide skin cancer rates have increased over the last three decades [4]. Populations which previously had low skin cancer rates may present the biggest challenge for public health officials due to the lack of established preventative measures. The rise in the incidence of skin cancer is becoming a significant public health problem in China. Between the years of 1990 and 1999, the rate of basal cell carcinoma (BCC) in the nearly doubled

from 16.0 to 31.8 per 10,000 new cases, contributing to 60% of newly diagnosed skin cancers [5]. Squamous cell carcinoma (SCC) is the second most diagnosed type of skin cancer among the Chinese population [5]. Also reflected in the overall number of cutaneous malignancies is the increased mortality rate from melanoma between 1988 and 2007 in the cities of Shanghai and Beijing [6].

The majority of the Chinese population have fair skin along with increased exposure to ultraviolet B (UVB) rays from the sun—creating a heightened risk for the development of skin cancer diseases [7, 8]. Specifically, BCC is linked with short-term burning incidents or long-term exposure of the head and neck; SCC is often related to extended periods of short- and long-term sun exposure [9]. Thus, skin cancer rate reduction warrants use of sun protective strategies to lower UV absorption. Examples of modifiable behaviors include using sunscreen, limiting direct sun exposure, and wearing protective clothing. Therefore, addressing attitudes and perceptions related to skin cancer within the Chinese population can lead to the initiation and continuation of sun protective behaviors.

Local governments in China distribute treatment expenditures but typically fail to provide money for preventative medicine [10]. Since 2004, the central government has worked to increase cancer prevention funding [10]. As China's rapidly aging population continues to strain its healthcare system financially, preventative measures are of utmost importance due to their cost-saving benefits. The importance of these actions extends beyond the elderly of China's population.

A study conducted on staff and volunteers from seven different Olympic event locations in Beijing found that 79.3% were aware of the association between UV exposure and skin cancers. Nevertheless, only 49.3% of participants wore protective clothing, 45.3% used sunglasses, and 58.8% applied sunscreen [11]. In another study, sunscreen usage rates were as low as 23.1% among college-age Chinese residents [12]. These findings suggest that more intervention regarding sun safety should be provided to young Chinese adults. Education is especially important due to a significant risk of SCC from early age exposure in males and lifetime sun exposure in females [9].

This article presents a narrative review on the knowledge, attitudes, and practices (KAP) related to skin cancers within the Chinese population. Based on this framework, recommendations of preventative public health strategies to engage the population have been made.

2. Methods

In the initial search, a systematic, computer-based literature search was conducted using MEDLINE (PubMed), Cumulative Index to Nursing and Allied Health Literature (CINAHL), and ScienceDirect. The search was performed in these electronic databases using combinations of the following terms: "China", "Chinese", "skin cancer", "melanoma", "sun protection", "sun behaviors", "knowledge", "attitudes", "beliefs", "perceptions", "sunscreen", "prevention", "practices", and "behaviors". Results of the initial literature search conducted in August 2017 included reviews of abstracts and titles with exclusion of off-topic articles.

Analyses of further studies updated in October 2017 were performed by reviewing reference lists of the articles of interest, along with searches in Google Scholar. The search was not limited by date of publication or language. Both English and Chinese language studies that contained digital and searchable English abstracts and keywords were included.

To the best of the reviewers' knowledge, all manuscripts published in peer-reviewed journals in the selected databases were considered for inclusion in this review. Research studies that measured skin cancer or sun protection related

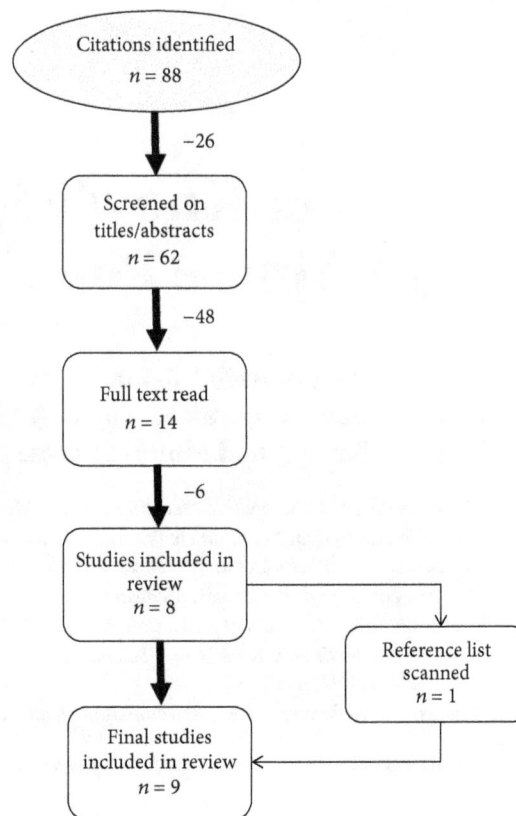

FIGURE 1: Chart of literature review.

knowledge, attitudes, beliefs, and behaviors in China were included. Exclusion criteria for the articles included the following: (1) irrelevant topics to review article aim, (2) articles that focused on treatment of skin cancers instead of preventative practices, and (3) comparable studies conducted on similar groups not indigenous to China. The literature search was conducted by four independent reviewers. Any disagreement regarding inclusion criteria was resolved via discussion until consensus was reached.

3. Results

Electronic searches identified a total of 88 citations. After removing duplicates ($n = 26$), the remaining 62 articles were screened based on titles and abstracts. After screening, the remaining 14 articles were read in their entirety to determine inclusion criteria eligibility. In summary, a total of nine articles met the eligibility criteria and were included in the review (Figure 1).

Table 1 provides details of the literature review pertaining to skin cancer knowledge, attitudes, and practices among the Chinese population. The first column displays the senior author of each corresponding article, as well as the date and location of the study. Column two includes the methodologies used for data collection and sample size (n) for each study, along with the gender and age of the participants. Extracted data regarding knowledge, attitudes, and beliefs of the participants are located within the third column. Only preintervention data were extracted and included in the

TABLE 1: Summary of included studies.

First author, date, and location	Data collection method, sample size (n), gender, and age	Knowledge, attitudes, and beliefs	Skin cancer prevention practice
Cheng, 2008, and Beijing [21]	Questionnaire, $n = 720$ (patients and hospital staff) 424 females, mean age = 37 years (SD = 27.5), age range = 14–72 years	49.3% knew that sunscreen could protect people from both UVA and UVB radiation Groups within the populations of males, middle-aged, elderly, low-education, and people with skin phototype I and II had misunderstandings of sunscreen's recognition and application	Sunscreen application Use sunscreen very often: 40% Reapply sunscreen in burning sun: 43.3%
Yang, 2009, and Nanjing [15]	Direct observation, $n = 39$ (dermatologists, 28 attending, 11 residents), 21 females, mean age = 35.3 years, age range = 27–48 years $n = 41$ (photosensitive patients), 23 females, mean age = 49 years, age range = 19–72	Fluorescent agent detection according to skin site Dermatologists: Hairline of forehead = 51.3%, forehead = 92.3%, temples = 74.4%, cheek = 100%, nose = 92.3%, perioral = 82.1% (male = 61% female = 100% $p < 0.01$), ears, neck, hands, and wrists: 0% Photosensitive patients: Hairline of forehead = 36.6%, forehead = 100%, temples = 41.5% (male = 28% female = 57% $p < 0.05$), cheek = 100%, nose = 75.6%, perioral = 73.2%, ears = 2.4%, neck = 0%, hand and wrists = 4.9% Density of fluorescent agent (mg/cm^2) Dermatologists: Hairline of forehead: male = 0.5 (SD = 0.31), female = 0.5 (SD = 0.38), forehead: male = 1.0 (SD = 0.38), female = 1.5 (SD = 0.02), temples: male = 0.5 (SD = 0.41), females = 1.0 (SD = 0.29), cheek: male = 1.0 (SD = 0.29), female = 1.0 (SD = 0.25), nose: male = 0.5 (SD = 0.35), female = 1.0 (SD = 0.21), perioral: male = 0.5 (SD = 0.32), female = 1.0 (SD = 0.17), ears: 0% Neck/V area of the chest = 0%, Hand and wrist: 0% Photosensitive patients: Hairline of forehead: male = 0.5 (SD = 0.47), female = 0.5 (SD = 0.44), forehead: male = 1.0 (SD = 0.33), female = 1.5 (SD = 0.36), temples: male = 0.5 (SD = 0.27), female = 0.2 (SD = 0.31), cheek: male = 1.0 (SD = 0.28), female = 1.0 (SD = 0.23), nose: male = 0.5 (SD = 0.26), female = 0.5 (SD = 0.35), perioral: male = 0.5 (SD = 0.36) female = 0.5 (SD = 0.25), ears: 0% Neck/V area of the neck: 0%, Hand and wrist: male = 0.1, female = 0	Sunscreen cream application Dermatologists: 28.2% put cream on the tip of finger 71.8% put cream in the palm of the hand and rubbed the hands together before applying to target skin sites Photosensitive patients: 17.1% put cream on the tip of finger 82.9% put cream in the palm of the hand and rubbed the hands together before applying to target skin sites

TABLE 1: Continued.

First author, date, and location	Data collection method, sample size (*n*), gender, and age	Knowledge, attitudes, and beliefs	Skin cancer prevention practice
Cheng, 2010, and Beijing [11]	Questionnaire, *n* = 623 (volunteers), 61.8% female, mean age = 24.6 (SD = 6.7), age range = 18–60 years	Total knowledge score of types of UV that can damage the skin = 29.7%, men = 12.6%, women = 40.3% Total knowledge score that people should take precautions from the sun in the morning or at nightfall = 73.0%, men = 58.4%, women = 82.1% Total knowledge score that people should take precautions from the sun on a cloudy day = 58.8%, men = 44.5%, women = 67.5% Total knowledge score that UV-induced skin damage is accumulative = 80.3%, men = 71.4%, women = 85.7% Meaning of SPF total knowledge score = 61.2%, men = 51.3%, women = 67.3% Meaning of PA total knowledge score = 34.4%, men = 31.5%, women = 36.1% Know how to use sunscreen correctly 74.2%, men = 58.8%, women = 83.6% Awareness score of what types of skin damage the sun causes: burn (total = 81.2%, men = 70.2%, women = 88.1%), skin cancer (total = 79.3%, men = 73.1%, women = 83.1%), tan (total = 52.0%, men = 40.8%, women = 59.0%), skin aging (total = 65.8%, men = 53.8%, women = 73.3%), blemishes (total = 73.4%, men = 60.9%, women = 81.0%), do not know (total = 2.4%, men = 5.0%, women = 0.8%)	Sunscreen = 58.8%, men = 28.2%, women = 77.7% Protective clothing = 49.3%, men = 59.7%, women = 42.9% Hat = 42.2%, men = 39.5%, women = 43.9% Parasol (sun umbrella) = 45.4%, men = 14.3%, women = 64.7% Sunglasses = 45.3%, men = 42.9%, women = 46.8% No protection = 9.0%, men = 16.4%, women = 4.4% Have ever used sunscreen before = 80.3%, men = 59.2%, women = 93.2% Correct sunscreen use among those who have ever used sunscreen before = 45.0%, men = 14.9%, women = 56.8% Mean SPF value of sunscreen used = 27.7 (SD = 9.2), men = 30.7 (SD = 11.2), women = 26.7 (SD = 8.2) Mean Protection Grade (PA) value of sunscreen used = 2.3 (SD = 0.6), men = 2.6 (SD = 0.7), women = 2.3 (SD = 0.6)
Fan, 2012, and Hefei [22]	Questionnaire, *n* = 1501 (freshmen military cadets), 1488 males, mean age = 20.35 (SD = 2.13), age range = 15–29	78.8% and 81.7% of the subjects did not know that the UV consists of three parts and the meaning of the PA and SPF, respectively.	Sunscreen: 61.6% Long-sleeved clothing and pants: 48% Umbrella and hat: 61.8% Sunglasses: 63.8% 32.7% had been taken protective measures, and only 50 cases did a professional skin examination.
He, 2012, and Beijing and Ningxia [23]	Questionnaire, *n* = 217 (all females) 66.4% females from Beijing and 33.6% from Ningxia, mean age = 32 years (SD = 9.7), age range = 17–59 years	Despite the difference in cognition degrees between the two groups, both groups have high degrees of cognition on the damage of UV to skin Both groups have low basic UV knowledge 24.9% of the two groups have correct knowledge about types of UV 22.6% of the participants were aware that sun protection should be started as early as in one's infancy People get access to knowledge of sunburn and sun protection from the same sources: television 40.2%, magazines 27.6% 27.6% knew the meaning of SPF 6.3% knew the mean of PA	Walking in shadows: 63.6% Avoiding going out at noon: 60.8% Sunscreen: 62.2% Wearing long-sleeved t-shirts: 18.4% Hats: 26.7% Umbrellas: 53% Sunglasses: 30.9%

TABLE 1: Continued.

First author, date, and location	Data collection method, sample size (n), gender, and age	Knowledge, attitudes, and beliefs	Skin cancer prevention practice
Yan, 2015, and Shanghai [12]	Questionnaires, n = 5964 (residents), 53.2% females, mean age = 43.2 years and age range = 20–60 years	Knowledge about UV-induced risk by gender Premature aging: male = 59.7%, female = 73.3% Immune suppression: male = 47.8%, female = 58.5% Skin cancer: male = 50.3%, female = 59.5% Sun protection attitudes by gender Need sun protection in winter: male = 27.8%, female = 43.1% Need sun protection indoors or in the vehicle: male = 21.9%, female = 32.6% Tanning attitudes by gender Appears healthy: male = 11%, female = 10.2% Looks attractive: male = 5.7%, female = 4.3% Not favorable: male = 13.7%, female = 38.1%	Sun exposure behavior by gender Avoid outdoor actives in strong sunlight: male = 71.2%, female = 82% Avoid extensive exposure in sunny midday: male = 72.2%, female = 84.2% Average daily sun exposure time (min) by gender 7AM–5PM: male = 111.8 (SD = 105.7), female = 82.2 (SD = 64.7) 10AM–2PM: male = 31.1 (SD = 45.1), female = 20.1 (SD = 28.9) 21.3% of the participants have applied sunscreen with 93.3% of respondents female
Zhou, 2015, and Nanjing [13]	Questionnaire, n = 253 (college students) standard care group = 126, self-regulation group = 127, 97.6% females, mean age = 21.26 years (SD = 1.34), and age range = 18–24 years	Intention to use sunscreen mean score Standard care group: 2.64 (SD = 1.41) Self-regulation group: 2.71 (SD = 1.09) Sunscreen action planning mean score Standard care group: 1.79 (SD = 0.89) Self-regulation group: 1.87 (SD = 0.86) Sunscreen coping planning mean score Standard care group: 1.83 (SD = 0.90) Self-regulation group: 1.74 (SD = 0.81)	Mean sunscreen use: Standard care group: 1.77 (SD = 1.15) Self-regulation group: 1.95 (SD = 1.21)
Zhou, 2016, and Nanjing [24]	Questionnaire, n = 515 (medical students), 73.2% females	Mean knowledge score of men = 2.41 (SD = 1.51) and women = 2.56 (SD = 1.38) out of maximum total score of 6, no gender difference among scores $p = 0.31$ Highest rate of correct responses 68.0%, lowest rate 9.6% Students that thought sun exposure was enough = 67.5% Students with negative sun exposure response = 32.5% Most common reasons among 44 male students for inadequate sun exposure: 43.2% avoiding dark skin, 18.2% no desire to go out, 13.6% skin cancer Most common reasons among 124 female students for inadequate sun exposure: 75.0% avoiding dark skin, 16.1% skin cancer, 12.1% accelerated aging Student knowledge of Vitamin D obtained from: media = 59.9%, health professionals = 43.3%, classmates and friends = 25%, parents = 8.8% 68% of students correctly knew that the human body can get vitamin D through sun exposure 3.0% of students had no desire to learn about vitamin D Female students had greater desire to learn compared to male students (88.3% versus 78.5%) Male students had greater indifferent attitude than female students (18.5% versus 8.7%)	Most students lacked sun exposure because they did not want to get tan Length of sun exposure: <15 mins/d = 6.8% 15–30 mins/d = 31.8% 30–45 min/d = 27.4% Not in sun for >45 min/day = 34.0% 82.7% of students used some sun protections Frequency of sun protection use Never: male = 49.3%, female = 5.6% Rarely: male = 29.4%, female = 23.0% Sometimes: male = 13.2%, female = 36.1% Often: male = 8.1%, female = 30.2% Always: male = 0%, female = 5.1% Types of sun protection Sunscreen: male = 33%, female = 75% Hats; male = >50%, female = 42% Umbrellas: male = 20%, female = 72%

TABLE 1: Continued.

First author, date, and location	Data collection method, sample size (n), gender, and age	Knowledge, attitudes, and beliefs	Skin cancer prevention practice
Wan, 2016, and Guangzhou City [14]	Questionnaire, $n = 3083$ (parents/guardians and their children), 51.6% male children, children mean age = 7.70 years (SD = 2.78), children age range = 3–13 years, mean rent/guardian age = 36.72 years (SD = 5.95), 70.5% female	Reasons why parents supported their children in preventing sun exposure: 50.9% protecting from suntan, 75.6% protecting from sunburn, 15.3% preventing skin photoaging, 4.9% unclear, 3.1% other Reasons why parents did not support their children in preventing sun exposure: 23.2% UV is beneficial to the child's skin, 11.7% UV is no harm to the child's skin, 30.7% benefits of UV to the child's skin are greater than its harm, 52.5% the child's skin does not need sun protection Parent's opinions on using a different sunscreen for children than for parents: 69.7% the child's skin is different from the parent's skin, 27.7% the child's skin is easily allergic, 2.6% other Parent's opinions on the nonuse sunscreen for children: 44.4% sunscreen is not suitable for children, 27.9% do not know how to choose the sunscreen for children, 28.2% use alternative sun protection methods, 44.3% worried that the child's skin is allergic to sunscreen, 9.2% other Sources of sun protection information for increasing parents/guardians knowledge: 52% television advertisements 37.6% newspapers, 37% magazines, 31.1% friends, 28.2% books, 17.5% beauty parlors, 16.2% family members, 12.4% radio advertisements, 10.3% relatives, 10% dermatologist, 12.5% others	Mean time spent in the sunshine per day: <2 h: 49.8%, male = 47.7%, female = 52.1% 2–4 h: 43.9%, male = 44.6%, female = 43.1% >4 h: 6.3%, male = 7.7%, female = 4.8% Weather in which protective measures were taken: Sunny day: 93.6% Cloudy day: 8.3% Rainy day: 8.4% Cloudy to sunny day: 17.5% Occasions for sun protection: Travel: 57.8% Outdoor leisure activities: 56.4% Swimming: 36.5% Playing ball: 16.1% Physical education: 9.8% Others: 3.2% Stayed under shade: 12.8%, male = 12.3%, female = 13.4% Sunscreen: 38.2%, male = 30.2%, female = 46.6% Long-sleeved shirt: 27.6%, male = 23.8%, female = 31.7% Hat: 61.9%, male = 60.7%, female = 63.2% Umbrella: 53.2%, male = 40.8%, female = 66.4% Sunglasses: 26.8%, male = 25%, female = 28.7%

table for studies utilizing experimental design. Prevention practices of participants in each study are described in the last column.

4. Discussion

The purpose of this article was to conduct a narrative review to summarize the knowledge, attitudes, and practices (KAP) related to skin cancers within the Chinese population. The Chinese are generally fair-skinned thus making them vulnerable to cutaneous cancers. The other primary modifiable preventative risk factor for skin cancers is exposure to UVB radiation, especially from the sun. The best protective measure, therefore, is limiting exposure to sunlight, particularly during the peak hours between 10 am and 2 pm. Other methods suggested to reduce skin cancer incidence include covering the skin with protective clothing—sunglasses, long sleeves, and hats—and the regular application of sunscreens with a sufficiently high sun protection factor (SPF) [8]. Sunscreen use was found to be a popular method of skin protection due to its enhanced affordability in an improving Chinese economy [11]. However, these findings were not in agreement with the results from a survey conducted among 11 communities in Shanghai, where only 21.3% utilized sunscreen, while the majority of the other participants preferred shade or hats as their primary means of skin protection [12].

While the prevalence of skin cancer is lower in China relative to some of the Western countries [11], BCC and SCC remain common cancers; therefore, skin protection remains important for public health [12]. One possible explanation for the reduced incidence of skin cancer may be that the average complexion among the Chinese populace is not as fair as that found in Western countries. One study found that the majority of the Chinese population is skin type IV on the Fitzpatrick scale, making them amenable to easy tanning and rare burning [12]. Darker-skinned populations have a lower incidence of skin cancer in general but are likely to be diagnosed with more advanced stages of the disease, if it does develop [12]. Another possible explanation may be that, in contrast to Western populations, many Chinese citizens find paler complexions more desirable and are therefore more likely to avoid unnecessary sunlight exposure and tanning [13].

Studies have found educational programs to reduce rates of sunburn and skin aging in the general population [11]. However, based on this review we found that such initiatives are rather few in China, with the effects of UVB being largely ignored [12]. Furthermore, knowledge and attitudes pertaining to UVB radiation have been found to be somewhat deficient among many Chinese communities. Among men and women, one study found that only 55.2% knew that UV radiation causes skin cancer [12]. Similar to Western populations, women scored higher on skin protective knowledge tests than men [11, 12]. Men were found to be less likely to care for their skin regularly compared to women, with many men expressing that sunscreen and umbrella usage are women's activities. Men were also less willing to participate in educational programs about skin protection [11]. Additional efforts should be made to improve the

population's perspective, particularly men, on skin cancer prevention and to increase their involvement.

Sun exposure during childhood has been correlated with skin cancer development later in life [14]. The percentage of children with a history of experiencing a sunburn increases as age increases. Therefore, it is imperative for educational programs to be introduced at an early age before multiple sunburns have been manifested. Interestingly, a large percentage (93.6%) of parents reported utilizing sunscreen for skin protection on their children (including 38.2% who are less likely to utilize the same methods for themselves), citing sunburn prevention as the main reason [14]. Involving parents in their children's educational program presents a possible avenue for improving adult attitudes as well.

The appropriate application of sunscreens is another area of concern. Frequently, inadequate amounts of sunscreens were found to be used in addition to inconsistent methods of application, i.e., some areas of the body received more sunscreen, leaving other areas at risk. An application density of 2 mg/cm^2 has been found to be most appropriate to receive the full SPF of the sunscreen [15]. Parents who did not use sunscreens on their children were fearful either that the products were unhealthy or that they would cause an allergic reaction, but among those who did use this preventative measure, nearly half did not follow the recommended reapplication rate of every 2-3 hours or used a product strength that was often less than 30 SPF [14].

Before introducing UVB awareness and skin protection programs to the Chinese population, modifications should be made to assure cultural and ethical appropriateness. One such concern is the risk of vitamin D deficiency, which Asian adults face due to their complexion [16]. In terms of disseminating knowledge and awareness to the public at large, television advertisements were selected by parents as an important medium for sun protection information (52% agreement) [14]. This finding suggests that the Chinese population is receiving a substantial portion of its medical information from nonmedical sources. Mass media campaigns, therefore, should attempt to involve medical professionals in their creation to improve the broad dissemination of effective skin protective strategies.

Knowledge alone has not been found to be a strong predictor of behavioral change [13]. The level of health literacy was a significant factor in the relationship between knowledge and behavior. For example, in the context of vitamin D absorption and sun exposure, individuals with high health literacy were more likely to discern appropriate amounts of sun exposure to maximize the amount of vitamin D absorption; unfortunately, poor attitudes counteracted the benefits of health literacy [17]. This suggests that any educational initiative should not only focus on increasing knowledge and health literacy, but also on improving societal attitudes, which insure the initiation and continuation of healthy behavioral changes related to skin protection and sun exposure. Thus, evidence-based theoretical approaches need to be instituted to foster effectual behavior change [18]. In present day context, fourth generation behavior changes that utilize multiple theories are in vogue [19]. One such utilization is through the multi-theory model (MTM) of health behavior change that breaks down behavior change into initiation and sustenance [20]. For initiation of sun protection behaviors attitudes that underscore advantages over disadvantages of such behavior change and behavioral confidence to use sun protection behaviors along with the changes in physical environment that support sun protection are important. In order to sustain sun protective behaviors, one needs to promote conversion of emotions toward goals for adhering to and continually practicing these behaviors, as well as mobilizing changes in social environment.

5. Limitations

There are limitations in the construct and the included studies of this narrative review. Some of the studies are susceptible to measurement biases due to self-reported data collection methods. Additionally, the data collected via questionnaires are subject to the recall bias. Although some of the studies were in Chinese with abstracts in English, the search was conducted solely using English language accessible electronic databases; therefore it is possible that some relevant articles were missed. Furthermore, we omitted searches within the grey literature. Finally, caution should be exercised when making generalizations of findings to the Chinese population since this review included only nine studies from six locations.

6. Conclusions

The findings of this study indicate a need for increasing awareness and knowledge among the Chinese population about skin cancer risk factors and institute effectual changes and interventions that promote sun protection behaviors. More research is needed with this population to gain a better understanding of attitudes and beliefs and how they could be adjusted into meaningful skin cancer prevention practices. Future studies must attempt to develop evidence-based theoretical interventions to help individuals to initiate and sustain sun protection behaviors in order to decrease their future skin cancer risk. Finally, research should take into consideration behavior change differences between gender, age, and socioeconomic status with regard to sun protection behaviors.

References

[1] F. Xiang, R. Lucas, S. Hales, and R. Neale, "Incidence of non-melanoma skin cancer in relation to ambient UV radiation in white populations, 1978–2012: empirical relationships," *JAMA Dermatology*, vol. 150, no. 10, pp. 1063–1071, 2014.

[2] J. Ferlay, E. Steliarova-Foucher, J. Lortet-Tieulent et al., "Cancer incidence and mortality patterns in Europe: estimates for 40 countries in 2012," *European Journal of Cancer*, vol. 49, no. 6, pp. 1374–1403, 2013.

[3] A. Lomas, J. Leonardi-Bee, and F. Bath-Hextall, "A systematic review of worldwide incidence of nonmelanoma skin cancer,"

British Journal of Dermatology, vol. 166, no. 5, pp. 1069–1080, 2012.

[4] J. Yu, X. Luo, H. Huang, Z. Zhai, Z. Shen, and H. Lin, "Clinical characteristics of malignant melanoma in southwest China: A Single-Center Series of 82 consecutive cases and a meta-Analysis of 958 reported cases," *PLoS ONE*, vol. 11, no. 11, Article ID e0165591, 2016.

[5] S. Y. Cheng, N. M. Luk, and L. Y. Chong, "Special features of non-melanoma skin cancer in Hong Kong Chinese patients: 10-year retrospective study," *Hong Kong medical journal*, vol. 7, no. 1, pp. 22–28, 2001.

[6] H. M. Zeng, S. W. Zhang, R. S. Zheng et al., "Analysis of incidence and mortality of cutaneous melanoma from 2003 to 2007 in China," *China Cancer*, vol. 3, pp. 183–189, 2012.

[7] M. A. Linares, A. Zakaria, and P. Nizran, "Skin Cancer," *Primary Care—Clinics in Office Practice*, vol. 42, no. 4, pp. 645–659, 2015.

[8] Skin Cancer Facts & Statistics, "Skin Cancer Foundation website," http://www.skincancer.org/skin-cancer-information/skin-cancer-facts#general.

[9] C. Pelucchi, A. Di Landro, L. Naldi, and C. La Vecchia, "Risk factors for histological types and anatomic sites of cutaneous basal-cell carcinoma: An Italian case-control study," *Journal of Investigative Dermatology*, vol. 127, no. 4, pp. 935–944, 2007.

[10] X. Ma, C. Lin, and W. Zhen, "Cancer care in China: A general review," *Biomedical Imaging and Intervention Journal*, vol. 4, no. 3, 2008.

[11] S. Cheng, S. Lian, Y. Hao et al., "Sun-exposure knowledge and protection behavior in a North Chinese population: a questionnaire-based study," *Photodermatology, Photoimmunology & Photomedicine*, vol. 26, pp. 177–181, 2010.

[12] S. Yan, F. Xu, C. Yang et al., "Demographic Differences in Sun Protection Beliefs and Behavior: A Community-Based Study in Shanghai, China," *International Journal of Environmental Research and Public Health*, vol. 12, no. 3, pp. 3232–3245, 2015.

[13] G. Zhou, L. Zhang, N. Knoll, and R. Schwarzer, "Facilitating Sunscreen Use Among Chinese Young Adults: Less-Motivated Persons Benefit from a Planning Intervention," *International Journal of Behavioral Medicine*, vol. 22, no. 4, pp. 443–451, 2015.

[14] M. Wan, R. Hu, Y. Li et al., "Attitudes, Beliefs, and Measures Taken by Parents to Protect Their Children from the Sun in Guangzhou City, China," *Photochemistry and Photobiology*, pp. 753–759, 2016.

[15] H. P. Yang, K. Chen, M. Ju, B. Z. Chang, L. Y. Wang, and H. Gu, "A study of the way in which dermatologists and photosensitive patients apply sunscreen in China," *Photodermatology, Photoimmunology & Photomedicine*, vol. 25, no. 5, pp. 245–249, 2009.

[16] Q. Gao, G. Liu, and Y. Liu, "Knowledge, attitude and practice regarding solar ultraviolet exposure among medical university students in Northeast China," *Journal of Photochemistry and Photobiology B: Biology*, vol. 140, pp. 14–19, 2014.

[17] A. Y. M. Leung, M. K. T. Cheung, and I. Chi, "Supplementing vitamin D through sunlight: Associating health literacy with sunlight exposure behavior," *Archives of Gerontology and Geriatrics*, vol. 60, no. 1, pp. 134–141, 2015.

[18] M. Sharma, *Theoretical Foundations of Health Education and Health Promotion*, Jones and Bartlett Learning, Burlington, MA, USA, 2017.

[19] M. Sharma, "Trends and prospects in public health education: A commentary," *[Editorial]. Social Behavior Research & Health*, vol. 1, no. 2, pp. 67–72, 2017.

[20] M. Sharma, "Multi-theory model (MTM) for health behavior change," *WebmedCentral Behaviour*, vol. 6, no. 9, Article ID WMC004982, 2015.

[21] S. W. Cheng, F. Liu, M. Cao et al., "Knowledge and the Use of about Sunscreen Among Chinese Population in Beijing," *The Chinese Journal of Dermatovenereology*, vol. 22, no. 9, pp. 566–569, 2008.

[22] D. Z. Fan, S. Liu, T. Yang, J. L. Wand, K. Ye, and F. M. Pan, "The Investigation and Analysis on the Awareness of Sun Protection Knowledge and the Use of Sunscreen Among Cadets in Hefe," *China Medical Abstract of Dermatology*, pp. 6–9, 2012.

[23] R. He, "A questionnaire-based study on sun-exposure knowledge and protection behavior in women from North China," *Ningxia Medical Journal*, pp. 12–031, 2012.

[24] M. Zhou, W. Zhuang, Y. Yuan, Z. Li, and Y. Cai, "Investigation on Vitamin D knowledge, attitude and practice of university students in Nanjing, China," *Public Health Nutrition*, vol. 19, no. 1, pp. 78–82, 2016.

7

Evaluation of Lipid Profile in Patients with Cherry Angioma: A Case-Control Study in Guilan, Iran

Abbas Darjani,[1] **Rana Rafiei** ⓘ**,**[2] **Sareh Shafaei,**[1] **Elahe Rafiei,**[3] **Hojat Eftekhari,**[1] **Narges Alizade,**[1] **Kaveh Gharaei nejad,**[1] **Behnam Rafiee,**[4] **and Sara Najirad**[5]

[1]*Skin Research Center, Dermatology Department, Guilan University of Medical Sciences, Razi Hospital, Sardare Jangal Street, Rasht, Iran*
[2]*Fellowship of Dermatopathology, Skin Research Center, Dermatology Department, Guilan University of Medical Sciences, Razi Hospital, Sardare Jangal Street, Rasht, Iran*
[3]*Razi Clinical Research Development Center, Guilan University of Medical Sciences, Rasht, Iran*
[4]*Department of Pathology, NYU Winthrop Hospital, 222 Station Plaza, No. 620, Mineola, NY 11501, USA*
[5]*Department of Internal Medicine, Nassau University Medical Center, 2201 Hempstead Turnpike, East Meadow, NY 11554, USA*

Correspondence should be addressed to Rana Rafiei; rafieirana@yahoo.com

Academic Editor: Luigi Naldi

Background. Cherry angioma is the most common type of acquired cutaneous vascular proliferation which would increase with aging due to some angiogenic factors but the exact pathogenesis is unknown. Usually angiogenic factors are synthesized in human body to compensate occlusive effects of atherogenic agents such as serum lipids. Our hypothesis was that increased levels of these angiogenic factors could be a trigger for development of cherry angioma. This study has been designed to compare frequency of dyslipidemia in subjects with and without cutaneous cherry angioma. *Methods*. In this case-control study, 122 cases with cherry angioma and 122 control subjects without cherry angioma were enrolled. Demographic characteristics, number of the cherry angioma lesions, and serum lipid profile were collected for all subjects. The data was analyzed using SPSS 18 software. *Results*. Mean levels of the total cholesterol, triglyceride, low-density lipoprotein, and high-density lipoprotein were higher in patients with cherry angioma compared to control subjects in which differences were significant for total cholesterol, low-density lipoprotein, and triglyceride ($P < 0.05$) but not for high-density lipoprotein level. *Conclusion*. Serum lipids may have a role in producing angiogenic factors and development of cherry angioma and it seems logical to evaluate lipid profile in these cases.

1. Introduction

Cherry angioma (CA) or senile angioma is the most common type of acquired benign vascular proliferation which usually presents as nonblanching red papules on the acral and truncal areas [1]. CA has been seen in 2% of children, 50% of adults, and 50%–75% of people aged older than 75 years [1–4]. It has a polygenic mode of inheritance. These lesions often have no symptoms and patients are always concerned about the increasing number of the lesions, risk of malignancy, and their cosmetic aspects [1]. CA develops due to abnormal proliferation of well differentiated endothelial cells [5]. The exact pathogenesis is unknown. Hyperprolactinemia, pregnancy, human herpesvirus 8 (HHV-8) infection, mustard

gas poisoning, immunosuppression induced by cyclosporine, underlying malignancy, some chemokines, and bromide and 2-butoxyethanol exposure all have been incriminated [6–11]. These agents would be associated with eruptive form of CA but in noneruptive form of CA; the lesions gradually increase with aging and they are more and larger in diabetic patients [1, 12]. Our hypothesis was that some angiogenic factors are synthesized in the body to compensate occlusive effects of atherogenic agents. These angiogenic factors could be a trigger for development of CA. Serum lipids are one of the most important atherogenic agents [11, 13].

This research was designed to determine possible association between CA and dyslipidemia. If we could find any association, CA might be considered as a cutaneous marker of dyslipidemia and these patients should be screened earlier to prevent cardiovascular diseases.

2. Materials and Methods

This study was designed as an age-matched case-control study at Skin Research Center of Guilan University of Medical Sciences, Razi Hospital, Rasht, from June 2016 to March 2017.

This study included 244 volunteers, 122 cases with CA and 122 healthy control subjects without CA, randomly selected from our patients who visited the hospital for aesthetic reasons. Final sample size was calculated after a primary pilot study. Both groups were frequency-matched in age groups (30–39; 40–49; 50–59; . . ., 80–89 years).

All patients aged ≥30 years who did not meet our exclusion criteria and had consent for body examination and doing laboratory evaluation were included.

We excluded some cases as follows to decrease confounding factors that may affect serum lipid levels: patients with drug history of agents which could be able to change lipid profile such as statin group, fibrate group, beta blockers, steroidal hormones, contraceptive pills, cyclosporine, oral retinoids, and diuretics; pregnancy or lactation, smoking, alcoholism, diabetes, history of mustard gas poisoning, hypertension, underlying malignancy, thyroid dysfunction, eruptive form of CA; patients who had very high lipid levels in the form of familial dyslipidemia; and patients with chronic inflammatory skin diseases such as lichen planus or psoriasis.

CA was diagnosed based on the physical examination performed by an individual dermatologist without skin biopsy.

Demographic characteristics of participants (age, sex, and Fitzpatrick skin phototype) and number of the cherry lesions were recorded in the first visit. Lipid profile including triglyceride (TG), cholesterol (CHOL), low-density lipoprotein (LDL), and high-density lipoprotein (HDL) level was collected for both groups. Lipid profile was evaluated in venous blood samples drawn after 12 h fasting in an individual laboratory by Hitachi analyzer 717 made in Japan.

Examination of the patients was conducted according to the declaration of Helsinki principles with informed consent. For patient comfort, scalp and genital area were not examined. This research project was approved by Ethics Committee of Guilan University of Medical Sciences (Code: IR.GUMS.REC.1395.204). The data of our manuscript is available.

Dyslipidemia was defined as TG level ≥ 150 mg/dl (hypertriglyceridemia) or total cholesterol level ≥ 200 mg/dl (hypercholesterolemia) or LDL level ≥ 130 mg/dl or HDL level < 40 mg/dl for men and <50 mg/dl for women, so if a patient had one or more of these abnormalities, they were categorized as having dyslipidemia [14].

Quantitative variables were described using mean and standard deviation and qualitative data were reported by number and percentage. For the comparison of frequencies, the chi-square test or Fisher's exact test was used and, for the comparison of continuous variables, Mann–Whitney

TABLE 1: Characteristics of participants in the case and control groups.

Variable[*]	Case $N = 122$	Control $N = 122$	P value
Age (year)	43.98 ± 9.11	43.48 ± 11.55	0.21[**]
Sex			
Male	33 (27%)	44 (36.1%)	0.13[***]
Female	89 (73%)	78 (63.9%)	
Skin phototype			
2	12 (9.8%)	8 (6.6%)	
3	54 (44.3%)	50 (41%)	0.476[α]
4	52 (42.6%)	62 (50.8%)	
5	4 (3.3%)	2 (1.6%)	
Levels of serum lipids (mg/dl)			
Triglyceride	167.37 ± 86.38	144.8 ± 105.40	0.004[×]
Cholesterol	200.39 ± 43.21	175.05 ± 38.15	<0.001[×]
LDL	117.52 ± 29.31	100.64 ± 31.30	<0.001[×]
HDL	50.24 ± 25.28	45.58 ± 13.52	0.096[×]

[*]Variables were described by number (percent) or mean ± standard deviation; [**]Mann-Whitney, [***]Chi square, [α]Fisher's exact test, [×]Kruskal-wallis.

and Kruskal–Wallis test were applied in both groups. All statistical tests were performed in SPSS 18 software. All P values were two-sided; significance level was set at $P < 0.05$.

3. Results

A total of 122 cases with CA and 122 control subjects without CA were enrolled in this study. Mean age and sex distribution and Fitzpatrick skin phototype of the participants were not significantly different in two groups which have been shown in Table 1.

Mean levels of the total cholesterol, TG, LDL, and HDL were higher in patients with CA compared to control group in which differences were significant for total cholesterol, LDL, and TG ($P < 0.05$) but not for HDL level ($P = 0.096$) (Table 1).

Frequency of dyslipidemia, hypertriglyceridemia, hypercholesterolemia, high LDL levels, and low levels of HDL in the participants has been summarized in Table 2. There was no significant difference in frequency of dyslipidemia between two groups ($P = 0.27$) but there was significant difference in frequency of hypertriglyceridemia, hypercholesterolemia, and high LDL levels between two groups ($P < 0.05$).

Patients with CA were allocated into three subgroups on the basis of CA count: (A) <5 lesions, (B) 5–10 lesions, and (C) >10 lesions; then mean age in these subgroups was compared. In paired comparison, there was a significant difference in mean age between subgroups A and C (Table 3).

Mean levels of total cholesterol, triglyceride, HDL, and LDL were not significantly different in these subgroups ($P > 0.05$).

TABLE 2: Lipid profile of participants in case and control groups.

Lipid profile	Case Number (%)	Control Number (%)	Total subjects Number (%)	P value*
Dyslipidemia				
No	22 (18)	29 (23.8)	51 (20.9)	0.27
Yes	100 (82)	93 (76.2)	193 (79.1)	
Hypertriglyceridemia				
No	61 (50)	82 (67.2)	143 (58.6)	0.006
Yes	61 (50)	40 (32.8)	101 (41.4)	
Hypercholesterolemia				
No	70 (57.4)	91 (74.6)	161 (66)	0.005
Yes	52 (42.6)	31 (25.4)	83 (34)	
High LDL				
No	86 (70.5)	103 (84.4)	189 (77.5)	0.009
Yes	36 (29.5)	19 (15.6)	55 (22.5)	
Low HDL				
No	60 (49.2)	52 (42.6)	112 (45.9)	0.304
Yes	62 (50.8)	70 (57.4)	132 (54.1)	

*Chi-square.

TABLE 3: Mean age in subgroups of patients with cherry angioma.

Subgroups of case group	Number of patients	Mean age (year) ± standard deviation	P value*
A (<5 lesions)	71	41.82 ± 8.38[a]**	
B (5–10 lesions)	23	44.09 ± 8.26[ab]	0.002
C (>10 lesions)	28	49.36 ± 9.58[b]	

*Kruskal–Wallis. **Similar characters represent nonsignificant differences of mean age in subgroups.

4. Discussion

Senile hemangioma or CA is a vascular tumor which consists of proliferated small vascular channels which have been originated from postcapillary venules in the upper dermis and it has been mentioned that CA should not be considered as a neovascularization [5]. Different etiologies and associations have been proposed for CA which include aging, genetic predisposition, hormonal changes, viral infection, immunosuppression, malignancy, hot climate, diabetes, and some chemical exposures [6–11, 15] but association with dyslipidemia has not been clearly mentioned in prior reports.

We found that hypertriglyceridemia, hypercholesterolemia, and high LDL levels were more frequent in patients with CA compared to control subjects. Mean age in patients with more than 10 CA lesions was significantly higher compared to patients with less than 10 CA lesions.

Increased levels of serum lipids in elderly could be as a triggering factor to release cytokines and chemokines which result in endothelial cell proliferation and CA lesions [11, 13]. Hypercholesterolemia is associated with endothelial cell dysfunction which may be due to toxic products derived from disintegration of lipoproteins [16]. Common pathogenic pathway could be incriminated for CA and dyslipidemia; for example, binding of Insulin-like Growth Factors (IGF) to their receptors results in proliferation of endothelial cells and hyperlipidemia [17]. It has been reported that CA are more and larger in patients with type 2 diabetes mellitus who have more IGF [12, 18] but CA has not been more prevalent in obese patients [19].

Mast cells (MC) may also have a potential role in development of CA and dyslipidemia. MC mediators are triggering factors in neovascularization and the number of mast cells increases in the CA lesions, but these new vascular proliferations may be due to degrading effects of MC mediators on dermal connective tissue [20]. On the other hand, angiogenic agents such as vascular endothelial growth factor (VEGF) have a chemotactic effect on the MC [20–22]. Interestingly it has been shown that MC may have a role in metabolic syndromes and dyslipidemia. It has been reported that chymase and tryptase of the MC could be able to actively degrade HDL. In animal models, it has been shown that mast cell-deficient mice had lower levels of serum triglycerides, total cholesterol, and phospholipids, so presenting a less atherogenic lipoprotein profile [22, 23]. Thus, it seems that MC might be incriminated in development of CA and dyslipidemia simultaneously.

CA has been associated with hypertension and varicosity in old ages [3] and hypertension by itself has been considered as a feature of metabolic syndrome [24] but we had to exclude hypertensive patients in our research because antihypertensive agents could be able to change lipid profile so it should be considered as a confounding factor. Also inflammatory factors decrease lipoprotein lipase activity in autoimmune skin diseases such as lichen planus, psoriasis, or pemphigus vulgaris which may result in dyslipidemia so we excluded these patients from this research [25].

Aging is associated with increasing in prevalence of dyslipidemia and CA, so we tried to have almost equal mean ages in both groups to minimize this confounding factor in our study.

We did not find any association between CA and skin phototype in this research. CA could be seen in any region of the body; thus it seems that sun exposure and skin phototype may not have major roles in development of CA. However it has been proposed that chronic sun exposure could be able to decrease skin tonicity and elasticity, so fragility of the blood vessels would be increased which results in the development of CA, telangiectasias, and senile purpura in elderly [26], but this theory could not justify development of CA on covered body areas and rejects the theory which says CA is a true vascular proliferation [5].

Frequency of hypercholesterolemia, hypercholesterolemia, and high levels of LDL was lower and frequency of low levels of HDL was higher in our study compared to estimated prevalence of dyslipidemia in Iranian people [14]. Unfortunately dyslipidemia has a higher prevalence among Iranian adults compared to US adults due to higher proportion of carbohydrates in Iranian diet [27].

In summary we think that CA lesions may be a sign of hypercholesterolemia or even a metabolic syndrome, but we had following limitations in our study: relatively small number of subjects was included which may not be fully representative of the general population. Also physical examination of genital and scalp areas was not done for patient's comfort which may result in control selection bias; many older patients were obligatorily excluded due to intake of antihypertensive and lipid lowering agents and other criteria for metabolic syndromes including body mass index were not considered.

5. Conclusion

Many different agents have been incriminated in development of CA. Although frequency of dyslipidemia was not significantly different in two groups, hypercholesterolemia and hypertriglyceridemia were more prevalent in patients with CA, so it seems logical to screen lipid profile in subjects with CA to prevent its atherogenic effect in the future.

Acknowledgments

This research project was derived from a residency thesis carried out at Skin Research Center of Guilan University of Medical Sciences. The authors would like to appreciate cooperation of Vice Chancellor of Research and Technology, Guilan University of Medical Sciences, as their funding source.

References

[1] A. Plunkett, K. Merlin, D. Gill, Y. Zuo, D. Jolley, and R. Marks, "The frequency of common nonmalignant skin conditions in adults in central Victoria, Australia," *International Journal of Dermatology*, vol. 38, no. 12, pp. 901–908, 1999.

[2] I. Inanir, M. Turhan Şahin, K. Gündüz, G. Dinç, A. Türel, and D. Serap Öztürkcan, "Prevalence of skin conditions in primary school children in Turkey: Differences based on socioeconomic factors," *Pediatric Dermatology*, vol. 19, no. 4, pp. 307–311, 2002.

[3] R. Reszke, D. Pełka, A. Walasek, Z. Machaj, and A. Reich, "Skin disorders in elderly subjects," *International Journal of Dermatology*, vol. 54, no. 9, pp. e332–e338, 2015.

[4] A. Darjani, Z. Mohtasham-Amiri, K. Mohammad Amini, J. Golchai, S. Sadre-Eshkevari, and N. Alizade, "Skin disorders among elder patients in a referral center in Northern Iran (2011)," *Dermatology Research and Practice*, vol. 2013, Article ID 193205, 2013.

[5] I. M. Braverman and A. Keh Yen, "Ultrastructure and three-dimensional reconstruction of several macular and papular telangiectases," *Journal of Investigative Dermatology*, vol. 81, no. 6, pp. 489–497, 1983.

[6] N. Askari, M.-R. Vaez-Mahdavi, S. Moaiedmohseni et al., "Association of chemokines and prolactin with cherry angioma in a sulfur mustard exposed population - Sardasht-Iran cohort study," *International Immunopharmacology*, vol. 17, no. 3, pp. 991–995, 2013.

[7] L. W. Raymond, L. S. Williford, and W. A. Burke, "Eruptive cherry angiomas and irritant symptoms after one acute exposure to the glycol ether solvent 2-butoxyethanol," *Journal of Occupational and Environmental Medicine*, vol. 40, no. 12, pp. 1059–1064, 1998.

[8] R. H. Barter, G. S. Letterman, and M. Schurter, "Hemangiomas in pregnancy," *American Journal of Obstetrics & Gynecology*, vol. 87, no. 5, pp. 625–635, 1963.

[9] A. D. Cohen, E. Cagnano, and D. A. Vardy, "Cherry angiomas associated with exposure to bromides," *Dermatology*, vol. 202, no. 1, pp. 52-53, 2001.

[10] I. De Felipe and P. Redondo, "Eruptive angiomas after treatment with cyclosporine in a patient with psoriasis [5]," *JAMA Dermatology*, vol. 134, no. 11, pp. 1487-1488, 1998.

[11] A. Borghi, S. Benedetti, M. Corazza et al., "Detection of human herpesvirus 8 sequences in cutaneous cherry angiomas," *Archives of Dermatological Research*, vol. 305, no. 7, pp. 659–664, 2013.

[12] B. Girisha and N. Viswanathan, "Comparison of cutaneous manifestations of diabetic with nondiabetic patients: A case-control study," *Clinical Dermatology Review*, vol. 1, no. 1, p. 9, 2017.

[13] J. Herrmann, L. O. Lerman, D. Mukhopadhyay, C. Napoli, and A. Lerman, "Angiogenesis in atherogenesis," *Arteriosclerosis, Thrombosis, and Vascular Biology*, vol. 26, no. 9, pp. 1948–1957, 2006.

[14] O. Tabatabaei-Malazy, M. Qorbani, T. Samavat, F. Sharifi, B. Larijani, and H. Fakhrzadeh, "Prevalence of dyslipidemia in Iran: A systematic review and meta-analysis study," *International Journal of Preventive Medicine*, vol. 5, no. 4, pp. 373–393, 2014.

[15] L. Requena and O. P. Sangueza, "Cutaneous vascular proliferation. Part II. Hyperplasias and benign neoplasms." *Journal of the American Academy of Dermatology*, vol. 37, no. 6, pp. 887–922, 1997.

[16] P. D. Henry, "Hyperlipidemic endothelial injury and angiogenesis," in *Arteriosclerosis*, Springer, Berlin, Germany, 1994.

[17] G. Akoglu, A. Metin, S. Emre, R. Ersoy, and B. Cakir, "Cutaneous findings in patients with acromegaly," *Acta Dermatovenerologica Croatica (ADC)*, vol. 21, no. 4, pp. 224–229, 2013.

[18] K. C. SHAH, A. C. SHAH, and P. C. SHAH, "CAMPBELL DE MORGAN'S SPOTS IN DIABETES MELLITUS.," *British Journal of Dermatology*, vol. 78, no. 8-9, pp. 493–495, 1966.

[19] L. García-Hidalgo, R. Orozco-Topete, J. Gonzalez-Barranco, A. R. Villa, J. J. Dalman, and G. Ortiz-Pedroza, "Dermatoses in 156 obese adults," *Obesity Research*, vol. 7, no. 3, pp. 299–302, 1999.

[20] K. Hagiwara, N. M. Khaskhely, H. Uezato, and S. Nonaka, "Mast cell 'densities' in vascular proliferations: a preliminary study of pyogenic granuloma, portwine stain, cavernous hemangioma, cherry angioma, Kaposi's sarcoma, and malignant hemangioen- dothelioma," *The Journal of Dermatology*, vol. 26, no. 9, pp. 577– 586, 1999.

[21] K. Aroni, E. Tsagroni, N. Kavantzas, E. Patsouris, and E. Ioanni- dis, "A study of the pathogenesis of Rosacea: how angiogenesis and mast cells may participate in a complex multifactorial process," *Archives of Dermatological Research*, vol. 300, no. 3, pp. 125–131, 2008.

[22] J. Zhang and G.-P. Shi, "Mast cells and metabolic syndrome," *Biochimica et Biophysica Acta (BBA) - Molecular Basis of Dis- ease*, vol. 1822, no. 1, pp. 14–20, 2012.

[23] P. T. Kovanen, "Mast cells: multipotent local effector cells in atherothrombosis," *Immunological Reviews*, vol. 217, no. 1, pp. 105–122, 2007.

[24] K. G. M. M. Alberti, P. Zimmet, and J. Shaw, "The metabolic syndrome—a new worldwide definition," *The Lancet*, vol. 366, no. 9491, pp. 1059–1062, 2005.

[25] C. Shenoy, M. M. Shenoy, and G. K. Rao, "Dyslipidemia in dermatological disorders," *North American Journal of Medical Sciences*, vol. 7, no. 10, pp. 421–428, 2015.

[26] N. Pustisek, N. Sikanic-Dugic, V. Hirsl-Hecej, and ML. Doml- jan, "Acute skin sun damage in children and its consequences in adults," *Collegium antropologicum*, vol. 34, no. 2, pp. 233–237, 2010.

[27] M. Kheirandish, S. Asgari, M. Lotfaliany et al., "Secular trends in serum lipid levels of a Middle Eastern adult population; 10 years follow up in Tehran lipid and glucose study," *Lipids in Health and Disease*, vol. 13, no. 1, article no. 20, 2014.

8

Factors Influencing Patient Decisions Regarding Treatments for Skin Growths: A Cross-Sectional Study

David G. Li,[1,2] **Fan Di Xia,**[3] **Jasmine Rana,**[4] **Grace J. Young,**[5] **Forootan Alizadeh,**[3] **Cara Joyce,**[6] **Shinjita Das,**[7] **and Arash Mostaghimi** ⓘ[1]

[1]*Department of Dermatology, Brigham & Women's Hospital, Harvard Medical School, Boston, MA, USA*
[2]*Tufts University School of Medicine, Boston, MA, USA*
[3]*Brigham & Women's Hospital, Harvard Medical School, Boston, MA, USA*
[4]*Santa Clara Valley Medical Center, San Jose, CA, USA*
[5]*Harvard Medical School, Boston, MA, USA*
[6]*Loyola University, Chicago, IL, USA*
[7]*Department of Dermatology, Massachusetts General Hospital, Harvard Medical School, Boston, MA, USA*

Correspondence should be addressed to Arash Mostaghimi; amostaghimi@bwh.harvard.edu

Academic Editor: E. Helen Kemp

Variations in treatment modalities for skin growths contribute substantially to overall healthcare spending within dermatology. However, little is known regarding factors impacting patient decision-making when choosing a treatment modality. In this survey-based, cross-sectional study (n = 375, 81.9% response rate), we asked patients to rate the importance of different treatment parameters for a nonfacial skin growth, further classified into five domains: efficacy, appearance, financial impact, visit duration, and productivity. Although patients generally prioritized treatment efficacy when selecting a treatment modality, they emphasized different aspects of the treatment experience as a function of age, gender, race, insurance status, and history of malignancy. Patients over age 50 were less likely to consider treatment impact on finances as being "important", but more so efficacy and visit duration. Women were more likely to value efficacy and appearance. Patients without private insurance were more likely to cite efficacy and impact on productivity as being "important". While the underlying reasons for these variations differ across patients, these findings help explain variations in treatment selection among patients choosing between treatments for skin growths and may ultimately lead to improved shared decision-making.

1. Introduction

Skin growths are a common presenting complaint in the outpatient dermatology setting, commonly manifesting as seborrheic keratoses, cysts, warts, lipomas, actinic keratoses, nonmelanoma skin cancers, benign nevi, and malignant melanomas [1, 2]. For each type of skin growth, existing treatment modalities confer different benefits and risks, necessitating individualized patient decision-making when selecting a treatment [3, 4].

Understanding patient characteristics associated with treatment preferences for skin growths may help promote shared decision-making to enhance patient experience and outcomes [5, 6]. Although variations in treatment modalities for skin growths contribute substantially to overall healthcare spending within dermatology, little is known about factors influencing patient decision-making when selecting a treatment modality [7]. In this cross-sectional study, we examined the factors underlying patient decision-making for treatment of skin growths.

2. Materials and Methods

We surveyed all patients aged ≥18 years at Brigham and Women's Hospital Dermatology over 5 days in August 2016. Patients were not required to have a history of skin conditions and participation was optional and uncompensated. Study

TABLE 1: Participant characteristics.

	Overall n = 375
Age, mean (SD)	51.4 (18.9)
Age ≤ 35	101 (26.9)
Female, n (%)	229 (61.1)
Race, n (%)	
White	306 (83.2)
Hispanic	25 (6.8)
African American	19 (5.2)
Asian	12 (3.3)
Other	6 (1.6)
Insurance, n (%)	
Private	231 (61.6)
Medicare	93 (24.8)
Medicaid	46 (12.3)
Self-insured/self-pay	4 (1.1)
Other/unknown	1 (0.3)
Dermatology visits in past 5 years, n (%)	
0-2	79 (21.1)
3-5	105 (28.0)
>5	191 (50.9)
Skin biopsies in past 5 years, n (%)	
0-2	329 (87.7)
3-5	35 (9.3)
>5	11 (2.9)
History of melanoma	42 (11.2)
History of SCC/BCC	98 (26.1)

staff provided a survey asking each patient to rate the importance of different treatment parameters for a nonfacial skin growth on a Likert scale between 1 and 5, with responses of 4 or 5 being categorized as "important". Treatment parameters were subsequently classified into five domains by study staff (DGL, AM): efficacy, appearance, financial impact, visit duration, and productivity (Supplemental Materials, available here). In addition, respondents were also asked to provide information on age, gender, insurance coverage, number of dermatology visits, number of biopsies in the past 5 years, and history of skin cancer.

Clinical and demographic information were reported descriptively using means (standard deviation) and percentages (Table 1). Percentage of respondents who rated each variable as 4 or 5 was calculated. Multivariable logistic regression analyses of patient characteristics associated with decision domains were performed. Statistical analyses were performed using SAS 9.4 (SAS Institute).

3. Results

458 surveys were administered, of which 375 surveys (81.9% response rate) were completed. Treatment efficacy was

considered an important factor by most (68.5%, n = 243) and visit duration (33.1%, n = 118) by the fewest. Patients over age 50 were less likely than those younger than 50 to consider treatment impact on finances (odds ratio [OR] 0.47 [95% CI 0.28-0.78]) as being "important", but more likely to consider efficacy (OR 1.78 [1.03-3.05]) and visit duration (OR 2.16 [1.26-3.71]) (Table 2). Women were twice as likely as men to value efficacy (OR 2.07 [1.27-3.36]) and appearance (OR 1.98 [1.23-3.19]). Non-white patients more frequently valued financial impact (OR 2.80 [1.49-5.29]) and visit duration (OR 2.60 [1.41-4.78]) than did white patients. Patients without private insurance were more likely than those with private insurance to cite efficacy (OR 2.11 [1.20-3.68]) and impact on productivity (OR 2.24 [1.35-3.71]) as being "important". Patients without a history of skin cancer emphasized appearance (OR 2.71 [1.56-4.73]), financial impact (OR 1.92 [1.11-3.32]), and visit duration (OR 2.34 [1.33-4.14]) over those with skin cancer history.

4. Discussion

This study highlights differences in prioritization among patients when deciding how to treat skin growths. Although patients overall prioritize treatment efficacy when making decisions, they emphasize different aspects of the treatment experience as a function of age, gender, race, insurance status, and history of malignancy.

While the underlying reasons for these variations differ across patients, many of these findings are consistent with known preferences. Patients over 50 are more likely to have a malignant skin growth compared to younger patients, thus being more likely to value treatment efficacy than their younger counterparts. Women's emphasis on appearance is consistent with greater use of plastic surgery cosmetic procedures, 92% of which are performed on female patients [8]. Non-white patients have been reported to earn less than their white counterparts, which may explain the greater emphasis on financial impact of treatment among non-white patients [9, 10]. Additionally, patients without private insurance may prefer treatment options minimizing the impact on productivity, as these patients may be more likely to be of lower socioeconomic status, thus necessitating an earlier return to work [11, 12].

These findings help explain variations in treatment choice among patients choosing between treatments that may have different treatment experiences and costs but similar clinical outcomes [13]. Although these differences impact treatment choice, they are overlooked in bundled payment models and may place patient preferences at odds with physician reimbursement [14]. While these results are specific to the treatment of skin growths in dermatology, these principles are applicable to medicine broadly, whenever patients have to choose between treatments with comparable clinical outcomes but differences in patient experience. These findings may therefore be broadly informative to patients and clinicians in explaining variations in treatment choices and support current efforts to use patient reported outcomes to capture more completely factors that influence patient decision-making.

TABLE 2: Adjusted odds ratios for patient characteristics associated with preferences about treatment approaches of skin growths.

	Treatment efficacy	Appearance	Financial impact	Visit Duration	Productivity
n responded	355	347	350	356	353
n (%) important	243 (68.5)	144 (41.5)	148 (42.3)	118 (33.1)	133 (37.7)
	Odds ratio (95% Confidence Interval)				
Age					
≤50	1 (reference)	1 (reference)	1 (reference)	1 (reference)	1 (reference)
>50	1.78 (1.03, 3.05)†	1.22 (0.72, 2.05)	0.47 (0.28, 0.78)‡	2.16 (1.26, 3.71)‡	0.84 (0.50, 1.43)
Gender					
Male	1 (reference)	1 (reference)	1 (reference)	1 (reference)	1 (reference)
Female	2.07 (1.27, 3.36)‡	1.98 (1.23, 3.19)‡	1.18 (0.74, 1.9)	1.06 (0.65, 1.72)	1.50 (0.93, 2.40)
Race					
White	1 (reference)	1 (reference)	1 (reference)	1 (reference)	1 (reference)
Non-White	1.77 (0.88, 3.56)	1.82 (0.98, 3.36)	2.80 (1.49, 5.29)‡	2.60 (1.41, 4.78)‡	1.67 (0.91, 3.04)
Insurance					
Private	1 (reference)	1 (reference)	1 (reference)	1 (reference)	1 (reference)
Public/self-pay	2.11 (1.20, 3.68)‡	0.91 (0.54, 1.51)	1.07 (0.64, 1.81)	1.37 (0.82, 2.28)	2.24 (1.35, 3.71)‡
History of skin cancer					
Yes	1 (reference)	1 (reference)	1 (reference)	1 (reference)	1 (reference)
No	1.03 (0.59, 1.80)	2.71 (1.56, 4.73)‡	1.92 (1.11, 3.32)†	2.34 (1.33, 4.14)‡	1.32 (0.77, 2.26)

†$p < 0.05$, ‡$p < 0.01$

Although this study contains a large sample size, our findings must be interpreted in the context of the study design. This study was conducted in a single academic medical center and study findings may not be generalizable to other patient populations. Additionally, because the survey does not specify the malignancy status associated with the hypothetical skin growth, respondents were free to assume the malignancy status, which may result in nondifferential misclassification bias owing to variable assumptions among survey respondents. Finally, although the study is cross-sectional in nature and survey-based, these results are unlikely to be subject to response bias given the high response rate (81.9%) among survey respondents.

5. Conclusion

Although treatment modalities for skin growths contribute considerably toward spending within dermatology, clinician understanding regarding factors impacting treatment selection is limited. These study findings are a step toward explaining variations in treatment selection among patients choosing between treatments for skin growths. Replication of these findings and a closer consideration of patient preferences across other spheres of care may help explain variations in practice.

Additional Points

Reprint Requests. Arash Mostaghimi, MD, MPA, MPH.

Authors' Contributions

David G. Li and Fan Di Xia contributed equally.

Acknowledgments

This study was supported by the TL1 Award (David G. Li) sponsored by the National Center for Advancing Translational Sciences, National Institutes of Health, Award no. TL1TR001062.

Supplementary Materials

(1) "ISCEP Survey: Skin Growths": (a) survey evaluating different domains of patient decision-making for the treatment of a nonspecific skin growth. (2) "Classification of Domains": (a) classification scheme identifying decision-making domains for survey questions. *(Supplementary Materials)*

References

[1] W Frank and G. S. Rogers, "Skin growths in the aged," *Treatment considerations Drugs Aging*, vol. 4, no. 3, pp. 194–206, 1994.

[2] M. C. Luba, S. A. Bangs, A. M. Mohler, and D. L. Stulberg, "Common benign skin tumors," *Am Fam Physician*, vol. 67, no. 4, pp. 729–738, 2003.

[3] K. Chitwood, J. Etzkorn, and G. Cohen, "Topical and intralesional treatment of nonmelanoma skin cancer: Efficacy and cost comparisons," *Dermatologic Surgery*, vol. 39, no. 9, pp. 1306–1316, 2013.

[4] O. Ibrahim, B. Gastman, and A. Zhang, "Advances in diagnosis and treatment of nonmelanoma skin cancer," *Annals of Plastic Surgery*, vol. 73, no. 5, pp. 615–619, 2014.

[5] F. D. Xia, J. Rana, G. J. Young et al., "Generational influence on patient learning preferences in dermatology," *Journal of the American Academy of Dermatology*, vol. 78, no. 6, pp. 1221–1223, 2018.

[6] A. G. Mulley, C. Trimble, and G. Elwyn, "Stop the silent misdiagnosis: patients' preferences matter," *BMJ*, vol. 345, no. nov07 6, pp. e6572–e6572, 2012.

[7] H. W. Lim, S. A. Collins, J. S. Resneck et al., "The burden of skin disease in the United States," *Journal of the American Academy of Dermatology*, vol. 76, no. 5, pp. 958–972.e2, 2017.

[8] "http://www.PlasticSurgery.org ASPS National Clearinghouse of Plastic Surgery Procedural Statistics 2016 Plastic Surgery Statistics," 9, 2018, https://www.plasticsurgery.org/.

[9] Pew Research Center, "On Views of Race and Inequality, Blacks and Whites Are Worlds Apart," Pew Research Center, 2016, 59, http://www.pewsocialtrends.org/2016/06/27/on-views-of-race-and-inequality-blacks-and-whites-are-worlds-apart/.

[10] "A Profile of the Working Poor," 2014, BLS Reports: U.S. Bureau of Labor Statistics, https://www.bls.gov/opub/reports/working-poor/2014/home.htm.

[11] "Eligibility," Medicaid.gov., https://www.medicaid.gov/medicaid/eligibility/index.html.

[12] "Key Facts about the Uninsured Population," The Henry J. Kaiser Family Foundation, https://www.kff.org/uninsured/fact-sheet/key-facts-about-the-uninsured-population/.

[13] M.-M. Chren, E. Linos, J. S. Torres, S. E. Stuart, R. Parvataneni, and W. J. Boscardin, "Tumor recurrence 5 years after treatment of cutaneous basal cell carcinoma and squamous cell carcinoma," *Journal of Investigative Dermatology*, vol. 133, no. 5, pp. 1188–1196, 2013.

[14] J. S. Kirby, A. Delikat, D. Leslie, and J. J. Miller, "Bundled payment models for actinic keratosis management," *JAMA Dermatology*, vol. 152, no. 7, pp. 789–796, 2016.

9

Effectiveness and Safety of Contrast Cryolipolysis for Subcutaneous-Fat Reduction

Marília Bueno Savacini,[1] Débora Tazinaffo Bueno,[1]
Ana Carolina Souza Molina,[1] Ana Caroline Almeida Lopes,[1] Caroline Nogueira Silva,[2,3,4]
Renata Gomes Moreira,[2,3] Stephani Almeida,[2,3] Renata Michelini Guidi,[2,3,5]
Estela Sant'Ana (ID),[2,3] and Richard Eloin Liebano[6]

[1]Ibramed Center for Education and Advanced Training (CEFAI), Amparo, Brazil
[2]Clinical Laboratory of the Ibramed Center for Education and Advanced Training (CEFAI), Amparo, Brazil
[3]Research, Development & Innovation Department IBRAMED, Ibramed Research Group (IRG), Amparo, Brazil
[4]Human Development and Technologies. Universidade Estadual Paulista (UNESP), Brazil
[5]Electrical Engineering Department, Faculty of Medical Sciences, University of Campinas (Unicamp), Brazil
[6]Department of Physiotherapy, Federal University of São Carlos, São Carlos, Brazil

Correspondence should be addressed to Estela Sant'Ana; profa_estelasantana@yahoo.com.br

Academic Editor: Craig G. Burkhart

Cryolipolysis is the noninvasive treatment of localized fat through cold-induced panniculitis. The purpose of the present study was to evaluate the safety and efficacy of contrast cryolipolysis for subcutaneous-fat reduction. Contrast cryolipolysis mixes the principles of conventional cryolipolysis and periods of heating in accordance with the contrast lipocryolysis process. Twenty-one subjects aged 34 ± 9 years were treated with contrast cryolipolysis in the regions of abdomen and flanks through the Polarys® device. Anthropometry, standardized photographs, measurements with a skinfold caliper, and diagnostic ultrasounds were performed at the baseline and during follow-ups at 30, 60, and 90 days after the treatment. The safety assessments included laboratory testing and monitoring of the adverse events. The level of significance for all tests was set at $P < 0.05$. No significant differences in weight and body mass index were found. The waist measurements at the baseline and 30-day follow-up had significant differences, as did the measurements at the 30-day and 60-day follow-ups. The skinfold and ultrasound measurements were significantly reduced in the treated areas in all the time points compared to the baseline. The laboratory results showed no significant changes from baseline. Temporary adverse effects were resolved spontaneously. This study confirmed that contrast cryolipolysis is safe and effective in reducing the fat layer and improving body contouring.

1. Introduction

Localized adiposity is an abnormal accumulation of fat in usual anatomical locations, and it is an important unaesthetic condition [1]. Liposuction has always been considered the standard treatment for body contouring; however, because of the potential complications associated with this procedure, new treatments were developed [2, 3]. Several treatments—including ultrasound, radiofrequency, and mesotherapy—have been developed to achieve adipocyte destruction [4–9]. Each technology employs a different

mechanism to cause the apoptosis or necrosis of the targeted adipocytes.

In recent years, a new technology for the noninvasive treatment of localized fat through cold-induced panniculitis—called cryolipolysis—appeared. This method is based on the concept that lipid-rich tissues are more susceptible to injury through cold than the surrounding water-rich tissue is [10]. On the other hand, studies [11–13] have shown that, when alternating low temperatures and cycles of heating, the lipids in the adipocytes crystallize more easily, which is similar to what happens in the tempering

CONVENTIONAL CRYOLIPOLYSIS   Total time = 60 min

0 min

60 min

CONTRAST CRYOLYPOLYSIS   Total time = 80 min

0 min

10 min

60 min

10 min

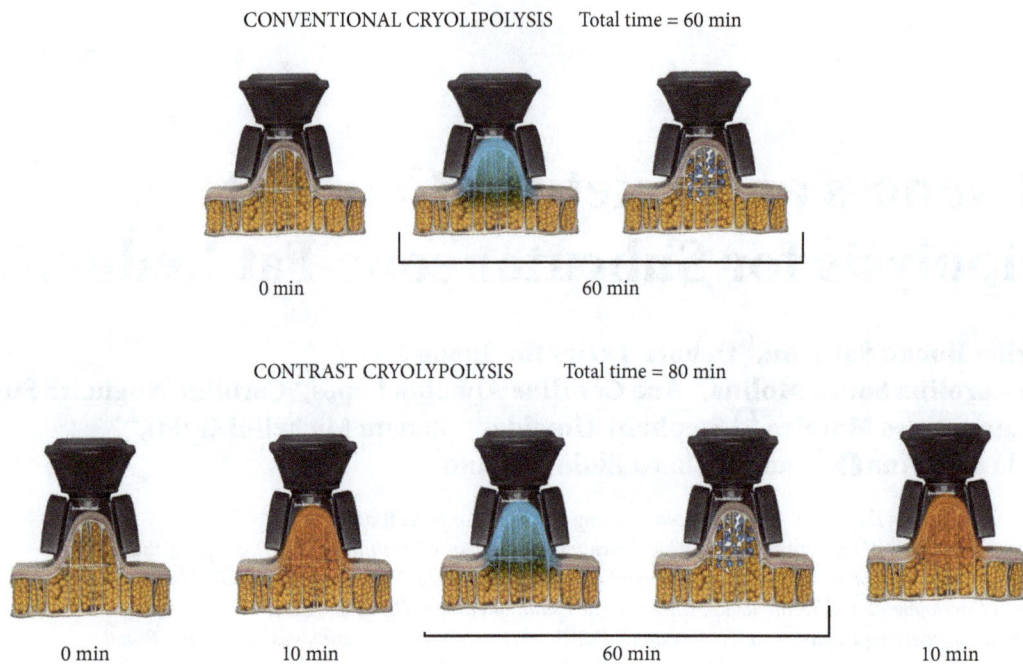

FIGURE 1: A comparison between conventional cryolipolysis and contrast cryolipolysis.

process of the food industry, and this process may improve the clinical outcome of the treatment. This method is known as contrast lipocryolysis. Based on both models (cryolipolysis and contrast lipocryolysis), a novel technology was conceived: contrast cryolipolysis. This technology differs from conventional cryolipolysis because it uses heating and cooling periods, and it differs from contrast lipocryolysis because it uses lower temperatures during cooling (Figure 1).

Although a large number of published studies on conventional cryolipolysis exist [14–24], studies assessing the effects of contrast cryolipolysis are still scarce. Therefore, the purpose of the present study was to evaluate the safe and efficacy of this method.

2. Materials and Methods

2.1. Subjects. This study included 21 healthy subjects aged between 18 and 50 years. The subject inclusion criteria were the presence of localized subcutaneous fat in the abdominal and flank regions and a body mass index (BMI) < 30. The subjects were excluded if they were in aesthetic treatment, had received some kind of treatment in the abdominal region in the 6 months before the start of this study, were pregnant or had experienced a recent pregnancy (within the past 6 months), or had a known history of cryoglobulinemia, cold urticaria, or paroxysmal cold hemoglobinuria.

The decision of which region to treat (i.e., the abdomen or the flanks) was made according to individual needs (Figure 2).

Assessments of body composition were performed at the baseline and during follow-ups 30, 60, and 90 days after the treatment.

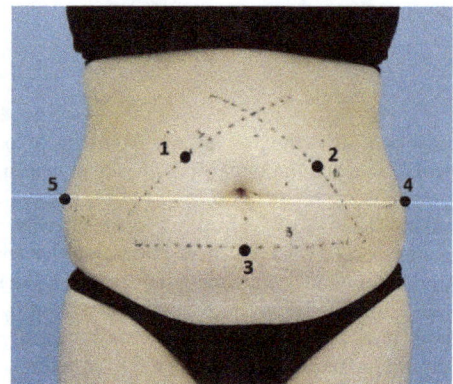

FIGURE 2: Points of evaluation and marked areas for the treatment. Each subject was treated at 1 or more areas for a total of up to 5 treatment areas; the areas were treated with either the medium or large applicator, based on the size of the localized fat area.

2.2. Ethical Aspects. The Research Ethics Committee: Institutions, Teaching, and Research approved this study: UNISEPE: CAAE: 61499416.5.0000.5490 (http://plataform-abrasil.saude.gov.br). All subjects signed informed consent forms, and the treatment was performed by trained physiotherapist in the Clinical Laboratory of the Ibramed Center for Education and Advanced Training CEFAI (Amparo, São Paulo, Brazil).

2.3. Sample Size. The sample size was calculated in consideration of a difference of 2.0 mm in the adipose layer, as evaluated by ultrasound. An estimated standard deviation of 2.0 mm was also considered, based on data from a previous study [25] on the effects of cryolipolysis on fat in the abdominal region of women. For a level of significance of 0.05 and power of 80%, the Minitab software calculated that 17 participants would be required (Minitab, v.17, StateCollege, PA). Thus, in order to avoid possible sample losses that would interfere with data analysis, 21 patients were recruited.

2.4. Treatment Protocol. The subcutaneous-fat layer in the regions of the abdomen and flanks was treated with contrast cryolipolysis. It was heated to 40°C for 10 minutes, cooled for 60 minutes (−8°C), and heated again to 40°C for 10 minutes with the cryolipolysis device Polarys® (Ibramed, Indústria Brasileira de Equipamentos Médicos EIRELI).

The subjects were treated at 1 or more areas for a total of up to 5 treatment areas in 1 or 2 sessions. Areas were treated with either the medium or large applicator, based on the size of the localized fat area and the anatomical limitations of the applicator placement. The treatment sessions were performed with the subjects comfortably positioned in the dorsal decubitus position with a 45° stretcher inclination or in the lateral decubitus position. The curved vacuum applicator was positioned in the center of the treatment area, and vacuum suction was initiated. The vacuum itself fixed the applicator over the treatment area, and pillows supported the applicator during the entire treatment.

2.5. Anthropometric Measurements. All the participants underwent anthropometric measurements that were performed at the baseline and during follow-ups 30, 60, and 90 days after the treatment. During assessments of their weight and height, the subjects wore only their underwear, without shoes. A classical mechanical stadiometer (model 110 CH, Welmy, São Paulo, Brazil) was used. The circumference of the abdomen was measured using a flexible measuring tape. Each measurement point was recorded at the baseline to ensure that subsequent measurements would be obtained from the same location.

2.6. Questionnaire. The patients completed a self-questionnaire that assessed the tolerability of the treatment. Volunteers indicated the tolerability of the treatment: selecting 1 for intolerable, 2 for tolerable, 3 for comfortable, and 4 for very comfortable.

2.7. Skinfold Caliper. A skinfold caliper (RMC, Amparo, SP, Brazil) was used to measure the site of greatest thickness within the treatment area for patients who were available for measurements at the baseline and during follow-ups 30, 60, and 90 days after the treatment.

2.8. Ultrasound Analysis. All the subjects underwent diagnostic ultrasound that was performed at the baseline and during follow-ups 30, 60, and 90 days after the treatment. Ultrasound assessment was performed using a linear transducer with a frequency of 6 to 18 MHz (MyLab™25 Gold; Esaote, Italy). Images were analyzed through quantitative measurements of the subcutaneous tissue between the

anatomic planes—the dermis and muscular fascia—and the thickness of the fat layer at the treatment area was measured in millimeters [26]. A single trained physiotherapist made the measurements. The probe was positioned on the previously demarcated points in the treatment area (Figure 2), with coupling gel and without tissue compression.

2.9. Standardized Photographs. Standardized digital photographs were taken with a digital camera (Canon EOS Rebel T3i, Canon USA Inc., Melville, NY, USA) at the baseline and during a follow-up 90 days after the treatment. All patients were photographed in standing positions in 3 views: the back view, right view, and left view; the image was taken at a distance of 1 m.

2.10. Safety Assessments. The safety assessments included laboratory testing and adverse-event monitoring. Blood collections were performed at the baseline and between 14 and 21 days after treatment for evaluations of the fasting glucose levels, lipid profiles, and liver function. Blood samples for all subjects were collected via venipuncture on a morning after overnight fasting of 12 to 14 hours. Immediately after the collection, the samples were processed and analyzed in a laboratory—São Francisco Laboratório de Análises Clínicas (Amparo, SP, Brazil). Serum lipid values were obtained for the following elements: cholesterol, triglycerides, very-low-density lipoprotein cholesterol, low-density lipoprotein cholesterol, and high-density lipoprotein cholesterol. Liver-related blood tests were obtained through the evaluation of the hepatic markers aspartate aminotransferase and alanine aminotransferase. Subjects with baseline laboratory values outside the reference range were excluded from this analysis. The occurrence of adverse events was monitored throughout the study.

2.11. Statistical Analysis. The statistical analysis was performed with Graph Pad Prism 6 (La Jolla, CA, USA). The normal-distribution assumption was assessed with a Shapiro-Wilk test. The differences between the beginning and posttreatment measurements were analyzed using an ANOVA and Tukey's multiple comparisons test or Friedman test and Dunn's multiple-comparisons test. For comparisons of glucose, the serum-liver test and serum-lipid values from the baseline and 3 weeks after the treatment were analyzed using the paired t-test or Wilcoxon signed-rank test. The level of significance for all tests was set at 0.05 ($P < 0.05$).

3. Results

Twenty-one subjects were enrolled and completed treatment (18 females and 3 males). The subjects were aged from 21 to 50 years, with a mean and standard deviation of 34 ± 9 years. Their weights ranged from 57.5 to 90.5 kg, with a mean and standard deviation of 70.3 ± 9; their BMI ranged from 21.8 to 30.0, with a mean and standard deviation of 25.7 ± 2. Weight and BMI did not undergo significant changes after treatment. The waist circumference data are presented in Figure 3. The measurements from the baseline and 30-day

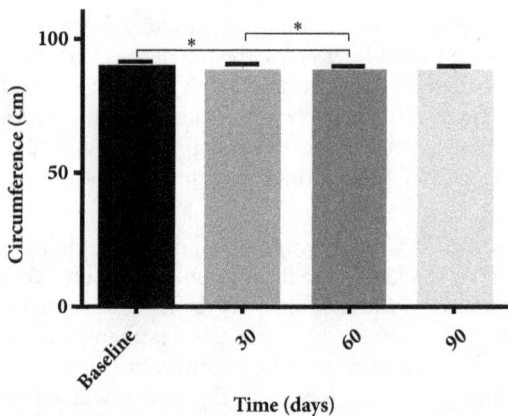

FIGURE 3: Means, with a standard error of the mean, of the waist circumference values before treatment (baseline) and after treatment (30, 60, and 90 days after treatment). $^*P < 0.05$.

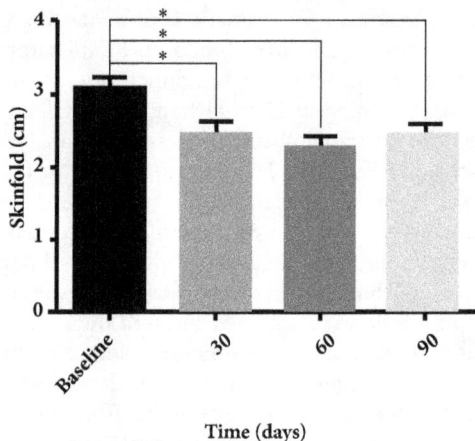

FIGURE 4: Means, with a standard error of the mean, of the abdominal length skinfold before treatment (baseline) and after treatment (30, 60, and 90 days after treatment). $^*P < 0.05$.

follow-up had statistically significant differences, as did those from the 30-day and 60-day follow-ups. However, we have not found differences between the measurements from the 90-day follow-up and the baseline.

The subjects tolerated the treatment well: 35% (N = 8) of the volunteers reported that it was tolerable, and 60% (N = 12) reported that it was comfortable. Only 1 volunteer (5%) considered the treatment intolerable.

The skinfold caliper data were analyzed to assess the treatment efficacy. The decrease in the skinfold-thickness values from the follow-ups and the baseline in the areas treated was statistically significant ($P < 0.05$) (Figure 4).

Ultrasound images were analyzed to calculate the fat-layer reduction. Figure 5 shows representative ultrasound images captured at the baseline and during follow-ups 30, 60, and 90 days after the treatment.

The reductions in the fat layer were statistically significant ($P < 0.05$) in both treated regions: the abdomen and flanks. The mean percentage of fat-layer reduction was 21.6% for the abdomen, and reductions of up to 50.1% were detected from

the baseline to 90 days after the treatment (Figure 6(a)). In the flanks, the mean reduction was 14.5%, and reductions of up to 43.2% were observed from the baseline to 90 days after the treatment (Figure 6(b)).

Figure 7 contains photographs that show that the sizes of the abdominal and flank areas visibly reduced between the baseline and 90-day follow-up.

The laboratory results are shown in Table 1. The mean values and standard deviations for the fasting glucose, liver-related tests, and serum lipids from the baseline were analyzed and compared with those from 3 weeks after the treatment. No significant changes were found.

4. Discussion

The purpose of the present study was to evaluate the safety and efficacy of contrast cryolipolysis: a method mixes the principles of conventional cryolipolysis and the contrast lipocryolysis process, which involves periods of heating.

The mechanism by which cryolipolysis induces damage to adipocytes is not well understood and remains an ongoing subject of research. The effectiveness and safety of this method has been widely established; however, it is important to highlight that the majority of published studies use a device that uses a cooling-intensity factor (CIF) and does not display the temperature in Celsius [27, 28]. The first study [29] with pigs that used a conventional cryolipolysis prototype were performed to investigate the effect of a controlled application of cold to the skin surface and the resulting selective damage to subcutaneous fat through the use of a cooled-fold metal plate. The skin surface areas were exposed to a cooling process with different temperatures (20°C, −1°C, −3°C, −5°C, and −7°C), and 20°C was considered the control temperature. The application time was 10 minutes. The authors observed that the apoptosis of fat cells started when the cooling panels were cooled to the temperature of −1°C. However, compared with the control, the most-intense results were obtained with the temperature of −7°C. In a subsequent study [30], also carried out with pigs, the researchers translated the temperature in degrees Celsius to milliwatts per centimeter squared and converted the result into CIF, a numerical value that defines heat extraction (cooling). The authors of this study observed a progressive inflammatory response to cold exposure. Immediately after treatment, no significant changes in subcutaneous fat were observed; however, 3 days after treatment, the presence of an inflammatory infiltrate was observed. The influx of inflammatory cells had increased when they were analyzed 7 and 14 days after treatment. After 30 days, the inflammatory process had begun to decline, and by 60 days, the thickness of the interlobular septa had apparently increased. The inflammatory process had weakened further by 90 days after treatment. The authors clearly showed that cryolipolysis induced subcutaneous panniculitis in response to cold exposure, with a decrease of the thickness of the fat layer, without affecting surrounding structures such as skin and water-rich tissue [24, 31]. These studies resulted in the development of the Coolsculpting™ device (Zeltiq Aesthetics, Inc., Pleasanton, CA) [30, 31]. Since then,

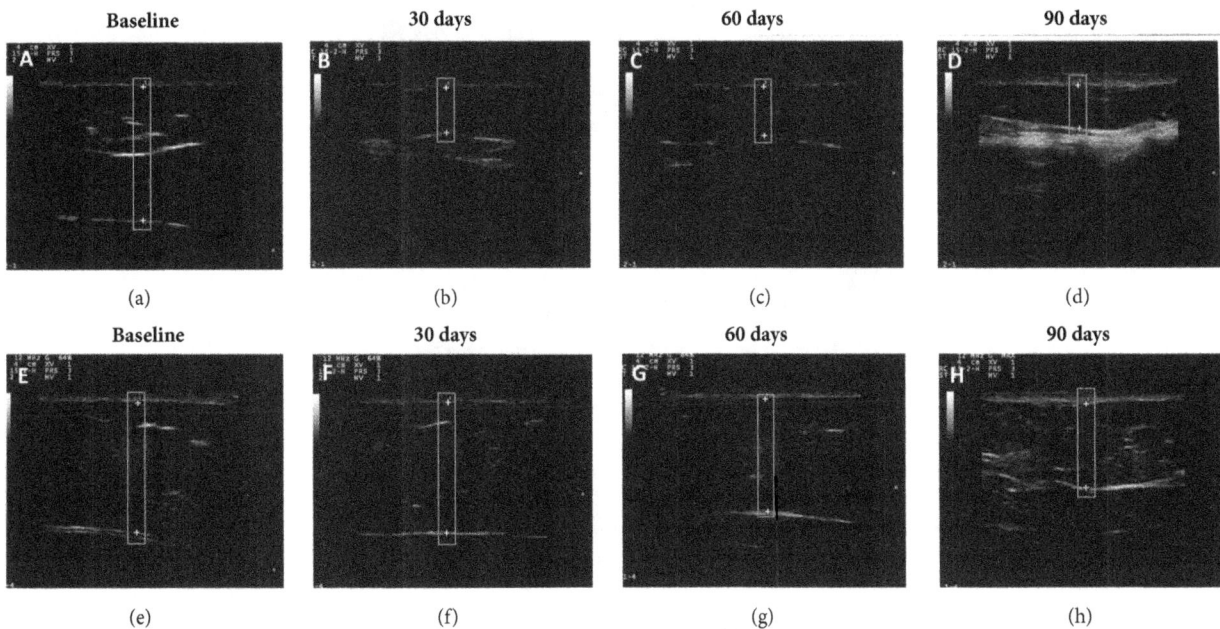

FIGURE 5: The thickness of the abdominal fat layer (a-d)—(a) at the baseline, (b) at the 30-day follow-up, (c) at the 60-day follow-up, and (d) at the 90-day follow-up—and the thickness of the flanks' fat layer (e-h): (e) at the baseline, (f) at the 30-day follow-up, (g) at the 60-day follow-up, and (h) at the 90-day follow-up. Note the hyperechoic areas—bright echoes and highly reflective structures (white = dermis fascia and fibrotic septa)—and hypoechoic areas: sparse echoes, reflection, or intermediate transmission (gray = adipose tissue and skeletal muscle). The boxes indicate the areas compared and the decrease of the thickness after the treatment.

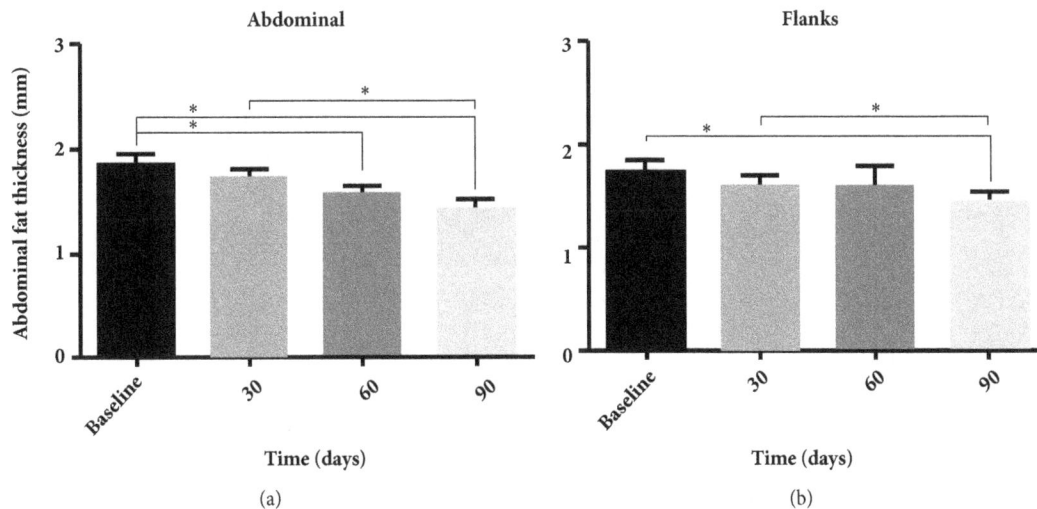

FIGURE 6: Means, with standard error of the mean, from an (a) abdominal fat-thickness assessment through diagnostic ultrasound before treatment (baseline) and after treatment (30, 60, and 90 days after treatment) and a (b) flank fat-thickness assessment through diagnostic ultrasound before treatment (baseline) and after treatment (30, 60, and 90 days after treatment). $^{*}P < 0.05$.

the publications that have used this device [28] have used values in CIF to express the rate of heat extraction. It is difficult to draw comparisons between the results of studies in general and the specific results of studies using Coolsculpting. Publications [20, 32] only recently provided the values of the treatment temperature in degrees Celsius.

A study involving another line of research (lipocryolysis) [33]—which used the isolated adipocyte suspension of Wistar

rats that were exposed to a temperature of 8°C for 0, 10, or 25 minutes—observed more crystallization when the exposure duration was increased. It was also observed that the crystals did not disappear when the samples were warmed at room temperature (22°C) for 2 hours. A subsequent study [12] applied several temperature patterns (heating and cooling) in isolated rat adipocytes and observed an increase in the crystallization process when using contrast temperatures:

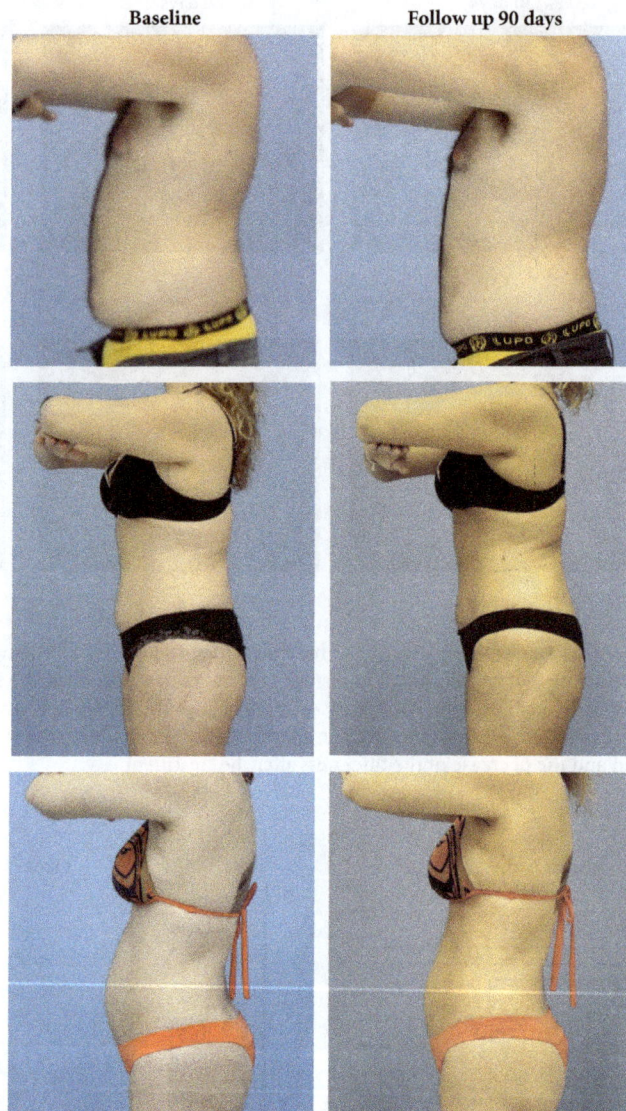

FIGURE 7: Comparison from the baseline and 90-day follow-up after the treatment with contrast cryolipolysis.

TABLE 1: Mean (SD) for fasting glycemia, serum liver test, and serum lipid values.

Analysis (units)	Reference	Time		P value
		Baseline	3 weeks later	
Glucose (mg/dL)[a]	70-100	85.71 ± 9.04	84.64 ± 10.99	0.862
AST (U/L)[a]	10 - 37 ♀ / 11 - 39 ♂	18.96 ± 5.83	21.27 ± 5.90	0.169
ALT (U/L)[a]	11 - 45 ♀ / 10 - 37 ♂	17.67 ± 11.96	21.27 ± 8.71	0.136
Cholesterol (mg/dL)[a]	< 200	176.4 ± 36.35	166.1 ± 25.54	0.491
Triglycerides (mg/dL)[b]	< 200	103 ± 63.16	89.18 ± 57.42	0.765
HDL Cholesterol (mg/dL)[a]	> 65	50.65 ± 12.01	47.09 ± 7.22	0.348
LDL Cholesterol (mg/dL)[a]	< 130	105.2 ± 30.49	101.2 ± 26.45	0.443
VLDL Cholesterol (mg/dL)[b]	< 40	20.59 ± 12.63	17.84 ± 11.48	0.765

ALT, alanine aminotransferase; AST, aspartate aminotransferase; HDL, high-density lipoprotein; LDL, low-density lipoprotein; VLDL, very-low-density lipoprotein.
[a]Paired t-test.
[b]Wilcoxon signed-rank test.
A P-value < 0.05 is considered statistically significant.

heating-cooling-heating. Both processes, cooling and contrast temperatures, showed high potential to induce the cellular death of adipocytes through lipid crystallization [11, 33]. This research contributed to the development of the Lipocryo® technology (Clinipro, S.L. Barcelona, Spain), and it is important to highlight that the technique of contrast lipocryolysis uses the extraction of temperatures up to 3°C [34].

A case report of a patient who went through a cryolipolysis treatment at −5°C with the Galeno device (South Korea) demonstrated, through diagnostic ultrasound, a reduction in the thickness of the fat layer. Histological analyses of the material collected during a later abdominoplasty showed significant adipocyte destruction [27].

In a study performed by Sasaki et al. [35], which used the Coolsculpting device, they inserted a temperature probe into the subcutaneous tissue in the treated area and revealed that the temperature in the tissues reached as low as 9°C.

Because studies use different nonsurgical devices that control cooling to decrease subcutaneous fat without damaging the surrounding tissues and each of them uses temperatures that range from the CIF index to 3°C, it is difficult to compare studies.

One fact is clear: cold-induced lipid crystallization (crystal-structure formation) of the adipocytes occurs at temperatures around 8°C to 10°C, and it is a condition dependent on time and temperature; this seems to be the key to the results [11–13, 33, 35].

In our study, all the participants were treated with a Polarys® device (Ibramed, Amparo, SP, Brazil) using the following protocol: initial heating of 40°C for 10 minutes, temperature extraction for 60 minutes (a cooling temperature of −8°C set in the device), and heating to 40°C for 10 minutes at the end of the cooling cycle. Extracting the temperature from the skin creates a thermal gradient. The superficial layers (skin surface) become cooler and deepen into the subcutaneous tissue (adipose layer) as the treatment proceeds [35]. The procedures were performed using vacuum-pressure applicators (medium or large size) for heating and extracting heat from both sides of a fold and reducing blood flow via tissue compression and cold-induced vasoconstriction. The total time of the treatment was 80 minutes for each area treated. Each subject received treatment in 3 to 5 areas: the abdomen or flanks, according to individual's needs. The treatment was performed in 1 or 2 visits.

During the treatment period, no significant changes in body weight or BMI occurred. However, compared to the baseline measurements, the waist circumferences were significantly reduced at the 30-day and 60-day follow-ups; the circumferences also decreased between the 30-day and 60-day follow-ups. No differences in waist circumference were observed at the 90-day follow-up (Figure 3). Despite the methodological accuracy, we believe that some factors may have affected the measurements at the 90-day follow-up [36]. This result contrasts measurements obtained through skinfold caliper (Figure 4) and diagnostic ultrasound (Figures 5-6).

The cold-induced metabolic stress during the treatment and the production of reactive oxygen species during the postischemia reperfusion that occurs immediately after the removal of the applicator have been the target of studies [37, 38]. From the beginning, in both preclinical and clinical studies, a cycle of massage (1-5 minutes) was applied immediately after procedure to facilitate the homogeneity of crystallization in the treatment area [29, 30, 37, 38]. It is believed that the process of reperfusion, after cooling of the tissue, can generate an increase in reactive oxygen species, the cytosolic calcium, and the activation of dependent and independent calcium proteolytic enzymes, including caspases that activate apoptotic pathways [35, 39]. In our study, the application time was 10 minutes of heating up to 40°C to increase reperfusion. This could explain our good results compared to those of other clinical studies that used ultrasound imaging to measure the abdominal fat layer. The averages for the fat-thickness reduction in these studies were 18.2% [24], 19.5% [28], and 19.6% [35] measured 6 months after the treatments. In our study, the mean percentage of fat-layer reduction was 21.6%, measured 3 months after treatment (Figure 6(a)). Reductions of up to 50.1% were detected at the baseline and after 3 months. The results were also effective in the flanks area; the mean percentage of reduction was 14.5%, and reductions of up to 43.2% were observed in comparisons of the measurements from the baseline and 3-month follow-up (Figure 6(b)). The results can be observed in the comparative photographs in Figure 7.

In terms of safety, we did not note any significant impact on fasting glucose, lipid levels, or liver function tests (aspartate aminotransferase and alanine aminotransferase) after contrast cryolipolysis treatments, as seen in Table 1. These results are similar to those obtained by Klein et al. [37], who used conventional cryolipolysis; the destruction of adipocytes does not significantly affect serum-lipid levels or liver-function tests.

In this study, 84 areas were treated with contrast cryolipolysis: 54 areas were treated with a medium applicator, and 30 areas were treated with a large applicator. The subjects reported mild to moderate discomfort at the treated site, especially during the contrast phase; however, the treatment was considered tolerable by 95% of the sample. The typical side effects of cryolipolysis procedures reported in clinical studies include erythema, edema, bruising, and transient neuralgia [40]. Subjects in this study experienced temporary adverse effects—such as redness, slight bruising, and numbness—that resolved spontaneously. The subjects did not report pain from neuralgia or burns.

5. Conclusion

Contrast cryolipolysis was safe and effective in the treatment of localized fat in the flanks and abdominal region. Even though the study was performed with a number of individuals greater than the number suggested by the sample calculation, we believe that studies with a larger sample should be performed.

Acknowledgments

The authors would like to thank São Francisco Laboratório de Análises Clínicas in Amparo, São Paulo, Brazil. The authors would also like to thank Ms. Marilia Lima, administrative assistant to CEFAI, for her help in the recruitment of the subjects. This study was partially funded by a research grant from IBRAMED, Indústria Brasileira de Equipamentos Médicos EIRELI, which covered the administrative costs to conduct the study.

References

[1] H. Pinto, "Local fat treatments: classification proposal," *Adipocyte*, vol. 5, no. 1, pp. 22–26, 2015.

[2] K. J. Stewart, D. A. Stewart, B. Coghlan, D. H. Harrison, B. M. Jones, and N. Waterhouse, "Complications of 278 consecutive abdominoplasties," *Journal of Plastic, Reconstructive & Aesthetic Surgery*, vol. 59, no. 11, pp. 1152–1155, 2006.

[3] Logan J. M., Ii G. B. Plastic Surgery: Understanding. 88(4):603–4, 2008.

[4] A. Fatemi, "High-Intensity Focused Ultrasound Effectively Reduces Adipose Tissue," *Seminars in Cutaneous Medicine and Surgery*, vol. 28, no. 4, pp. 257–262, 2009.

[5] J. Pumprla, K. Howorka, Z. Kolackova, and E. Sovova, "Non-contact radiofrequency-induced reduction of subcutaneous abdominal fat correlates with initial cardiovascular autonomic balance and fat tissue hormones: Safety analysis," *F1000Research*, vol. 4, 2015.

[6] W. Franco, A. Kothare, S. J. Ronan, R. C. Grekin, and T. H. McCalmont, "Hyperthermic injury to adipocyte cells by selective heating of subcutaneous fat with a novel radiofrequency device: Feasibility studies," *Lasers in Surgery and Medicine*, vol. 42, no. 5, pp. 361–370, 2010.

[7] M. A. Trelles and S. R. Mordon, "Adipocyte membrane lysis observed after cellulite treatment is performed with radiofrequency," *Aesthetic Plastic Surgery*, vol. 33, no. 1, pp. 125–128, 2009.

[8] O. Garcia Jr. and M. Schafer, "The effects of nonfocused external ultrasound on tissue temperature and adipocyte morphology," *Aesthetic Surgery Journal*, vol. 33, no. 1, pp. 117–127, 2013.

[9] P. T. Rose and M. Morgan, "Histological changes associated with mesotherapy for fat dissolution," *Journal of Cosmetic and Laser Therapy*, vol. 7, no. 1, pp. 17–19, 2005.

[10] M. M. Avram and R. S. Harry, "Cryolipolysis™ for subcutaneous fat layer reduction," *Lasers in Surgery and Medicine*, vol. 41, no. 10, pp. 703–708, 2009.

[11] H. Pinto and G. Melamed, "Contrast lipocryolysis," *Adipocyte*, vol. 3, no. 3, pp. 212–214, 2014.

[12] H. Pinto, D. Ricart-Jané, and E. Pardina, "Pre and post lipocryolysis thermic conditioning enhances rat adipocyte destruction," *Cryoletters*, vol. 35, no. 2, pp. 154–160, 2014.

[13] H. P. David Ricart Jane, "Isolated Rat Adipocytes are Still Capable of Inducing Lipolysis after a Lipocryolysis-Like Thermic Stimulus," *Journal of Glycomics & Lipidomics*, vol. 04, no. 04, 2014.

[14] C. C. Dierickx, J.-M. Mazer, M. Sand, S. Koenig, and V. Arigon, "Safety, tolerance, and patient satisfaction with noninvasive cryolipolysis," *Dermatologic Surgery*, vol. 39, no. 8, pp. 1209–1216, 2013.

[15] K. Chopra, K. K. Tadisina, and W. G. Stevens, "Interesting Case Series Cryolipolysis in Aesthetic Plastic Surgery," *Eplasty*, vol. 22, 2014.

[16] R. Wanitphakdeedecha, A. Sathaworawong, and W. Manuskiatti, "The efficacy of cryolipolysis treatment on arms and inner thighs," *Lasers in Medical Science*, vol. 30, no. 8, pp. 2165–2169, 2015.

[17] N. Krueger, S. V. Mai, S. Luebberding, and N. S. Sadick, "Cryolipolysis for noninvasive body contouring: Clinical efficacy and patient satisfaction," *Clinical, Cosmetic and Investigational Dermatology*, vol. 7, pp. 201–205, 2014.

[18] L. Garibyan, L. Cornelissen, W. Sipprell et al., "Transient Alterations of Cutaneous Sensory Nerve Function by Noninvasive Cryolipolysis," *Journal of Investigative Dermatology*, vol. 135, no. 11, pp. 2623–2631, 2015.

[19] W. G. Stevens and E. P. Bachelor, "Cryolipolysis conformable-surface applicator for nonsurgical fat reduction in lateral thighs," *Aesthetic Surgery Journal*, vol. 35, no. 1, pp. 66–71, 2015.

[20] S. L. Kilmer, "Prototype CoolCup cryolipolysis applicator with over 40% reduced treatment time demonstrates equivalent safety and efficacy with greater patient preference," *Lasers in Surgery and Medicine*, vol. 49, no. 1, pp. 63–68, 2017.

[21] M. T. Mahmoud ELdesoky, E. E. Mohamed Abutaleb, and G. S. Mohamed Mousa, "Ultrasound cavitation versus cryolipolysis for non-invasive body contouring," *Australasian Journal of Dermatology*, vol. 57, no. 4, pp. 288–293, 2016.

[22] J. L. Harrington and P. J. Capizzi, "Cryolipolysis for nonsurgical reduction of fat in the lateral chest wall post-Mastectomy," *Aesthetic Surgery Journal*, vol. 37, no. 6, pp. 715–722, 2017.

[23] E. F. Bernstein, "Long-term efficacy follow-up on two cryolipolysis case studies: 6 and 9 years post-treatment," *Journal of Cosmetic Dermatology*, vol. 15, no. 4, pp. 561–564, 2016.

[24] S. Y. Shek, N. P. Y. Chan, and H. H. Chan, "Non-invasive cryolipolysis for body contouring in Chinese-a first commercial experience," *Lasers in Surgery and Medicine*, vol. 44, no. 2, pp. 125–130, 2012.

[25] G. E. Boey and J. L. Wasilenchuk, "Enhanced clinical outcome with manual massage following cryolipolysis treatment: a 4-month study of safety and efficacy," *Lasers in Surgery and Medicine*, vol. 46, no. 1, pp. 20–26, 2014.

[26] L. R. Pianez, F. S. Custódio, R. M. Guidi, J. N. de Freitas, and E. Sant'Ana, "Effectiveness of carboxytherapy in the treatment of cellulite in healthy women: A pilot study," *Clinical, Cosmetic and Investigational Dermatology*, vol. 9, pp. 183–190, 2016.

[27] P. F. Meyer, R. M. V. da Silva, G. Oliveira et al., "Effects of Cryolipolysis on Abdominal Adiposity," *Case Reports in Dermatological Medicine*, vol. 2016, Article ID 6052194, 7 pages, 2016.

[28] C. D. Derrick, S. M. Shridharani, and J. M. Broyles, "The safety and efficacy of cryolipolysis: A systematic review of available literature," *Aesthetic Surgery Journal*, vol. 35, no. 7, pp. 830–836, 2015.

[29] D. Manstein, H. Laubach, K. Watanabe, W. Farinelli, D. Zurakowski, and R. R. Anderson, "Selective cryolysis: A novel method of non-invasive fat removal," *Lasers in Surgery and Medicine*, vol. 40, no. 9, pp. 595–604, 2008.

[30] H. R. Jalian and M. M. Avram, "Cryolipolysis, a historical perspective and current clinical practice," *Seminars in Cutaneous Medicine and Surgery*, vol. 32, no. 1, pp. 31–34, 2013.

[31] B. Zelickson, B. M. Egbert, J. Preciado et al., "Cryolipolysis for noninvasive fat cell destruction: initial results from a pig model," *Dermatologic Surgery*, vol. 35, no. 10, pp. 1462–1470, 2009.

[32] S. L. Kilmer, A. J. Burns, and B. D. Zelickson, "Safety and efficacy of cryolipolysis for non-invasive reduction of submental fat," *Lasers in Surgery and Medicine*, vol. 48, no. 1, pp. 3–13, 2016.

[33] H. Pinto, E. Arredondo, and D. Ricart-Jané, "Evaluation of adipocytic changes after a simil-lipocryolysis stimulus," *Cryoletters*, vol. 34, no. 1, pp. 100–105, 2013.

[34] H. R. Pinto, E. Garcia-Cruz, and G. E. Melamed, "A study to evaluate the action of lipocryolysis," *Cryoletters*, vol. 33, no. 3, pp. 177–181, 2012.

[35] G. H. Sasaki, N. Abelev, and A. Tevez-Ortiz, "Noninvasive selective cryolipolysis and reperfusion recovery for localized natural fat reduction and contouring," *Aesthetic Surgery Journal*, vol. 34, no. 3, pp. 420–431, 2014.

[36] J. A. Bernritter, J. L. Johnson, and S. L. Woodard, "Validation of a novel method for measuring waist circumference," *Plastic Surgical Nursing*, vol. 31, no. 1, pp. 9–13, 2011.

[37] K. B. Klein, B. Zelickson, J. G. Riopelle et al., "Non-invasive cryolipolysis™ for subcutaneous fat reduction does not affect serum lipid levels or liver function tests," *Lasers in Surgery and Medicine*, vol. 41, no. 10, pp. 785–790, 2009.

[38] E. F. Bernstein, J. D. Bloom, L. D. Basilavecchio, and J. M. Plugis, "Non-invasive fat reduction of the flanks using a new cryolipolysis applicator and overlapping, two-cycle treatments," *Lasers in Surgery and Medicine*, vol. 46, no. 10, pp. 731–735, 2014.

[39] M. J. Ingargiola, S. Motakef, M. T. Chung, H. C. Vasconez, and G. H. Sasaki, "Cryolipolysis for fat reduction and body contouring: safety and efficacy of current treatment paradigms," *Plastic and Reconstructive Surgery*, vol. 135, no. 6, pp. 1581–1590, 2015.

[40] W. Grant Stevens, L. K. Pietrzak, and M. A. Spring, "Broad overview of a clinical and commercial experience with coolsculpting," *Aesthetic Surgery Journal*, vol. 33, no. 6, pp. 835–846, 2013.

10

Potential Use of Essential Oil Isolated from *Cleistocalyx operculatus* Leaves as a Topical Dermatological Agent for Treatment of Burn Wound

Gia-Buu Tran ⓘ, Nghia-Thu Tram Le, and Sao-Mai Dam

Institute of Biotechnology and Food Technology, Industrial University of Ho Chi Minh City, 12 Nguyen Van Bao Street, Go Vap District, Ho Chi Minh City, Vietnam

Correspondence should be addressed to Gia-Buu Tran; giabuu06cs@gmail.com

Academic Editor: Craig G. Burkhart

Several herbal remedies have been used as topical agents to cure burn wound, one of the most common injuries in worldwide. In this study, we investigated the potential use of *Cleistocalyx operculatus* essential oil to treat the burn wound. We identified a total of 13 bioactive compounds of essential oil, several of which exhibited the anti-inflammatory and antimicrobial activities. Furthermore, the essential oil showed the antibacterial effect against *S. aureus* but not with *P. aeruginosa*. The supportive effect of essential oil on burn wound healing process also has been proven. Among three groups of mice, wound contraction rate of essential oil treated group (100%) was significantly higher than tamanu oil treated (79%) and control mice (71%) after 20 days (0.22 ± 0.03 versus 0.31 ± 0.02 cm^2, resp., $p < 0.05$). Histological studies revealed that burn wounds treated with essential oil formed a complete epidermal structure, thick and neatly arranged fibers, and scattered immune cells in burn wound. On the contrary, saline treated burn wound formed uneven epidermal layer with necrotic ulcer, infiltration of immune cells, and existence of granulation tissue. This finding demonstrated *Cleistocalyx operculatus* essential oil as promising topical dermatological agent to treat burn wound.

1. Introduction

Burn, one of the most common household injuries, is defined as a type of damage of skin or other tissues caused by exposure to heat, chemicals, electric currents, flame, hot liquid, hot metal or object, steam, radiation from X-ray, sunlight, ultraviolet, and so forth. Among them, the thermal injuries are leading cause of burn (86%), followed by electrical sources (4%) and contacting with chemical sources (3%), and other sources of burns (7%) [1]. Note that flame and scald burns account for the majority of burns in children and adults. Thermal burn causes not only a small or local injury which can be treated at home or outpatient but also the severe and fatal injuries which require the in-hospital treatment. The World Health Organization estimates that thermal burns account for approximated 6.6 million injuries and 300 thousand deaths annually over the world [1]. Furthermore, Kemp et al. (2017) also suggest that 25,000 children who suffered from burns or scald require the Emergency Department admission in English and Wales each year, of which 3,800 patients must receive in-hospital treatment [2]. The severity of burn is evaluated by the extent and the depth of burn. The extent of burn is estimated through total body surface area burn (% TBSA) whereas the depth of burn is estimated by the deep extent of injury into the epidermis or dermis. If the burn extent involves only the epidermis, thus it is classified as superficial burn (first degree). When the burn involves epidermis and dermis, it is categorized as partial thickness burn (second degree). The other burn is full-thickness burn (third degree) which extend into subcutaneous fat or deeper. Thermal burns resulted in both local injuries and a systemic response, in case of severe burn (% TBSA > 20%). Deep and widespread burns may cause many complications such as infection, hypovolemia, hypothermia, blood clotting, scarring, joint mobility problem, and posttraumatic stress disorder. In superficial and partial thickness of burns, topical antibacterial regimes with antibiotic ointments or cream and/or absorbent dressing to cover the burn wound are recommended. Otherwise, in deep partial and full thickness of burns, the surgical excision of damaged tissue and skin grafting are performed to cure the wound.

Several medical plants exerting antibacterial activity and/ or wound healing potential have been applied for treating burn injuries such as *Aloe vera*, *Achillea millefolium*, *Carica papaya*, and *Datura alba* [10]. Herbal preparations may be obtained from a variety of parts of plants (fruit, leaf, bulb, stem, root, pollen, whole plant, and seed) and extraction forms (oil, acetone, methanol, ethanol, hydroalcoholic, and aqueous extract). In Polynesia and Southeast Asia, tamanu oil which is produced from *Calophyllum inophyllum* is the well-known and common use product to heal thermal burn wound. Tamanu oil has been proven as promising topical remedy which exerts acceleration of skin healing process, antineuralgic, antioxidant, anti-inflammatory, and antimicrobial effects [11]. Note that the number of researches using vegetable oil and essential oil to treat burn wound has been increased. Dursun et al. (2003) suggested that thymus essential oil could reduce NO level induced by burn and enhance the formation of new tissue in burn wound [12]. The beneficial effect of *Nigella sativa* seed oil on burn wound healing process also was proven [13]. Furthermore, Khedir et al. (2016) observed that *Pistacia lentiscus* fruit oil accelerated wound contraction in CO_2 laser burned wound model [14]. These findings consolidate the idea using the vegetable and vegetable oils for treating burn wound.

Cleistocalyx operculatus (Roxb.) Merr & Perry is a well-known medicinal plant in Asia. It is grown and widely spread in Vietnam, China, Malaysia, Myanmar, Thailand, Sri Lanka, India, Nepal, and other tropical countries. Leaves and buds are two parts of *C. operculatus* commonly used for treating gastrointestinal disorder and dermatophytic infection for many years [15]. Furthermore, the other beneficial effects of *C. operculatus* such as anticancer, antihyperglycemic hypolipidemic, and cardiotonic effects are well documented [16, 17]. In addition, Dũng et al. (1994) have analyzed the chemical composition of essential oil isolated from *Cleistocalyx operculatus* leaves [18]. Recently, Dosoky et al. (2015) proved that essential oil of *Cleistocalyx operculatus* leaves possessed a strong antimicrobial effect and cytotoxicity to cancer cell lines [19]. However, application of essential oil isolated from *Cleistocalyx operculatus* leaves on wound healing, especially in thermal injury, has not been elucidated yet. Therefore, we investigated the effect of essential oil isolated from *Cleistocalyx operculatus* leaves on burn wound model in this study.

2. Materials and Methods

2.1. Collection and Preparation of Cleistocalyx operculatus Essential Oil. *Cleistocalyx operculatus* leaves were purchased from local herbal supplier in Go Vap District, Ho Chi Minh City, Vietnam (Thanh Binh Medicinal Plants and Herbals Co., Vietnam). Air-dried and ground leaves were subjected to hydrodistillation for 4 hours at 100°C in 15% NaCl solution using a Clevenger apparatus [20]. The essential oils were collected over aqueous phase amd transferred into 1.5 mL tube, after which essential oil was stored in dark chamber at 4°C prior to GC/MS analysis and bioactivities testing.

2.2. Gas Chromatography-Mass Spectrometry (GC-MS) Analysis. The GC-MS analysis of the essential oil was performed at Department of Analytical Chemistry, University of Science, Vietnam National University of Ho Chi Minh City with the given protocol. Briefly, chemical compositions of essential oil were analyzed on a GC-MS Aligent 6890 system equipped with a splitless mode injector and DB–5MS column (30 m × 0.25 mm ID, film thickness 0.25 μm from Aligent Technologies, USA). The GC injector temperature was set at 250°C. A 1 mL volume of 2,000 ppm oil solution (1 hot water: 10 methanol) was injected. Helium in constant pressure was used as carrier gas at flow rate of 1.0 mL/min. The oven initial temperature was maintained 60°C for 1 min and heated at 10°C/min until oven temperature reached 200°C, and the oven was kept in this temperature for 5 min. Then oven was heated at 20°C/min to 280°C and then kept for 1 min. The temperature of transfer line was set at 280°C. For GC-MS analysis, an electron ionization with ionization energy of 1700 eV was used, covering a mass range from 40 to 450 mz. The compounds were identified by NIST MS Search version 2.0.

2.3. Antimicrobial Activity. The antimicrobial activity of essential oil was determined by the agar diffusion method. The following bacterial strains *Staphylococcus aureus* ATCC 6538 and *Pseudomonas aeruginosa* ATCC 9027, which are considered as two common opportunistic bacteria in skin and mucous membrane [21], were employed for screening the antimicrobial activity of *C. operculatus* essential oil. Briefly, the tested microorganisms (0.1 ml of 1×10^8 CFU/ml) were inoculated on LB agar. Then the sterilized filter paper discs (6 mm in diameter) were impregnated with 20 μL of *Cleistocalyx operculatus* essential oil or tamanu oil. The discs were placed in LB agar plates, after which the plates were incubated at 37°C for 24 hours. The commercial antibiotic discs (Gentamycin, Nam Khoa Biotek Co.) and tamanu oil (Inopilo, Binh Minh Pharmaceutical Joint Co. Ltd.) were used as positive controls. The diameters of inhibition zones were measured in millimeters.

2.4. Establishment of Burned Mouse Model. Eight-week-old male Swiss albino mice were obtained from Pasteur Institute of Ho Chi Minh City, weighing approximately 30–32 g. The animals were randomly divided into polycarbonate cages with 4 mice for each cage. They were housed under standard husbandry conditions with 12 h light-dark cycle (8:00–20:00) for at least 1 week to acclimate with laboratory environment. They were supplied ad libitum with standard chow and distilled water. The experimental procedure was strictly in compliance with the Declaration of Helsinki (1964). Briefly, twelve healthy mice were randomly divided into 3 groups with 4 mice per group and treated as the protocol of Tavares Pereira et al. (2012) with some modifications [22]. Mice were anesthetized with diethyl ether for 3 min, then the hair on back of mice was removed using razor. The dorsal proximal region was antisepsis with polyvinyl pyrrolidone iodine. Thermal lesion was generated by a massive aluminum bar 10 mm in diameter preheated to $100 \pm 5°C/10$ min. The probe was kept to contact with mouse skin for 15 sec. After that,

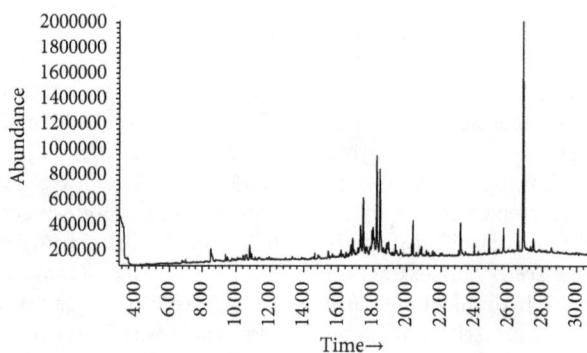

FIGURE 1: *GC/MS chromatogram of essential oil extracted from Cleistocalyx operculatus leaves.* A total of 13 compounds were identified in CLO: 6-camphenol; isopinocarveol; p-cymen-8-ol; (−)-myrtenol; I-verbenone; cis-carveol; ethaneperoxoic acid, 1-cyano-4,4-dimethyl-1-phenylpentyl ethaneperoxate; (+)-carotol; caryophyllene oxide; (−)-globulol; 2-(4a,8-dimethyl-2,3,4,4a,5,6-hexahydronaphthalen-2-yl)propan-1-; and longipinocarvone. Among them, many bioactive compounds identified in CLO exhibited antimicrobial and/or anti-inflammatory activities. This finding supports the idea of using *Cleistocalyx operculatus* essential oil as topical agent for treatment of burn wound, at least to prevent the infection and sepsis.

the burn wound was treated with an indicated volume of saline, tamanu oil, or diluted *C. operculatus* essential oil (50 μl/lesion) once per day for 20 days. Tamanu oil (Inopilo, Binh Minh Pharmaceutical Joint Co. Ltd.) was used as reference treatment. Diluted *C. operculatus* essential oil (1% solution) was prepared by dissolving the essential oil in 0.1% DMSO and Tween 20 solution. The burned area of mice was measured after 10 days and 20 days and the results were presented as square centimeter (cm^2).

2.5. Histological Study. At the end of experiment (20 days), all mice were anesthetized with diethyl ether and then euthanized by carbon dioxide. The skin of burned area was collected and preserved in 10% formalin. The sample was processed for histological studies with Hematoxylin and Eosin staining in Division of Pathological Anatomy, the Cancer Diagnosis and Treatment Centre of Military Hospital 175 with given protocol [23].

2.6. Statistical Analysis. All experiments were repeated in triplicate. Statistical analysis was performed using Statgraphics Centurion XVI software (Statpoint Technologies Inc., Warrenton, Virginia, USA). The data were presented as mean ± standard deviation. Differences between means of different groups were analyzed using ANOVA variance analysis followed with multiple range tests, and the criterion of statistical significance was set as $p < 0.05$.

3. Results and Discussions

3.1. Screening Bioactive Compounds of C. operculatus Essential Oil. *C. operculatus* leaves essential oil (CLO) has yellowish color and fragrant odor, with 0.1% yield. The presence of some active compounds in CLO was determined by GC-MS analysis, and data were recorded in Figure 1 and Table 1. Briefly, a total of 13 compounds were identified in CLO: 6-camphenol; isopinocarveol; p-cymen-8-ol; (−)-myrtenol;

I-verbenone; cis-carveol; ethaneperoxoic acid, 1-cyano-4,4-dimethyl-1-phenylpentyl ethaneperoxate; (+)-carotol; caryophyllene oxide; (−)-globulol; 2-(4a,8-dimethyl-2,3,4,4a,5,6-hexahydronaphthalen-2-yl) propan-1-; and longipinocarvone. Most of bioactive compounds identified in CLO exhibited antimicrobial and/or anti-inflammatory activities, such as isopinocarveol, (−)-myrtenol; I- verbenone; cis-carveol; (+)-carotol; caryophyllene oxide; (−)-globulol. This finding indicated that CLO may be used as topical treatment, at least as the anti-infective and antiseptic agent, for burn wound. Therefore, the next question has been raised whether CLO could inhibit the growth and/or eliminate some common bacteria inhabited on burn wound or not.

3.2. Screening of Antibacterial Activity of C. operculatus Essential Oil. In previous report, Livimbi and Komolafe (2007) suggested that *S. aureus* was the most common bacteria isolated from burn wound, followed by *P. mirabilis, Streptococci* spp., *P. aeruginosa, E. coli, Salmonella*, and *Klebsiella* spp. [21]. Therefore, we investigated antibacterial activity of *C. operculatus* essential oil against two bacteria commonly found on burn wound such as *S. aureus* and *P. aeruginosa* to prove the anti-infective efficiency of *C. operculatus* essential oil (CLO). Furthermore, *S. aureus* and *P. aeruginosa* also represent two types of bacteria, Gram positive and Gram negative bacteria, respectively. We found that both CLO and commercial tamanu oil exhibited antibacterial activity against *S. aureus* whereas they did not exhibit antibacterial activity against *P. aeruginosa* (Figure 2). The diameter of inhibition zones of gentamicin (positive control) against *S. aureus* was highest (11.37 ± 0.15 mm), followed by tamanu oil (9.03 ± 0.31 mm) and CLO (7.17 ± 0.12 mm, $p < 0.05$). On the contrary, only gentamicin showed the antibacterial activity against *P. aeruginosa* (12.07 ± 0.15), but *P. aeruginosa* was resistant with commercial tamanu oil and CLO (diameters of inhibition zones = diameter of dishes, 6 mm). These results were identical with previous reports [19, 24, 25]. In previous study, Nguyen et al. (2017) suggested that methanol extract of

TABLE 1: Identification of some bioactive compounds in essential oil of *Cleistocalyx operculatus* leaves.

Number	RT (min)	Compound name	Formulas	M.W.	NIST ref.	Bioactivities
(1)	9.498	Camphenol, 6-	$C_{10}H_{16}O$	152	141039	
(2)	9.767	Isopinocarveol	$C_{10}H_{16}O$	152	292836	Antimicrobial, anti-inflammatory, antioxidant [3]
(3)	10.416	p-Cymen-8-ol	$C_{10}H_{14}O$	150	290794	
(4)	10.595	(−)-Myrtenol	$C_{10}H_{16}O$	152	334014	Anti-inflammatory, antinociceptive [4]
(5)	10.785	I-Verbenone	$C_{10}H_{14}O$	150	141212	Antibacterial, anti-inflammatory, anticonvulsive [5]
(6)	10.897	cis-Carveol	$C_{10}H_{16}O$	152	291523	
(7)	15.416	Ethaneperoxoic acid, 1-cyano-4,4-dimethyl-1-phenylpentyl ethaneperoxate	$C_{16}H_{21}NO_3$	275	66383	
(8)	16.098	(+)-Carotol	$C_{15}H_{26}O$	222	42544	Antifungal [6]
(9)	16.154	Caryophyllene oxide	$C_{15}H_{24}O$	220	156329	Analgesic, anti-inflammatory [7], anticancer [8]
(10)	17.273	(−)-Globulol	$C_{15}H_{26}O$	222	109228	Antimicrobial [9]
(11)	17.418	2-(4a,8-Dimethyl-2,3,4,4a,5,6-hexahydronaphthalen-2-yl)propan-1-	$C_{15}H_{24}O$	220	189031	
(12)	17.418	6-Isopropenyl-4,8a-dimethyl-1,2,3,5,6,7,8,8a-octahydro-naphthalen-2-ol	$C_{15}H_{24}O$	220	189102	
(13)	19.331	Longipinocarvone	$C_{15}H_{22}O$	218	151871	

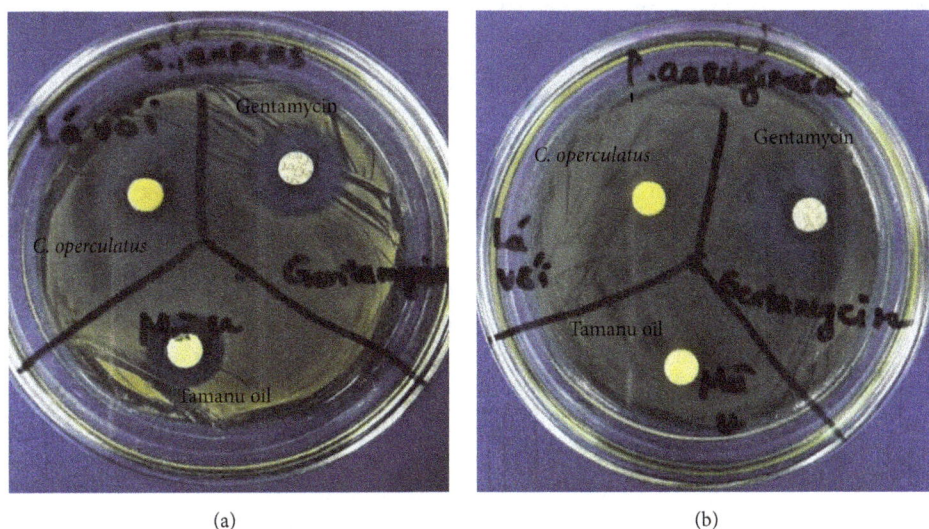

(a)   (b)

FIGURE 2: *Antimicrobial activity of C. operculatus essential oil.* Both CLO and commercial tamanu oil exhibited antibacterial activity against *S. aureus* whereas they did not inhibit the growth of *P. aeruginosa*. The diameter of inhibition zones against *S. aureus* of gentamicin (positive control) was highest (11.37 ± 0.15 mm), followed by tamanu oil (9.03 ± 0.31 mm) and CLO (7.17 ± 0.12 mm). On the contrary, only gentamicin showed the antibacterial activity against *P. aeruginosa* (12.07 ± 0.15 mm); both tamanu oil and CLO did not affect the growth of *P. aeruginosa*. This finding implies the potential use of CLO as anti-infective agent for burn wound treatment. The experiments were triplicated, and results were presented as mean ± standard deviation.

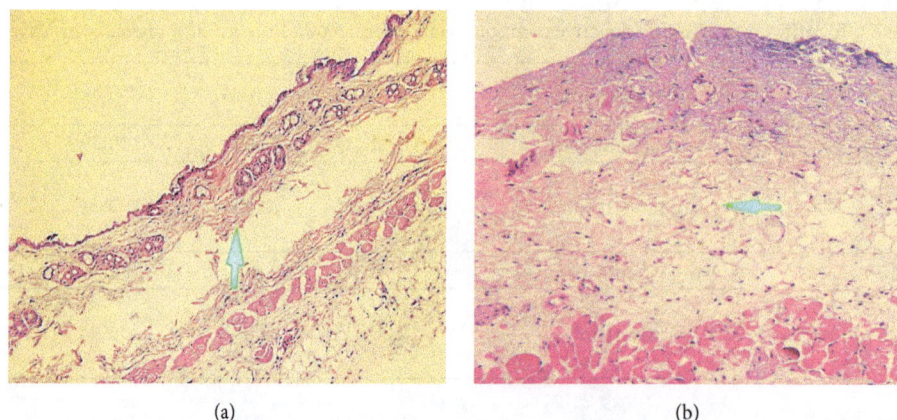

(a)

(b)

FIGURE 3: *Establishment of second-degree burn wound models*. Histological analysis showed that injury of burn wound was extended into both epidermis and dermis. In normal skin section, thick squamous epithelium covered the epidermis, and both of epidermis and dermis had the normal structure with several hair follicles and sebaceous glands (a). In burn wound skin section, epidermis and dermis lost their normal structure. Of note, squamous epithelium layer was removed, and epidermis was necrotized. Moreover, the underlying stromal tissue was swollen and congestive (b). These results indicated that the second-degree burn model was successfully established in experimental mice. The arrows indicated the border between the dermis and hypodermis.

C. operculatus leaves could inhibit *S. aureus* but not hinder *P. aeruginosa* growth [24]. Furthermore, the antimicrobial activity of essential oil of *C. operculatus* leaves from Nepal against *S. aureus* has also been demonstrated [19]. However, Dung et al. (2008) indicated that essential oil of *C. operculatus* isolated from flower buds could inhibit both *S. aureus* and *P. aeruginosa* [16]. It may be explained that different parts of *C. operculatus* possess a variety of bioactive compounds which account for different antimicrobial activities of essential oils isolated from different parts of *C. operculatus*. In addition, although tamanu oil is effective remedy for burn wound treatment, *P. aeruginosa* is also resistant with commercial tamanu oil [25]. From these results, we suggested that CLO has antimicrobial activity against *S. aureus*, the most common skin wound opportunistic bacterium, but the effectiveness of CLO is lower than commercial tamanu oil. This finding implies the potential use of CLO as anti-infective agent for burn wound treatment. Next we investigated the wound contractive ability of *C. operculatus* essential oil on second-degree burn wound model.

3.3. Establishment of Second-Degree Burn Wound Model. The second-deep-degree burn is characterized by the extent of injury through the epidermis and into the dermis with painful, red, blistered, moist wound [1]. To confirm severity of burn wound, the histological examination of burned skin collected from burn lesion was performed with pathological experts from Division of Pathological Anatomy, the Cancer Diagnosis and Treatment Centre of Military Hospital 175. Histological analysis showed that injury of burn wound was extended into both epidermis and dermis. In normal skin section, thick squamous epithelium covered the epidermis, and both of epidermis and dermis had the normal structure with several hair follicles and sebaceous glands. In burn wound skin section, epidermis and dermis lost their normal structure. Of note, squamous epithelium layer was removed,

and epidermis was necrotized. Moreover, the underlying stromal tissue was swollen and congestive. These results indicated that the second-degree burn model was successfully established in experimental mice (Figure 3).

3.4. Supportive Effect of C. operculatus Essential Oil on Burn Wound Model. We found that both tamanu oil and essential oil accelerated the wound contraction rate of burn wound after 10 days and 20 days ($p < 0.05$). At the beginning of the experiment, all burn wounds were of similar sizes in three groups. In day 10, burn wound areas of tamanu oil and CLO treated mice (0.57 ± 0.04 and 0.43 ± 0.03 mm^2, accordingly) were smaller than saline treated group (0.73 ± 0.04 cm^2), and the significant difference of wound contraction between tamanu oil and essential oil treated mice was observed ($p < 0.05$). Furthermore, essential oil group was fully recovered whereas the burn areas of tamanu oil treated and control groups remained after 20 days. Of note, wound healing process of tamanu oil treated mice was also significantly higher than control mice at this time-point (0.22 ± 0.03 versus 0.31 ± 0.02 cm^2, respectively, $p < 0.05$). These results implied that *C. operculatus* essential oil has supportive effect on wound healing process and its efficiency was higher than the commercial tamanu oil (Table 2, Figure 4).

For reconfirmation of efficiency of essential oil on wound healing process, we investigated the microscopic structure of skin from burn wounds treated with essential oil, tamanu oil, and saline via histological examination (Figure 5). Histology studies revealed that burn wounds treated with essential oil developed complete epidermal structure: squamous epithelium covered on epidermis, the stratum spinosum keratinized, observation of matured hair follicles, thick and neatly arranged fibers, and scattered immune cells. That proved that burn wound treated with essential oil was fully recovered. In tamanu oil treated mice, wounds were partially recovered with existence of coagulative necrosis region on epidermis

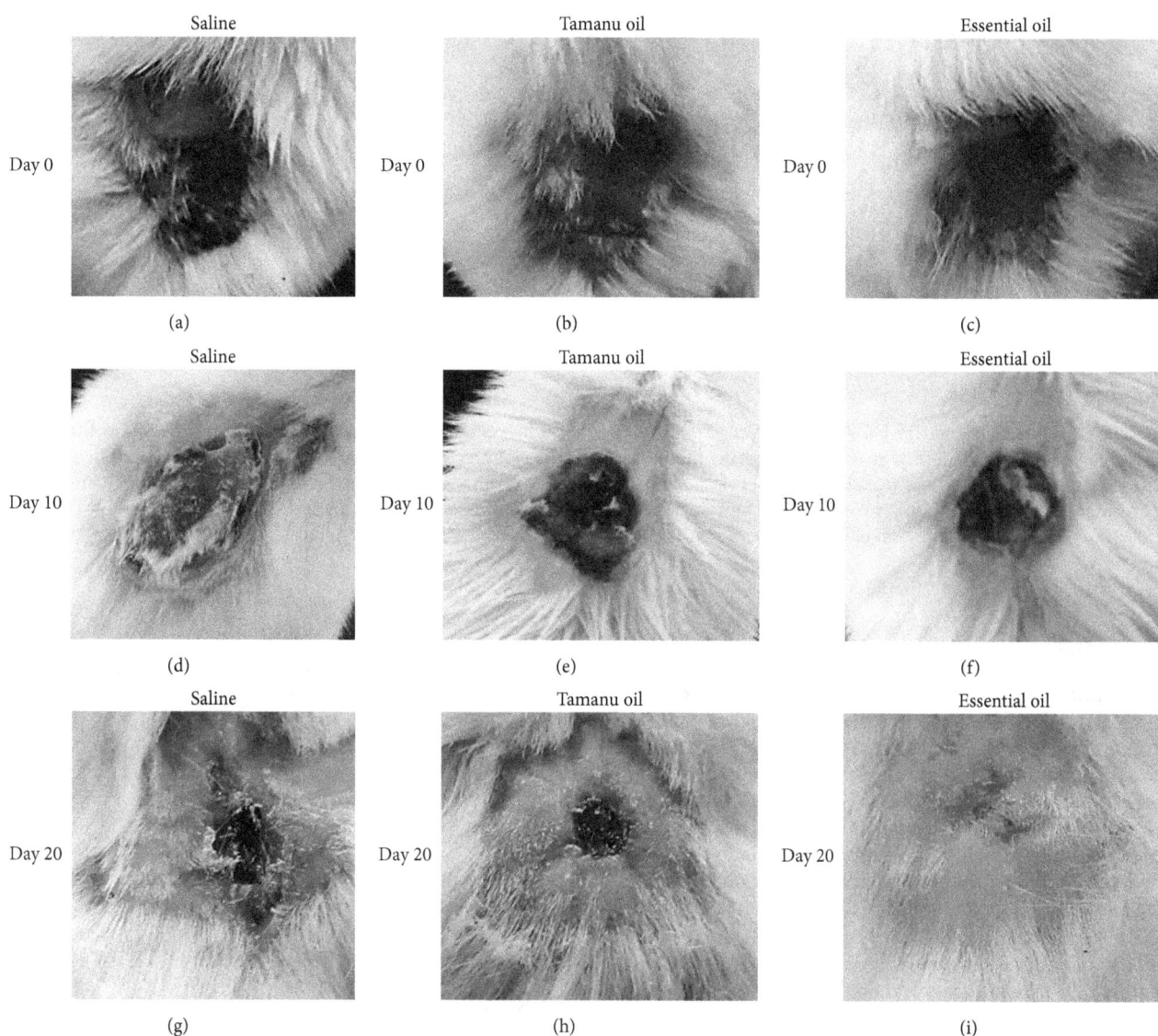

FIGURE 4: *Evaluation of the healing rate of burn wound in experimental mice.* At the beginning of experiment, all burn wounds were of similar sizes in three groups (a, b, c). In day 10, burn wound areas of tamanu oil (e) and essential oil treated mice (f) were smaller than saline treated group (d), and the significant difference of wound contraction between tamanu oil and essential oil treated mice was observed ($p < 0.05$). Furthermore, we found that burn wounds of essential oil treated mice were fully recovered (i). Burn wound contraction rate of tamanu oil treated mice (h) was significantly higher than that of saline treated groups (g) after 20 days. These results implied that *C. operculatus* essential oil has supportive effect on wound healing process and its efficiency was higher than the commercial tamanu oil.

TABLE 2: Burn wound areas of experimental mice after 10 days and 20 days.

Day	Remaining burned skin area (cm^2)		
	Saline	Tamanu oil	Essential oil
0	1.08 ± 0.10^a	1.07 ± 0.06^a	1.05 ± 0.06^a
10	0.73 ± 0.04^a	0.57 ± 0.04^b	0.43 ± 0.03^c
20	0.31 ± 0.02^a	0.22 ± 0.03^b	0.00 ± 0.00^c

a,b,c Values with different letters within the rows are significantly different ($p < 0.05$).

and vascular congestion, swollen stromal tissue, and no matured hair follicles. On the contrary, saline treated mice formed uneven epidermal layer with the necrotic ulcer on epidermis layer, infiltration of lymphocytes, plasmatocytes and multinuclear leukocytes, existence of granulation tissue, and fibrosis region. These results suggested that *C. operculatus* essential oil did not only accelerate the wound healing rate but also helped the wound recovery with normal structure.

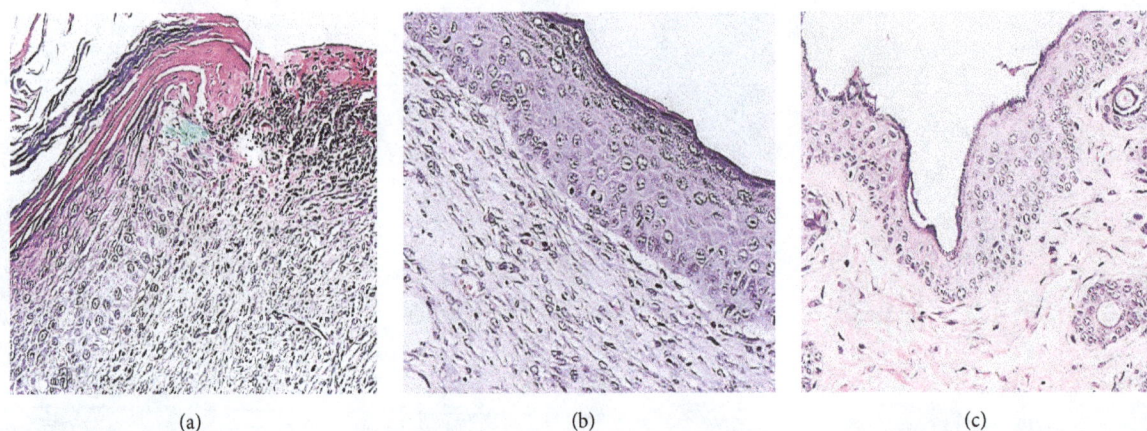

(a)   (b)   (c)

FIGURE 5: *Microscopic changes in burn wounds of experimental mice.* Histology studies revealed that burn wounds treated with essential oil developed complete epidermal structure (c). In tamanu oil treated mice, wounds were partially recovered with existence of coagulative necrosis region on epidermis and vascular congestion, swollen stromal tissue, and no matured hair follicles (b). On the contrary, saline treated mice formed uneven epidermal layer with the ulcer on epidermis layer and infiltration of immune cells (a). The highlighted part in (a) pointed out the ulcer region with infiltration of lymphocytes and multinuclear leukocytes.

4. Conclusion

We identified a total of 13 bioactive compounds of essential oil, several of which exhibited the anti-inflammatory and antimicrobial activities. Furthermore, the essential oil showed the antibacterial effect against *S. aureus*, the common pathogen bacterium in skin. The supportive effect of essential oil on burn wound healing process also has been proven. Of note, wounds of essential oil treated group were fully recovered. Furthermore, we found that wound contract rate of tamanu oil treated mice was higher than control mice (0.22 ± 0.03 and $0.31 \pm 0.02 \, \text{cm}^2$, respectively) after 20 days. Histological studies revealed that burn wounds treated with essential oil formed a complete epidermal structure. On the contrary, tamanu oil and saline treated burn wounds were partially recovered. Therefore, these data prove that essential oil exerts the supportive effect for wound healing process not only in acceleration of wound contraction rate but also in recovery of normal epidermis and dermis structure. This finding demonstrates the utilization of *Cleistocalyx operculatus* leaf essential oil as promising topical agent. Furthermore, it also sheds light on the application of aromatherapy from by-product of tropical plants for treating the dermatological trauma.

Authors' Contributions

Gia-Buu Tran conceived and designed the study and drafted the manuscript. Gia-Buu Tran and Nghia-Thu Tram Le performed the experiments. Sao-Mai Dam handled the research data and conducted the statistical analysis of the data. Gia-Buu Tran interpreted the result, revised the manuscript, and resolved the queries of reviewers. All authors read and approved the final manuscript.

Acknowledgments

The authors would like to thank their colleagues from Division of Pathological Anatomy, the Cancer Diagnosis and Treatment Centre of Military Hospital 175 and Department of Analytical Chemistry, University of Science, Vietnam National University of Ho Chi Minh City for their assistance during this project.

References

[1] T. J. Schaefer, K. D. Szymanski, and Burns., "Burns, Evaluation and Management," in *StatPearls*, StatPearls Publishing, Treasure Island, Fla, USA, 2017, https://www.ncbi.nlm.nih.gov/books/NBK430741/.

[2] A. M. Kemp, S. Jones, Z. Lawson, and S. A. Maguire, "Patterns of burns and scalds in children," *Archives of Disease in Childhood*, vol. 99, no. 4, pp. 316–321, 2014.

[3] N. M. Sahi, "Evaluation of insecticidal activity of bioactive compounds from eucalyptus citriodora against tribolium castaneum," *International Journal of Pharmacognosy and Phytochemical Research*, vol. 8, no. 8, pp. 1256–1270, 2016.

[4] R. O. Silva, M. S. Salvadori, F. B. M. Sousa et al., "Evaluation of the anti-inflammatory and antinociceptive effects of myrtenol, a plant-derived monoterpene alcohol, in mice," *Flavour and Fragrance Journal*, vol. 29, no. 3, pp. 184–192, 2014.

[5] C. G. F. de Melo, P. R. R. Salgado, D. V. da Fonsêca et al., "Anticonvulsive activity of (1S)-(−)-verbenone involving RNA expression of BDNF, COX-2, and c-fos," *Naunyn-Schmiedeberg's Archives of Pharmacology*, vol. 390, no. 9, pp. 863–869, 2017.

[6] I. Jasicka-Misiak, J. Lipok, E. M. Nowakowska, P. P. Wieczorek, P. Młynarz, and P. Kafarski, "Antifungal activity of the carrot seed oil and its major sesquiterpene compounds," *Zeitschrift fur Naturforschung*, vol. 59, no. 11-12, pp. 791–796, 2004.

[7] M. J. Chavan, P. S. Wakte, and D. B. Shinde, "Analgesic and anti-inflammatory activity of Caryophyllene oxide from *Annona squamosa* L. bark," *Phytomedicine*, vol. 17, no. 2, pp. 149–151, 2010.

[8] Z. Pan, S.-K. Wang, X.-L. Cheng, X.-W. Tian, and J. Wang, "Caryophyllene oxide exhibits anti-cancer effects in MG-63 human osteosarcoma cells via the inhibition of cell migration, generation of reactive oxygen species and induction of apoptosis," *Bangladesh Journal of Pharmacology*, vol. 11, no. 4, pp. 817–823, 2016.

[9] M. Tan, L. Zhou, Y. Huang, Y. Wang, X. Hao, and J. Wang, "Antimicrobial activity of globulol isolated from the fruits of *Eucalyptus globulus* Labill," *Natural Product Research (Formerly Natural Product Letters)*, vol. 22, no. 7, pp. 569–575, 2008.

[10] R. Bahramsoltani, M. H. Farzaei, and R. Rahimi, "Medicinal plants and their natural components as future drugs for the treatment of burn wounds: an integrative review," *Archives of Dermatological Research*, vol. 306, no. 7, pp. 601–617, 2014.

[11] C. Kilham, "Tamanu oil: a tropical topical remedy," *HerbalGram*, vol. 63, pp. 26–31, 2004.

[12] N. Dursun, N. Liman, I. Özyazgan, I. Güneş, and R. Saraymen, "Role of Thymus Oil in Burn Wound Healing," *Journal of Burn Care & Rehabilitation*, vol. 24, no. 6, pp. 395–399, 2003.

[13] I. Yaman, A. S. Durmus, S. Ceribasi, and M. Yaman, "Effect of Nigella sativa and silver sulfadiazine on burn wound healing in rat," *Veterinarni Medicina*, vol. 55, no. 12, pp. 619–624, 2010.

[14] S. B. Khedir, S. Bardaa, N. Chabchoub, D. Moalla, Z. Sahnoun, and T. Rebai, "The healing effect of Pistacia lentiscus fruit oil on laser burn," *Pharmaceutical Biology*, pp. 1–8, 2016.

[15] T. L. Do, *Vietnamese Medicinal Plants and Remedies*, Medical Publishing House, Hanoi, Vietnam, 2004, In Vietnamese.

[16] N. T. Dung, J. M. Kim, and S. C. Kang, "Chemical composition, antimicrobial and antioxidant activities of the essential oil and the ethanol extract of Cleistocalyx operculatus (Roxb.) Merr and Perry buds," *Food and Chemical Toxicology*, vol. 46, no. 12, pp. 3632–3639, 2008.

[17] T. T. Mai, N. Fumie, and N. Van Chuyen, "Antioxidant activities and hypolipidemic effects of an aqueous extract from flower buds of Cleistocalyx operculatus (Roxb.) Merr. and Perry," *Journal of Food Biochemistry*, vol. 33, no. 6, pp. 790–807, 2009.

[18] N. X. Dũng, H. Van Luu, T. T. Khôi, and P. A. Leclercq, "GC and GC/MS analysis of the leaf oil of Cleistocalyx operculatus Roxb. Merr. et Perry (Syn. Eugenia operculata Roxb.; Syzygicum mervosum DC.)," *Journal of Essential Oil Research*, vol. 6, no. 6, pp. 661-662, 1994.

[19] N. S. Dosoky, S. K. Pokharel, and W. N. Setzer, "Leaf essential oil composition, antimicrobial; and cytotoxic activities of Cleistocalyx operculatus from Hetauda, Nepal," *American Journal of Essential Oils and Natural Products*, vol. 3, no. 1, pp. 34–37, 2015.

[20] T. C. Nguyen, T. N. Nguyen, K. N. C, D. P. Do, T. K. Duong, and T. T. Nguyen, "Chemical composition and anti-microbial activity of essential oil from leaves of Piper betel L," *Can Tho University Journal of Science*, vol. 45, pp. 28–32, 2016, In Vietnamese.

[21] O. M. Livimbi and I. O. Komolafe, "Epidemiology and bacterial colonization of burn injuries in Blantyre," *Malawi Medical Journal*, vol. 19, no. 1, pp. 25–27, 2007.

[22] D. D. S. Tavares Pereira, M. H. M. Lima-Ribeiro, N. T. De Pontes-Filho, A. M. D. A. Carneiro-Leão, and M. T. D. S. Correia, "Development of animal model for studying deep second-degree thermal burns," *Journal of Biomedicine and Biotechnology*, vol. 2012, Article ID 460841, 7 pages, 2012.

[23] R. Bahramsoltani, M. H. Farzaei, A. H. Abdolghaffari et al., "Evaluation of phytochemicals, antioxidant and burn wound healing activities of Cucurbita moschata Duchesne fruit peel," *Iranian Journal of Basic Medical Sciences*, vol. 20, no. 7, pp. 799–806, 2017.

[24] P. T. M. Nguyen, N. Schultze, C. Boger, Z. Alresley, A. Bolhuis, and U. Lindequist, "Anticaries and antimicrobial activities of methanolic extract from leaves of Cleistocalyx operculatus L," *Asian Pacific Journal of Tropical Biomedicine*, vol. 7, no. 1, pp. 43–48, 2017.

[25] H. H. Nguyen and T. M. T. Tran, "Chemical composition analysis and antibacterial-anti-inflammatory activity test of tamanu seed oil extract by supercritical fluid technology," *Journal of Science and Technology Development*, vol. 19, no. 6, pp. 145–153, 2016.

11

From Localized Scleroderma to Systemic Sclerosis: Coexistence or Possible Evolution

Giuggioli Dilia ⓘ, Colaci Michele ⓘ, Cocchiara Emanuele, Spinella Amelia, Lumetti Federica ⓘ, and Ferri Clodoveo

Scleroderma Unit, Chair of Rheumatology, University of Modena and Reggio Emilia, Modena, Italy

Correspondence should be addressed to Giuggioli Dilia; diliagiuggioli@hotmail.com

Academic Editor: Jag Bhawan

Background. Systemic sclerosis (SSc) and localized scleroderma (LoS) are two different diseases that may share some features. We evaluated the relationship between SSc and LoS in our case series of SSc patients. *Methods.* We analysed the clinical records of 330 SSc patients, in order to find the eventual occurrence of both the two diseases. *Results.* Eight (2.4%) female patients presented both the two diagnoses in their clinical histories. Six developed LoS prior to SSc; in 4/6 cases, the presence of autoantibodies was observed before SSc diagnosis. Overall, the median time interval between LoS and SSc diagnosis was 18 (range 0–156) months. *Conclusions.* LoS and SSc are two distinct clinical entities that may coexist. Moreover, as anecdotally reported in pediatric populations, we suggested the possible development of SSc in adult patients with LoS, particularly in presence of Raynaud's phenomenon or antinuclear antibodies before the SSc onset.

1. Introduction

Systemic sclerosis (SSc) is a connective tissue disease characterized by different degrees of skin fibrosis and visceral organ involvement. The etiology of SSc remains obscure; the disease appears to be the result of a multistep and multifactorial process, including immune system alterations, under the influence of genetic and exogenous (toxic or infectious) factors [1].

Morphea, also known as localized scleroderma (LoS), is a distinctive inflammatory disease involving the skin and the subcutaneous tissue, characterized by excessive collagen deposition that ultimately leads to fibrosis. Differently from SSc, Raynaud's phenomenon, typical autoantibodies, and visceral involvement are generally absent.

The incidence of LoS is around 0.3 to 3 cases per 100.000 inhabitants/year [2]. It affects commonly Caucasian women, with a women/men ratio of 2–4/1, a similar prevalence in children and adults with a peak in the fifth decade of life in adults, whereas 90% of children are diagnosed between 2 and 14 years of age [3, 4].

Etiology of LoS is unknown, even if the probable trigger is a vascular injury that culminates in increased collagen production and decreased collagen destruction [5].

Plaque morphea lesions have an initial inflammatory (or active) stage of erythematous to lilaceous dusky patches or plaques; over time, the center becomes white and sclerotic, and the borders take on a characteristic "lilaceous ring." When the active stage ends, white sclerotic plaques with postinflammatory hyperpigmentation may be found. LoS is classified according to clinical presentation: the most widely used classification in literature is the "Mayo Clinic Classification" [6, 7].

Plaque morphea is the most common presentation in adults, unlike the linear morphea that is more common in children and it often presents with fibrosis of underlying tissues up to bone. The subcutaneous tissue and the muscular fascia are targeted by the deep morphea. Finally, the generalized and the bullous morphea are rare clinical entities [3].

Though LoS is known as a dermatologic disease, it has also been reported in literature the possibility of visceral involvement, in the case of overlap with other autoimmune diseases or as possible evolution towards a systemic form; the latter possibility was described anecdotally in pediatric cases [8, 9].

Despite distinct clinical entities, SSc and LoS present analogue histopathological findings [3–5]; furthermore, the presence of autoantibodies or Raynaud's phenomenon (RP) could be reported also in LoS [3]. In this perspective they might represent two extremities of the same spectrum of disease.

The aim of our study was to retrospectively evaluate a large SSc cohort in order to investigate the relationship between SSc and LoS.

2. Patients and Methods

We retrospectively studied 330 patients fulfilling the ACR/EULAR criteria for SSc [10] referring to our university-based Rheumatology Unit from January 2003 to July 2017.

The eventual coexistence of LoS and SSc diagnosis was searched for each patient in the medical records. The clinical, laboratory, and instrumental features were available for all patients, from the first visit at our referral center and throughout the follow-up. In every patient, the description of cutaneous sclerosis was registered, for the purpose of an early SSc diagnosis or to document the progression of the cutaneous sclerosis.

In case of LoS, the lesions were described as regards number, site of localization, macroscopic aspects, and histological features obtained by skin biopsy, which is routinely prescribed for new patients. In these cases, the referral to our center was indicated by the dermatologist who first evaluated the subjects.

Systemic symptoms and signs evocative for SSc, such as presence of RP or acrocyanosis, telangiectasias or calcinosis, visceral involvement such as interstitial lung disease, or esophagus dyskinesia were always reported. Skin disorders different from morphea were also included in the records.

Laboratory blood tests, including erythrocyte sedimentation rate, c-reactive protein, blood cell counts, liver, kidney, and thyroid function assessments, were routinely registered. Moreover, spirometry, lung diffusion for carbon monoxide test, chest high-resolution computed tomography, echocardiography, nailfold videocapillaroscopy, and esophagus X-ray were carried out in all patients at the baseline and during the follow-up, according to patients' clinical conditions.

Possible exogenous toxic agents, such as cigarettes smoking, occupational and environmental exposures, and the eventual presence of comorbidities, were reported.

Finally, therapies administered for both localized and systemic scleroderma were registered.

3. Results

In total, 8/330 (2.4%) SSc patients presented also LoS (Table 1). Six SSc female patients (1.8%) had a clinical history of LoS prior to SSc diagnosis (all limited SSc subtype). The mean age at the time of LoS onset in these 6 cases was 43.5 years and the median time interval between Los and SSc diagnosis was 18 (range 0–156) months.

Other 2 SSc patients (50 F, 70 F) developed LoS after 5 and 10 years of follow-up, at the trunk and left pretibial area, respectively; both patients were anticentromere positive and with limited skin SSc subset.

Skin biopsies confirmed the diagnosis of LoS, showing nonspecific inflammatory infiltrate, collagen fiber deposition, and dermis sclerosis.

In the 6 patients with LoS before SSc, RP preceded LoS in 2 cases of 48 and 4 months, respectively; in the remaining 4 patients RP occurred after LoS onset, along with other SSc systemic symptoms.

Cutaneous involvement was represented by patches of skin sclerosis localized in limbs, trunk, or face; in one case linear LoS was reported. A single lesion was found in 3/6 patients, while the remaining cases presented multiple lesions.

Cutaneous limited SSc was diagnosed in all patients. During the follow-up, 4/8 patients developed digital ulcers (pitting scars and ulcers on calcinosis), 4/8 esophagopathy confirmed with barium swallow test and only 1/8 interstitial lung disease. No cardiac or renal involvements were reported; moreover, 5/8 patients complained arthromyalgias in absence of arthritis or myositis.

All patients underwent a nailfold videocapillaroscopy test evidencing a typical SSc pattern [11] in 6/8 patients (active pattern in 3, early pattern in 3 cases).

Serum antinuclear antibodies were detected in all patients: 4 anticentromere, 2 antinucleolar, 1 anti-Scl70, and 1 ANA speckled. Of interest, the positivity of ANA was observed in 4/6 LoS patients before the diagnosis of SSc.

No patient reported exposure to toxic substances or cigarettes smoke; autoimmune thyroiditis was a comorbidity in 2/8 patients.

Finally, no local treatment was employed for LoS, while low dosage of systemic steroids was administered.

4. Discussion

In the present study, we retrospectively evaluated a large cohort of SSc patients, in order to find the cases who presented also LoS; eight patients (2.4%) were found.

LoS and SSc are two distinct clinical entities that may share some features, such as the histopathological findings in the skin and the possible presence of antinuclear autoantibodies. In this perspective they might represent two ends of a unique disease spectrum [8].

LoS and SSc cannot be differentiated by histopathological examination because they share the same aspects: lymphocytic perivascular infiltration in the reticular dermis and swollen endothelial cells in the early phase, followed by thickened collagen bundles infiltrating the entire dermis and extending into subcutaneous fat in the late phase, with loss of eccrine glands and blood vessels, and "fat trapping." Therefore, skin biopsy does not allow making differential diagnosis per se; conversely, the global evaluation of the clinical picture is fundamental for the diagnosis. LoS is characterized by the absence of sclerodactyly, RP, and nailfold capillary changes; moreover, even if patients with LoS commonly have nonspecific systemic symptoms, such

TABLE 1: Summary of the patients of our series with LoS associated with SSc.

Number	Age/sex	First diagnosis	Clinical picture at the 1st rheumatologic visit	Time to 2nd disease onset (months)	Second diagnosis	Clinical picture at the 2nd diagnosis	Other SSc features during the follow-up
(1)	26 F	LoS	Morphea at right leg from 2 years; RP onset 4 years before, new telangiectasias, nondiagnostic alterations at VC, ANoA with ENA neg.	24	SSc	RP, sclerodactyly and sclerodermic face, ACA plus anti-SSA, DU, "early" SSc pattern at VC	Esophagopathy
(2)	60 F	LoS	Morphea at the abdomen from 2 years, ANoA, nonspecific pattern at VC	48	SSc	ANoA, "active" SSc pattern at VC, Esophagopathy	RP, sclerodactyly and sclerodermic face, ILD
(3)	33 F	LoS	Recent onset of morphea at right arm and face, ANA speckled, SSc pattern at VC, 2 episodes of RP	7	SSc	RP, puffy hands, ANA speckled, "early" SSc pattern at VC	- (pregnancy complicated by IUGR)
(4)	69 F	LoS	Recent onset of morphea at dorsum, previous RP, puffy hands, Scl70, DU, "active" SSc pattern at VC	contemporary	SSc	-	Sclerodermic face
(5)	50 F	LoS	Recent onset of morphea at trunk and right thigh, doubtful very mild sclerodactyly, ANA speckled, aspecific pattern at VC	12	SSc	RP, sclerodactyly, ANoA, aspecific pattern at VC	Esophagopathy
(6)	83 F	LoS	Morphea at dorsum from 13 years, RP, ACA	156	SSc	RP, mild sclerodactyly, ACA, "early" SSc pattern at VC, sicca syndrome, DLCO 68%	DLCO further reduction (56%)
(7)	70 F	SSc	RP, sclerodactyly, ACA, DU, Esophagopathy	120	LoS	Left pretibial linear LoS	-
(8)	50 F	SSc	RP, sclerodactyly, ACA, DU, "early" SSc pattern at VC, melanodermia, calcinosis	60	LoS	Morphea at trunk	-

Legend. In the first 6 cases LoS was the first diagnosis made by a dermatologist; successively, these patients referred to ourRheumatology Unit because of the suspect of an unrecognized SSc. After a variable period, SSc diagnosis was formulated in presence of a SSc-specific clinical picture. During the follow-ups, eventual new features of the disease appeared; in the 7th and 8th case (italic rows) Los developed in the course of a definite SSc, in patients referring to our Rheumatology Unit. The second diagnosis (LoS) was confirmed by the dermatologist.

as malaise, fatigue, arthralgias, and myalgias, as well as the presence of autoantibodies, the typical features of SSc visceral involvement are absent [3, 12].

Even if the course of LoS is usually benign, with slow resolution of the skin lesions, there are data in literature suggesting that LoS is not an exclusively cutaneous disease [13]. There is evidence of possible internal organs involvement and association with other connective tissue disease, and the evolution towards SSc was reported in pediatric population [8, 9].

In this study, we documented the close onset of both LoS and SSc in 3 patients and the apparent "evolution" from LoS to SSc in other 3 cases. Nonetheless, the appearance of LoS *after* SSc diagnosis (2 of our patients and others described in literature) raises the hypothesis of mere coexistence of LoS and SSc. The presence of RP and serum ANA positivity or typical videocapillaroscopic alterations can be considered "red flags" of SSc onset in patients with LoS, consistently

with what is reported in the literature regarding pediatric population [8].

Interestingly, in our study, ANA positivity was reported in 4/6 individuals before the diagnosis of SSc. Otherwise, the presence of a scleroderma pattern at videocapillaroscopy was a useful finding for the formulation of SSc diagnosis [1, 11].

The coexistence of SSc and LoS was already described in 3.2–6.7% of SSc patients [14–19]. Toki et al. [16] found 9 cases (M/F 3/6) of LoS out of 135 SSc patients, and 6 were ANA negative. In the study by Maricq [14] only 1 case out of 12 developed SSc 6 months after the onset of morphea, while the 2 diseases presented contemporary in other 4 patients; in all these cases the limited SSc subset was described. Chen et al. [15] described 8 patients with LoS out of 220 SSc case series, and in 3 patients LoS preceded the onset of SSc. Again, negative ANA were significantly prevalent in the overlap subjects. Interestingly, considering all the SSc/LoS cases described in the literature [14–19] plus

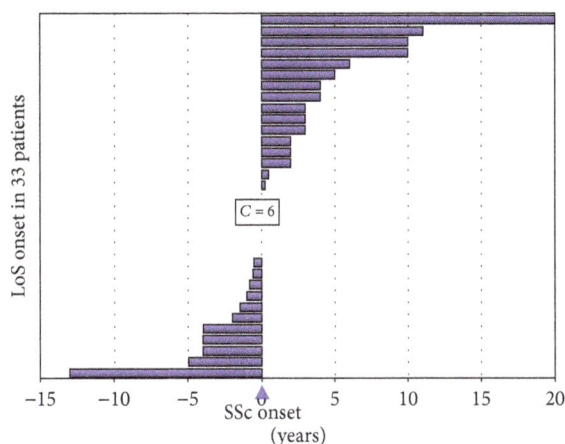

FIGURE 1: Graphical representation of the LoS onset in 33 patients (25 cases from the literature plus our 8 cases) concerning SSc onset (coloured bars correspond to the time spans between LoS and SSc beginnings). LoS may appear before or after SSc diagnosis, mainly in a time period between −5 and +5 years from SSc onset (27/33, 81.8%). To note, in 5 patients LoS and SSc presented contemporarily ("C = 6").

our 8 patients, the LoS and SSc onsets are generally very close (mean LoS-SSc difference time: 1.5 ± 5.7 years; Figure 1). Indeed, the occurrence of two or more distinct autoimmune disorders suggest the presence of a common autoimmunity-prone background.

On the other hand, a prospective multicentre study performed in four French academic dermatology departments [20], including 76 patients with morphea and 101 age- and sex-matched controls, did not find predictive signs for SSc evolution in LoS patients, in comparison with controls. Indeed, the authors concluded that SSc and LoS are not likely as 2 entities belonging the same disease spectrum.

The main limit of our study is the small number of patients who presented both LoS and SSc. However, the coexistence of these 2 disorders seems to be quite rare; therefore it is difficult to recruit large case series. Therefore, the findings of this preliminary study should be confirmed in multicentre large cohort-based surveys.

In conclusion, LoS and SSc are 2 distinct clinical entities with autoimmune origin, and they are infrequently associated with each other. The possible onset of SSc in LoS patients should be considered, particularly in the cases that present features suggestive for SSc development, such as RP, presence of SSc-specific autoantibodies, or videocapillaroscopic abnormalities; in these cases, a careful clinical and laboratory follow-up is recommended.

Authors' Contributions

Giuggioli Dilia and Colaci Michele equally contributed to this article.

Acknowledgments

An earlier version of this work was presented as a poster at the Annual European Congress of Rheumatology, EULAR 2017, with the same title. Therefore, the authors thank Dr. Carmela Esposito and Dr. Vincenzo Raimondo for their scientific contribution given to the realization of the aforementioned poster.

References

[1] C. Ferri, M. Sebastiani, A. Lo Monaco et al., "Systemic sclerosis evolution of disease pathomorphosis and survival. Our experience on Italian patients' population and review of the literature," *Autoimmunity Reviews*, vol. 13, no. 10, pp. 1026–1034, 2014.

[2] L. S. Peterson, A. M. Nelson, W. P. Su et al., "The epidemiology of Morphea (localized scleroderma) in Olmstead Country 1960-1993," *The Journal of Rheumatology*, vol. 24, pp. 73–80, 1997.

[3] N. Fett and V. P. Werth, "Update on morphea: Part I. Epidemiology, clinical presentation, and pathogenesis," *Journal of the American Academy of Dermatology*, vol. 64, no. 2, pp. 217–228, 2011.

[4] M. F. Careta and R. Romiti, "Localized scleroderma: Clinical spectrum and therapeutic update," *Anais Brasileiros de Dermatologia*, vol. 90, no. 1, pp. 62–73, 2015.

[5] L. Goldsmith, S. Katz, B. Gilchrest et al., *Flitzpatrick's Dermatology in General Medicine*, McGraw-Hill Education, 8th edition, 2012.

[6] L. S. Peterson, A. M. Nelson, and W. P. D. Su, "Classification of morphea (localized scleroderma)," *Mayo Clinic Proceedings*, vol. 70, no. 11, pp. 1068–1076, 1995.

[7] I. Bielsa Marsol, "Update on the Classification and Treatment of Localized Scleroderma," *Actas Dermo-Sifiliográficas (English Edition)*, vol. 104, no. 8, pp. 654–666, 2013.

[8] N. Birdi, R. M. Laxer, P. Thorner, M. J. Fritzler, and E. D. Silverman, "Localized scleroderma progressing to systemic disease. case report and review of the literature," *Arthritis & Rheumatism*, vol. 36, no. 3, pp. 410–415, 1993.

[9] F. J. Mayorquin, T. L. McCurley, and J. E. Levernier, "Progression of childhood linear scleroderma to fatal systemic sclerosis," *The Journal of Rheumatology*, vol. 21, pp. 1955–1957, 1994.

[10] F. van den Hoogen, D. Khanna, J. Fransen et al., "Classification criteria for systemic sclerosis: an American college of rheumatology/European league against rheumatism collaborative initiative," *Annals of the Rheumatic Diseases*, vol. 72, pp. 1747–1755, 2013.

[11] M. Cutolo, C. Pizzorni, M. Tuccio et al., "Nailfold videocapillaroscopic patterns and serum autoantibodies in systemic sclerosis," *Rheumatology*, vol. 43, no. 6, pp. 719–726, 2004.

[12] A. Gorkiewicz-Petkow and A. Kalinska-Bienias, "Systemic involvement in localized scleroderma/morphea," *Clinics in Dermatology*, vol. 33, no. 5, pp. 556–562, 2015.

[13] L. Dehen, J.-C. Roujeau, A. Cosnes, and J. Revuz, "Internal involvement in localized scleroderma," *Medicine (United States)*, vol. 73, no. 5, pp. 241–245, 1994.

[14] H. R. Maricq, "Capillary Abnormalities, Raynaud's Phenomenon, and Systemic Sclerosis in Patients with Localized Scleroderma," *JAMA Dermatology*, vol. 128, no. 5, pp. 630–632, 1992.

[15] J. K. Chen, L. Chung, and D. F. Fiorentino, "Characterization of patients with clinical overlap of morphea and systemic sclerosis:

A case series," *Journal of the American Academy of Dermatology*, vol. 74, no. 6, pp. 1272–1274, 2016.

[16] S. Toki, S.-I. Motegi, K. Yamada et al., "Clinical and laboratory features of systemic sclerosis complicated with localized scleroderma," *The Journal of Dermatology*, vol. 42, no. 3, pp. 283–287, 2015.

[17] Y. Soma, T. Tamaki, K. Kikuchi et al., "Coexistence of morphea and systemic sclerosis," *Dermatology*, vol. 186, no. 2, pp. 103–105, 1993.

[18] M. Hayashi, Y. Ichiki, and Y. Kitajima, "Coexistence of recurrent generalized morphea and systemic sclerosis," *Acta Dermato-Venereologica*, vol. 89, no. 3, pp. 329-330, 2009.

[19] Y. K. Sharma, M. P. Sawhney, and S. Srivastava, "Systemic sclerosis, localized morphea, en coup de sabre and aortic regurgitation: a rare association," *Indian Journal of Dermatology, Venereology and Leprology*, vol. 70, pp. 99–101, 2004.

[20] D. Lipsker, D. Bessis, A. Cosnes et al., "Prospective evaluation of frequency of signs of systemic sclerosis in 76 patients with morphea," *Clinical and Experimental Rheumatology*, vol. 33, Suppl. 91, no. 4, pp. S23–S25, 2015.

12

Histomorphometrical Study on Regional Variation in Distribution of Sweat Glands in Buffalo Skin

Debajit Debbarma, Varinder Uppal ⓘ, Neelam Bansal ⓘ, and Anuradha Gupta ⓘ

Department of Veterinary Anatomy, College of Veterinary Science, Guru Angad Dev Veterinary and Animal Sciences University, Ludhiana 141004, Punjab, India

Correspondence should be addressed to Varinder Uppal; v.uppal@yahoo.com

Academic Editor: Craig G. Burkhart

The study was conducted on skin of 24 buffaloes collected from slaughter house. The skin tissues were collected from dorsal, lateral, and ventral parts of head, neck, thorax, abdomen, and tail regions and fixed in 10% neutral buffered formalin. The tissues were processed for paraffin blocks preparation by acetone benzene schedule. The paraffin sections of 5-6 μm were cut with rotary microtome and stained with hematoxylin and eosin. The sweat glands in buffaloes were of saccular and simple coiled tubular type. Most of the sweat glands were associated with hair follicles and consisted of a coiled secretory portion (body) and a straight duct. The secretory portion was made up of glandular tubules, myoepithelium, and basement membrane. The duct portion had a narrow lumen and was lined by simple cuboidal epithelium. The glandular epithelium was simple squamous, simple cuboidal, or low columnar type depending upon their stage of secretary activity. Two types of sweat glands were observed, i.e., apocrine and merocrine. Large number of blood vessels and nerve fibers were observed in the vicinity of the sweat glands. In head, neck, and tail regions the maximum number of sweat glands/mm^2 was observed in dorsal side which did not vary significantly (p<0.05) from lateral and ventral side. In abdomen region the number of sweat glands/mm^2 was maximum on lateral region which varied significantly from ventral region (p<0.05). Overall, the maximum number of sweat glands/mm^2 was in head region followed by abdomen, thorax, neck, and tail but without any significant (p<0.05) difference. Maximum sweat gland diameter was found in abdomen region followed by thorax, head, neck, and tail region.

1. Introduction

The skin is one of the largest and the most important systems of the body and acts as a barrier between the external and internal environment [1]. It is a complex structure, being composed of different tissues. It is responsible for protection, thermoregulation, external sensory awareness, immunological defense, wound healing, perception, and excretion and is also an effective barrier which prevents desiccation of electrolytes and macromolecules from the body [2]. The skin is the multilayered organ comprising epidermis, dermis, and hypodermis and its layers get modified depending upon the species, habitat, and body region of the animal [3]. The hypodermis is crucial in controlling the temperature and nutrient storage, as well as secreting important hormones such as leptin [4].

Buffaloes are well adapted to diverse climatic conditions. Anatomically, buffalo skin is covered with a thick epidermis containing many melanin particles that give the skin surface its characteristic black colour. The melanin pigments trap ultraviolet rays and prevent them from penetrating through the dermis of the skin of lower tissue. Buffaloes exhibit great distress when exposed to direct solar radiation or when working in the sun during a hot weather. This is due to the fact that their bodies absorb a great deal of solar radiation because of dark skin and sparse coat of hair and in addition to that they possess a less efficient evaporative cooling system [5]. Also, histological knowledge of animal skin is very important to the tanner and leather chemist as it is important to know the changes that the structure undergoes when it is being converted into leather.

TABLE 1: Number of sweat glands/mm^2 and diameter of sweat glands in different body areas of different regions.

Body region	Area	No. of Sweat glands /mm^2	Sweat gland diameter (μm)
Head	Dorsal	1.1 ± 0.1[a]	114.90 ± 5.97[b]
	Lateral	0.71 ± 0.18[a]	156.28 ± 10.53[a]
	Ventral	0.91 ± 0.16[a]	125 ± 9.75[ab]
Neck	Dorsal	0.85 ± 0.14[a]	134.08 ± 7.08[a]
	Lateral	0.75 ± 0.13[a]	110.43 ± 6.99[a]
	Ventral	0.57 ± 0.09[a]	117.93 ± 7.49[a]
Thorax	Dorsal	0.62 ± 0.14[a]	109.7 ± 6.34[a]
	Lateral	0.82 ± 0.18[a]	132.51 ± 13.84[ab]
	Ventral	0.89 ± 0.2[a]	165.05 ± 8.44[a]
Abdomen	Dorsal	0.98 ± 0.17[a]	157.7 ± 14.92[a]
	Lateral	1.08 ± 0.08[a]	115.5 ± 12.15[b]
	Ventral	0.38 ± 0.17[b]	160.61 ± 6.15[a]
Tail	Dorsal	0.85 ± 0.28[a]	108.04 ± 3.77[b]
	Lateral	0.74 ± 0.11[a]	113.53 ± 5.04[ab]
	Ventral	0.44 ± 0.14[a]	132.75 ± 8.95[a]

Mean value with same superscript within column does not differ significantly (p> 0.05).

In literature histomorphochemical studies on skin are available in pig [6], sheep [7–11], goat [11, 12], camel [13], cattle, and buffalo [14–16] but scanty information is available regarding regional distribution of sweat glands in buffalo. So the present work was planned.

2. Materials and Methods

The study was conducted on skin of 24 buffaloes collected from slaughter house and postmortem hall of GADVASU, Ludhiana. The skin samples were collected from dorsal, lateral, and ventral regions of head, neck, thorax, abdomen, and tail. The tissues were fixed in 10% neutral buffered formalin. After the fixation, the tissues were processed for paraffin block preparation by acetone benzene schedule [17]. The blocks were prepared and sections of 5-6 μm thickness were cut with rotary microtome. These paraffin sections were stained with hematoxylin and eosin. The micrometrical observations on number of sweat glands/mm^2 and diameter of sebaceous glands were recorded in different regions of body on hematoxylin and eosin stained sections. The data obtained was statistically analyzed.

3. Results

The sweat glands in buffaloes were of saccular and simple coiled tubular type (Figures 5, 6, 7, 8, and 10). Most of the sweat glands were associated with hair follicles (Figures 5, 8, and 10). They were deeply situated into the reticular dermis. Buffalo sweat glands consisted of a coiled secretory portion (body) and a straight duct. The secretory portion was made up of glandular tubules, myoepithelium, and basement membrane. The myoepithelial cells were situated between the secretory cells and basement membrane (Figure 9). The duct portion had a narrow lumen and was lined by simple cuboidal epithelium. The upper ducts were lined by stratified

squamous epithelium. The supranuclear cytoplasm of the cell was more eosinophilic. The glandular epithelium was simple squamous, simple cuboidal, or low columnar. In the present study two types of sweat glands were observed i.e., apocrine and merocrine. The free surface of the cells in apocrine sweat glands had cytoplasmic protrusion indicating secretory activity and the merocrine sweat glands were made of tubules of cuboidal or flattened cells. Large number of blood vessels and nerve fibers were observed in the vicinity of the sweat glands. Myoepithelial cells were located between the lining epithelium and the basement membrane. Elastic and collagen fibers were seen around the secretory portion of the glands. The sweat glands were mostly associated with primary hair follicles in upper rows whereas hair follicles in the deepest layer were devoid of sweat glands and were of secondary type.

The distribution of sweat glands/mm^2 in different body areas of different regions has been summarized in Table 1 and Figure 1. In head region the maximum number of sweat glands/mm^2 was observed in head dorsal followed by head ventral and head lateral area but the difference was insignificant (p>0.05). In neck region, neck dorsal area had max. no. of sweat glands followed by neck lateral and neck ventral without any significant difference. In thorax region maximum number of sweat glands was observed in ventral area followed by lateral and dorsal areas without any significant difference (p>0.05). In abdomen maximum no. of sweat gland/mm^2 was observed in lateral side followed by dorsal and ventral areas. The number of glands in abdomen ventral area was significantly (p<0.05) less than abdomen dorsal and abdomen lateral areas. In tail region glands were maximum in tail dorsal followed by lateral and ventral areas but without any significant difference (p>0.05).

When the distribution of no. of sweat glands/mm^2 was observed among dorsal, lateral, and ventral areas of all regions, it was concluded that maximum number of sweat glands/mm^2 was observed in head dorsal followed by

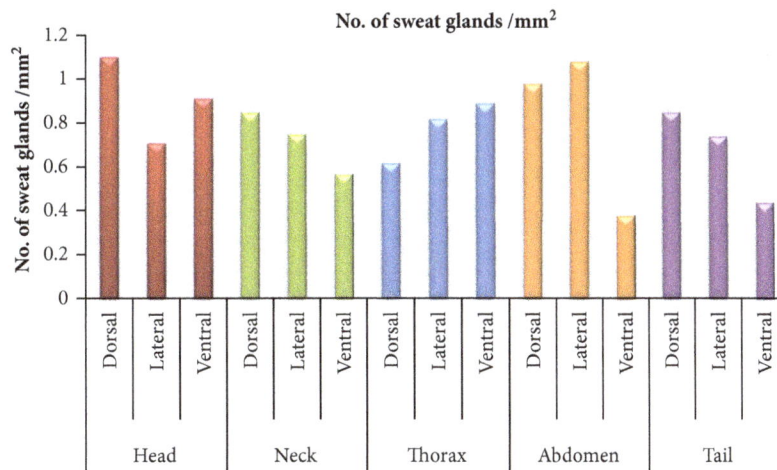

FIGURE 1: Graph showing distribution of no. of sweat glands/mm^2 in different areas of body regions.

TABLE 2: No. of sweat glands/mm^2 and diameter of sweat gland in different body regions.

Body region	No. of Sweat glands /mm^2	Sweat gland diameter (μm)
Head	0.93 ± 0.09[a]	132.30 ± 5.58[ab]
Neck	0.68 ± 0.10[a]	120.85 ± 4.28[b]
Thorax	0.76 ± .10[a]	135.80 ± 6.42[ab]
Abdomen	0.85 ± 0.10[a]	144.60 ± 7.14[a]
Tail	0.64 ± 0.12[a]	118.17 ± 3.84[b]

Mean value with same superscript within column does not differ significantly (p> 0.05).

abdomen dorsal, tail dorsal, neck dorsal, and thorax dorsal area without any significant difference (p>0.05). In lateral area among all the regions, maximum number of sweat gland was found in abdomen lateral region followed by thorax lateral, neck lateral, tail lateral, and head lateral region without any significant difference (p<0.05). In ventral side among all regions, maximum number of sweat glands/mm^2 was observed in head ventral followed by thorax ventral, neck ventral, tail ventral, and abdomen ventral areas without any significant (p>0.05) difference. The distribution of number of sweat glands/mm2 in different body regions has been summarized in Table 2 and Figure 2. The maximum number of sweat glands/mm2 was in head region followed by abdomen, thorax, neck, and tail region without any significant difference (p>0.05).

The diameter of sweat glands in different body areas of head, neck, thorax, abdomen, and tail has been summarized in Table 2 and Figure 3. In head region maximum diameter of sweat gland was observed in head lateral followed by head ventral areas with a significant difference (p<0.05) from head dorsal area. In neck region maximum diameter was in neck dorsal followed by neck ventral and neck lateral area but without any significant difference (p>0.05). In thorax maximum diameter was in ventral area followed by thorax lateral and thorax dorsal areas without any significant difference (p>0.05). In abdomen maximum diameter was in ventral area followed by abdomen dorsal and abdomen lateral. The diameter in abdomen ventral area was significantly higher (p<0.05) than diameter in abdomen lateral area. In tail region

maximum diameter was in tail ventral followed by tail lateral area with a significant difference (p<0.05) from tail dorsal area.

A comparison of sweat gland diameter in dorsal, lateral, and ventral areas of all the body regions concluded that in dorsal area the maximum diameter was observed in abdomen dorsal followed by neck dorsal, head dorsal, thorax dorsal, and tail dorsal areas but the difference was significant (p<0.05) in the head, thorax, and tail. In lateral area the maximum diameter was observed in head lateral area followed by thorax lateral, abdomen lateral, tail lateral, and neck lateral areas. The difference was significant (p<0.05) in all the regions except thorax. In ventral area, maximum diameter was observed in thorax ventral followed by abdomen ventral, tail ventral, head ventral, and neck ventral with a significant difference (p<0.05) in head and neck region only.

The sweat gland diameter in different body regions, i.e., head, neck, thorax, abdomen, and tail, has been summarized in Table 2 and Figure 4. The maximum sweat gland diameter was observed in abdomen region followed by thorax, head, neck, and tail but diameter in abdomen region was significantly higher (p<0.05) than in neck and tail regions.

4. Discussion

The sweat glands observed in present study were of saccular and simple coiled tubular type and most of them were associated with hair follicles as reported earlier by Taha and Abdalla [13], Goswami et al. [18] in camel, Schummer et al.

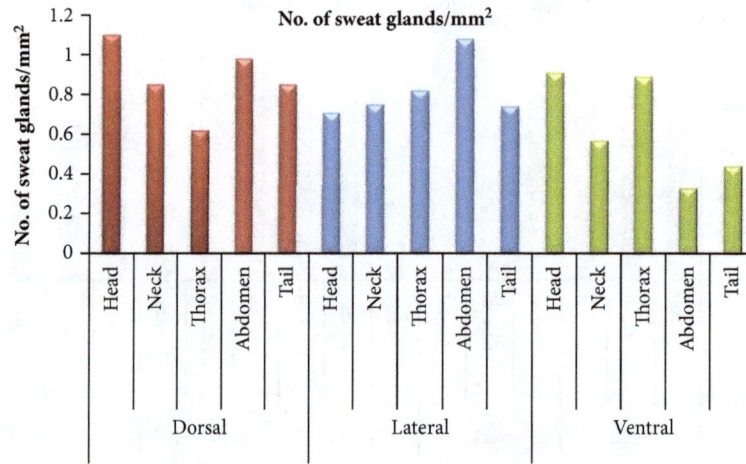

FIGURE 2: Graph showing distribution of no. of sweat glands/mm^2 in different body regions.

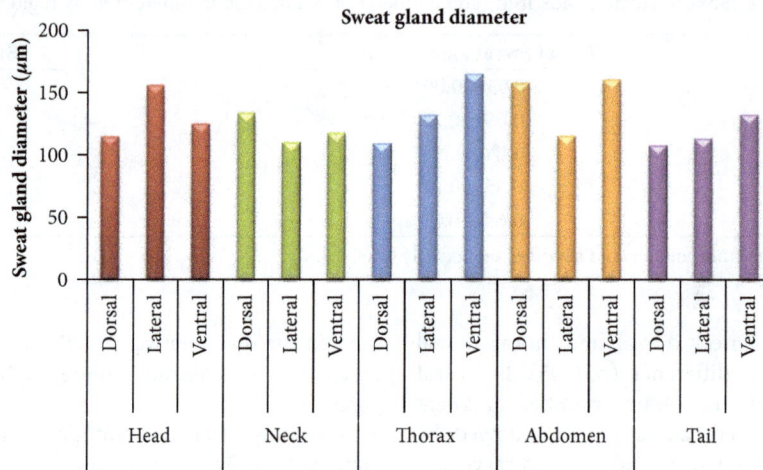

FIGURE 3: Graph showing diameter of sweat glands in different areas of body regions.

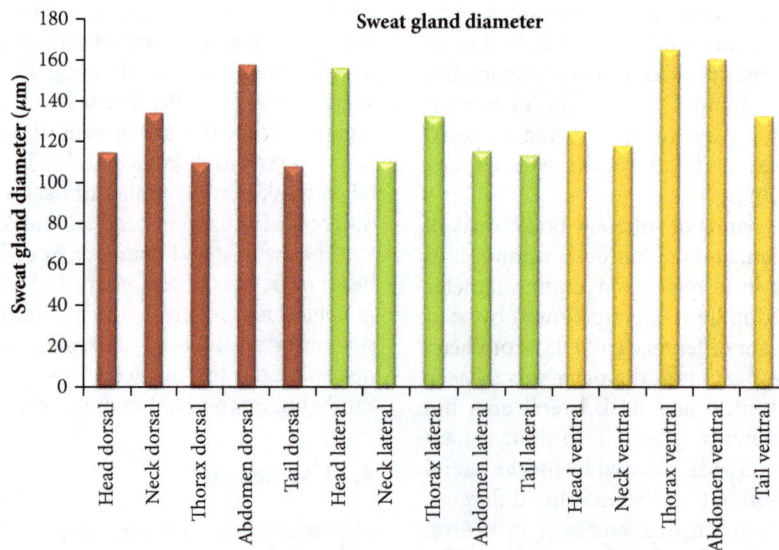

FIGURE 4: Graph showing a comparison of diameter of sweat glands in different areas of body regions.

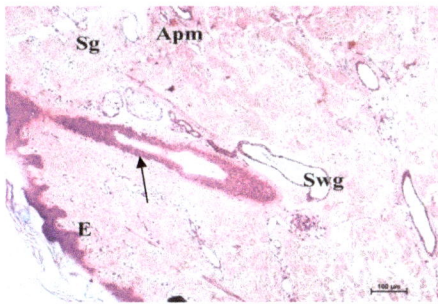

FIGURE 5: Photomicrographs from head ventral region skin showing epidermis (E), hair follicle (arrow), sweat gland (Swg), sebaceous gland (Sg), and arrector pili muscle (Apm). Hematoxylin and eosin X 100.

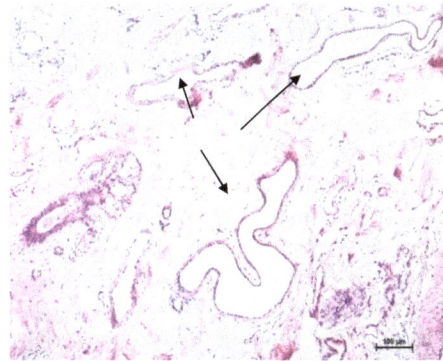

FIGURE 7: Photomicrographs from abdomen lateral region of skin showing sweat glands (arrow). Hematoxylin and eosin X 100.

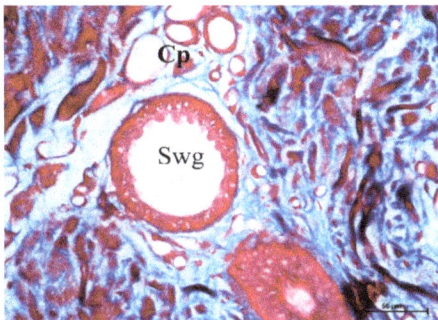

FIGURE 6: Photomicrographs from neck lateral region of skin showing sweat gland (Swg) and capillary Network (Cp). Masson, s trichrome X 400.

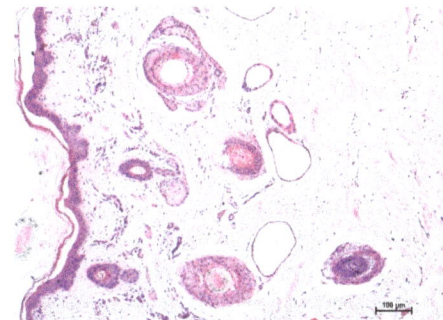

FIGURE 8: Photomicrographs from abdomen lateral region of skin showing epidermis (E), hair follicle (HF), sweat gland (Swg), and sebaceous gland (Sg). Hematoxylin and eosin X 100.

[19] in domestic animals, Baba et al. [20] in sheep, and Razvi et al. [11] in goat. The glandular epithelium was the same as that observed by Hafez et al. [21] in buffalo and cattle, Goldsberry and Calhoun [22] and Govindaiah et al. [23] in cattle, Dowling and Nay [24] in camel, Lyne and Hollis [25], Bhayani et al. [7], and Mandage et al. [26] in sheep, Razvi et al. [11] in goat, Singh et al. [14] in Buffalo calves and Taha and Abdalla [13] in camel, and Sumena et al. [6] in pig. The glandular epithelium depends upon their stage of secretary activity [3]. Hafez et al. [21] in Buffalo and cattle, Goldsberry and Calhoun [22] and Govindaiah et al. [23] in cattle, Dowling and Nay [24] in camel, Lyne and Hollis [25] and Mandage et al. [26] in sheep, Singh et al. [14] in buffalo calves, and Taha and Abdalla [13] in camel have also reported two types of sweat glands similar to those observed in the present study. Buffalo skin has one-sixth of density of sweat glands that cattle skin has so buffaloes dissipate heat poorly by sweating as earlier reported by Marai and Haeeb [5] in Buffalo. Sweat glands were found in clusters and mainly associated with primary hair follicles in camel [18], in sheep [20], and in goat [11, 27]. In the present study, sweat glands were mainly associated with primary hair follicles as observed in camel [18], in sheep [20], and in goat [11, 27]. Saravanakumar and Thiagarajan [28] reported that the mean diameter was 156.7 μm for Murrah, 155.3 μm for Surti, and 157.7 μm for nondescript type of buffaloes which was nearly in range with that of values of present study.

Govindaiah et al. [23] reported that number of sweat glands were more in neonatal cattle calves than young and adult animals. The depth of sweat glands increased with advancement of the age and highest density of sweat glands was observed in crossbred cattle below 12 months of age and lowest in adults of 96 months of age. These glands were maximum (10.40 ± 0.70) and minimum (2.10 ± 0.17) at dorsal and ventral regions of thorax, respectively, in neonatal age group. In young and adult age groups, the sweat glands were maximum at dorsal region of loin (5.00 ± 0.29 and 5.1 ± 0.27) and minimum in ventral region of thorax (1.60 ± 0.22 and 1.80 ± 0.20), respectively. Schummer et al. [19] observed that sweat glands were abundant in the skin of Large White Yorkshire pigs. At the neck dorsal and abdomen dorsal regions, the sweat glands were very large and lined by simple columnar epithelium whereas Sumena et al. [6] observed that the maximum number of sweat glands was observed in the snout region of Large White Yorkshire pigs. Razvi et al. [11] observed that density of sweat glands was maximum (10.40 ± 0.70) and minimum (2.10 ± 0.17) at dorsal and ventral regions of thorax, respectively. In young and adult age groups, the sweat glands were maximum at dorsal region of loin (5.00 ± 0.29 and 5.1 ± 0.27) and minimum at ventral region of thorax (1.60 ± 0.22 and 1.80 ± 0.20), respectively. Das et al. [29] reported in cattle that maximum number of sweat glands was in back region and minimum in abdomen. The

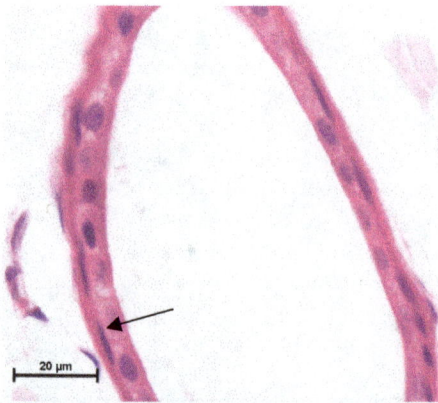

FIGURE 9: Photomicrograph from abdomen ventral region of skin showing myoepithelial cells (arrow) surrounding sweat gland. Hematoxylin and eosin X 1000.

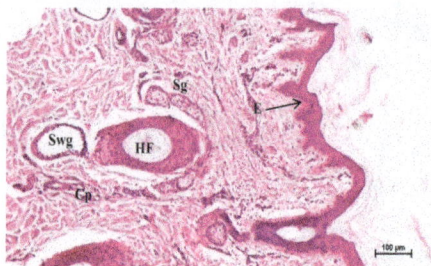

FIGURE 10: Photomicrograph from tail lateral region of skin showing Epidermis (E), hair follicle (HF), capillary network (Cp), sweat gland (Swg), and Sebaceous gland (Sg). Hematoxylin and Eosin X 100.

maximum sweat gland diameter was observed in abdomen region followed by thorax, head, neck, and tail but difference was significantly higher ($p<0.05$) than in neck and tail regions only as reported by Patil et al. [30] in cattle and Das et al. [29] in cattle and Yak.

References

[1] W. Montage, *The Structure and Function of Skin*, Academic press, New York, NY, USA, 2nd edition, 1960.

[2] M. Bhattacharya, I. U. Sheikh, and J. Rajkhowa, "Epidermal thickness in the skin of Yak (Poephagus poephagus," *Indian Journal of Veterinary Anatomy*, vol. 15, pp. 73–76, 2003.

[3] H. D. Dellmann, *Textbook of Veterinary Histology*, Lea and Febiger, Philadelphia, Pa, USA, 4th edition, 1993.

[4] S. Frank, B. Stallmeyer, H. Kämpfer, N. Kolb, and J. Pfeilschifter, "Leptin enhances wound re-epithelialization and constitutes a direct function of leptin in skin repair," *The Journal of Clinical Investigation*, vol. 106, no. 4, pp. 501–509, 2000.

[5] I. F. M. Marai and A. A. M. Haeeb, "Buffalo's biological functions as affected by heat stress - A review," *Livestock Science*, vol. 127, no. 2-3, pp. 89–109, 2010.

[6] K. B. Sumena, K. M. Lucy, J. J. Chungath, P. Kuttinarayanan, N. Ashok, and K. R. Harshan, "Regional Histology of the subcutaneous tissue and the sweat glands of large white Yorkshire pigs," *Tamilnadu Journal of Veterinary and Animal Sciences*, vol. 6, pp. 128–135, 2010.

[7] D. M. Bhayani, K. N. Vyas, A. M. Patel, and Y. L. Vyas, "Postnatal study on the sweat glands of Patanwadi and Marwari sheep," *Indian Journal of Animal Sciences*, vol. 74, no. 1, pp. 7–10, 2004.

[8] C. S. Mamde, N. S. Bhosle, R. R. Mugale, and S. B. Lambate, "Histological Studies of Skin in Sheep in relation with Age, Season and Region," *Indian Journal of Veterinary Anatomy*, vol. 22, pp. 5–7, 2010.

[9] M. S. Ahmad, O. R. Sathyamoorthy, and R. Geetha, "Regional variations in the microscopic structure of skin in postnatal Madras red sheep (Ovis aris)," *IndianJournal of Veterinary Anatomy*, vol. 22, pp. 33–39, 2010.

[10] B. Mobini, "Histology of the skin in an Iranian native breed of sheep at different ages," *Journal of Veterinary Advances*, vol. 2, pp. 226–231, 2012.

[11] R. Razvi, S. Suria, K. Sarma, and R. Sharma, "Histomorphological Study on the Sweat Glands in Bakerwali Goats," *Indian Journal of Veterinary Anatomy*, vol. 25, pp. 113-114, 2013.

[12] V. Pathak, R. Rajput, R. L. Bhardwaj, and R. K. Mandial, "Histological studies on the hair follicle and skin of Chegu goat," *Indian Journal of Small Ruminants*, vol. 18, pp. 275–277, 2012.

[13] A. A. Taha and A. B. Abdalla, "Light and Electron Microscopy of the Sweat Glands of the Dromedary Camel," *Acta Veterinaria Brno*, vol. 49, no. 1-2, pp. 31–35, 1980.

[14] L. P. Singh, J. Prasad, and R. C. P. Yadava, "Microscopic structure of sweat glands in the skin of paralumbar region of the Indian buffalo calves," *Bihar Journal of Veterinary Science and Animal Husbandry*, vol. 3, p. 10, 1976.

[15] M. R. Muralidharan and V. Ramesh, "Histological and Biochemical studies of the Skin of Cattle and Buffalo," *Indian Journal of Animal Research*, vol. 39, pp. 41–44, 2005.

[16] M. B. Hole, N. S. Bhosle, and P. J. Kapadnis, "Histological study of skin epidermis in red kandhari cows," *Indian Journal of Animal Research*, vol. 42, no. 1, pp. 69-70, 2008.

[17] L. G. Luna, *Mc Graw-Hill Book Company*, Mc Graw-Hill Book Company, New York, NY, USA, 3rd edition, 1968.

[18] S. K. Goswami, L. D. Dhingra, and S. K. Nagpal, "Histological and histochemical studies on sweat glands of camel," *Journal of Camel Practice and Research*, vol. 1, pp. 63–68, 1994.

[19] A. Schummer, H. Wilkens, B. Vollmerhaus, and K. Habermehl, *The Circulatory System, the Skin, and the Cutaneous Organs of the Domestic Mammals*, vol. 3, Verlag Paul Parey, Berlin, Germany, 1981.

[20] M. A. Baba, R. D. Sinha, R. Prasad, and J. Prasad, "Comparative histological and histochemical studies on the palpebral sweat glands of Goat and Sheep," *Indian Journal of Animal Sciences*, vol. 60, pp. 1203–1205, 1990.

[21] E. S. E. Hafez, A. L. Badreldin, and M. M. Shafei, "Skin structure of Egyptian buffaloes and cattle with particular reference to sweat glands," *The Journal of Agricultural Science*, vol. 46, no. 1, pp. 19–30, 1955.

[22] S. Goldsberry and M. L. Calhoun, "The comparative histology of the skin of Hereford and Aberdeen angus cattle," *American Journal of Veterinary Research*, vol. 20, pp. 61–68, 1959.

[23] M. H. Govindaiah, K. N. Sharma, and R. Nagarcenkar, "Density of sweat glands in Bos taurus x Bos indicus crossbred dairy cattle," *Indian Animal Genetics and Breeding*, vol. 2, pp. 25–30, 1980.

[24] D. F. Dowling and T. Nay, "Hair follicles and the sweat glands of the camel (camelus dromedarius)," *Nature*, vol. 195, no. 4841, pp. 578–580, 1962.

[25] A. G. Lyne and D. E. Hollis, "The skin of the sheep: a comparison of body regions.," *Australian Journal of Biological Sciences*, vol. 21, no. 3, pp. 499–527, 1968.

[26] S. T. Mandage, N. S. Bhosle, and P. J. Kapadnis, "Histomorphologic study on sweat gland of skin in Deccani sheep," *Indian Journal of Animal Research*, vol. 43, no. 2, pp. 133–135, 2009.

[27] M. H. A. Raheem and M. S. Al-Hety, "Histological and morphometrical study of the skin of black goat," *IraqiJournal of Veterinary Science*, vol. 10, pp. 59–71, 1997.

[28] V. R. Saravanakumar and M. Thiagarajan, "Comparison of sweat glands, skin characters and heat tolerance coefficients amongst Murrah, Surti and non-descript Buffaloes," *Indian Journal of Animal Sciences*, vol. 62, pp. 625-28, 1992.

[29] P. Das, R. Ranjan, and S. Paul, "A comparative histological study on the sweat gland of cattle (B. indicus) and Yak (P. poephagus)," *Exploratory Animal and Medical Research*, vol. 4, pp. 183–187, 2014.

[30] V. S. Patil, R. R. Mugale, and N. S. Bhosle, "Morphological variations in the sweat glands of intact and castrated Red kandhari cattle," *Indian Journal of Veterinary Anatomy*, vol. 14, pp. 35–38, 2002.

13

Clinical Features and Treatment Outcomes among Children with Stevens-Johnson Syndrome and Toxic Epidermal Necrolysis: A 20-Year Study in a Tertiary Referral Hospital

Susheera Chatproedprai (iD), **Vanvara Wutticharoenwong,
Therdpong Tempark, and Siriwan Wananukul**

*Department of Pediatrics, Faculty of Medicine, Chulalongkorn University and King Chulalongkorn Memorial Hospital,
Bangkok 10330, Thailand*

Correspondence should be addressed to Susheera Chatproedprai; susheera.c@chula.ac.th

Academic Editor: Luigi Naldi

Aim. To determine the probable causative factors, clinical features, and treatment outcomes of Stevens-Johnson syndrome (SJS), toxic epidermal necrolysis (TEN), and SJS-TEN overlap in children. *Methods.* A 20-year database review of all children diagnosed with SJS/TEN/SJS-TEN overlap at the King Chulalongkorn Memorial Hospital, Thailand. *Results.* 36 patients (M : F, 16 : 20) with the mean age of 9.2 ± 4.0 years were identified. There were 20 cases of SJS, 4 cases of SJS-TEN overlap, and 12 cases of TEN. Drugs were the leading cause for the diseases (72.3%); antiepileptics were the most common culprits (36.1%). Cutaneous morphology at presentation was morbilliform rash (83.3%), blister (38.9%), targetoid lesions (25.0%), and purpuric macules (2.8%). Oral mucosa (97.2%) and eye (83.3%) were the 2 most common mucosal involvements. Majority of the cases (77.8%) were treated with systemic corticosteroids, intravenous immunoglobulin, or both. Treatment outcomes between those who received systemic therapy and those who received only supportive care were comparable. Skin and eye were the principal sites of short-term and long-term complications. *Conclusions.* SJS/TEN are not common but are serious diseases which lead to significant morbidities in children. Early withdrawal of suspicious causes and meticulous supportive care are very important. This study found that the systemic therapy was not superior to supportive care because the treatment outcomes for both groups were comparable.

1. Introduction

Stevens-Johnson syndrome (SJS), toxic epidermal necrolysis (TEN), and SJS-TEN overlap are rare but serious diseases. They are considered to be the same spectrum of diseases, defined by the area of epidermal detachment. SJS is the mildest form affecting <10% of the body surface area (BSA). TEN is the most severe disease affecting >30% of the BSA. Total BSA involvement of 10–30% is defined as SJS-TEN overlap. The overall incidence of SJS and TEN was 0.4–6 cases per 1,000,000 persons [1, 2].

The optimal treatment for SJS/TEN is inconclusive. Meticulous skin care, hydration, pain control, early identification, and discontinuation of the probable culprit drug as well as an early admission to a specialised unit are the most important things in controlling the disease. Systemic corticosteroids (SCS) and/or intravenous immunoglobulin (IVIG) were proposed systemic treatments but their efficacy remains debatable. The mortality rate is high for SJS and significantly higher for TEN. The reported mortality rate in the Thai population was 7–50% [3] which is quite higher relative to other countries [4, 5].

This study assessed the probable causative factors, clinical features, and treatment outcomes in SJS/TEN/SJS-TEN overlap pediatric patients in a tertiary referral hospital.

2. Patients and Methods

This retrospective study was approved by the Institutional Review Board (IRB), Faculty of Medicine, Chulalongkorn University, and adheres to the provisions outlined in the Declaration of Helsinki (IRB number 316/55).

2.1. Participants. The database for all pediatric inpatients (<18 years old) diagnosed with SJS, TEN, or SJS-TEN, overlap by pediatric dermatologists and admitted to the King Chulalongkorn Memorial Hospital, Bangkok, Thailand, from January 1997 to December 2016 was retrospectively reviewed.

The following data were recorded: (1) history such as demographic data, comorbidity, past medical and allergic history, previous exposure to the inciting drug, and history of concurrent infection, (2) clinical features such as prodromal symptoms, cutaneous lesions (BSA involvement, pattern, and distribution of lesions), number and area of mucosal involvement, (3) treatment such as supportive care (wound care, hydration, and pain control) and/or systemic treatment (SCS and/or IVIG), and (4) outcomes such as duration of hospital stay, short-term complication, and long-term sequel. Long-term sequel was defined as observed end-organ failure after resolution of SJS/TEN, or the onset of another disease during the acute stage which did not resolve at least one month after the resolution of SJS/TEN [6]. Causative drugs were determined by considering the timeline of drug administration and disease occurrence. For the first time exposure, the interval between drug administration and the onset of symptoms should be within a week to a month and less than 2 weeks in the patients with history of re-exposure. In addition, the causative drugs were also identified by the result from the patch test if it was performed.

2.2. Statistical Analysis. Categorical data are presented as number and percentage. Continuous data are expressed as mean and standard deviation (SD). The statistical analysis was performed using Chi-Square test for proportion and Mann–Whitney U test for continuous data. All statistical analyses were done using the SPSS version 20 (IBM Corp, New York, NY, USA). P value < 0.05 was considered statistically significant.

3. Results

A total of 36 patients (male $n = 16$, 44.4%) with the mean age (SD) of 9.2 (4.0) years were identified for the study. The age ranged from 1 year 5 months to 15 years 10 months. There were 20 cases of SJS, 4 cases of SJS-TEN overlap, and 12 cases of TEN. The sample size for SJS-TEN overlap patients was small so the authors combined the patients from the SJS-TEN overlap group with the patients from the TEN group and reclassified them as overlap-TEN group.

3.1. Demographic Data. Fifteen patients (41.6%) were previously healthy. The remaining 21 cases had underlying diseases. Twelve (33.3%) of them had neurological diseases, followed by human immunodeficiency virus ($n = 3$, 8.3%), end-stage renal disease ($n = 2$, 5.6%), Wilson disease ($n = 2$, 5.6%), systemic lupus erythematosus ($n = 1$, 2.8%), and cyanotic heart disease ($n = 1$, 2.8%) (Table 1).

3.2. Causative Factors. For majority of the patients, the cause for the disease was prescription drugs ($n = 26$, 72.3%). The leading culprit was the antiepileptic drugs ($n = 13$, 36.1%), followed by antibiotics ($n = 9$, 25.0%). In the SJS group,

antibiotics (35.0%) were the leading cause for the disease. In the overlap-TEN group, the most common causes for the disease were antiepileptics (50.0%) followed by antibiotics (12.5%).

Almost all patients were investigated to exclude the possible infectious causative factors including *Mycoplasma pneumoniae* and/or herpes simplex virus and/or Epstein-Barr virus. The results were all negative except for 3 cases. For 1 case (5%) from the SJS group, infection was the possible cause for the disease but the organism could not be identified. In three cases (18.8%) from the overlap-TEN group, infections were the causes of the disease. Two of them had *Mycoplasma pneumoniae* infection and 1 case had Epstein-Barr virus infection. All of them had no previous history of any drug exposure prior to the lesions. On the other hand, of 36 cases, we could not identify causes of the disease in 6 cases (16.6%) (Table 1).

Concerning the timeline for considering a drug as suspicious, duration from drug administration to disease occurrence was 12.6 ± 3.9 days (7–21 days) for patients with history of first-time exposure and 3.3 ± 3.8 days (1–10 days) for those with previous exposure ($P < 0.001$). However, the duration was comparable between SJS group (8.6 ± 6.6 days) and overlap-TEN group (9.4 ± 5.0 days).

3.3. Clinical Features. Seventy-five percent of SJS group and 68.8% of overlap-TEN group had prodromal symptoms. Fever was the main complaint, ranging from 1 to 7 days with the mean duration (SD) of 1.3 (1.5) days, followed by stinging eyes and sore throat. The most common cutaneous morphology at the presentation was morbilliform rash, including maculopapular rash and exanthematous rash (95.0% in SJS; 68.8% in overlap-TEN); there were significant differences between the SJS and overlap-TEN groups for morbilliform rash ($P = 0.036$). Purpura was found in only 1 case (5.0%) from the SJS group. Five patients (25%) from the SJS group and 4 cases (25%) from the overlap-TEN had both blister and morbilliform rash.

The 2 most common areas of mucosal involvement in this study were oral ($n = 35$, 97.2%) and eye ($n = 30$, 83.3%) but this was not statistically significant for both groups (Table 2). The number of sites with mucosal involvement varied between 2, 3, and 4 sites. For SJS cases, 45.0% ($n = 9$) involved 2 mucosal sites, 40.0% ($n = 8$) involved 3 mucosal sites, and 15.0% ($n = 3$) involved 4 mucosal sites. For overlap-TEN cases, 50.0% ($n = 8$) involved 2 mucosal sites, 31.2% ($n = 5$) involved 3 mucosal sites, and 18.8% ($n = 3$) involved 4 mucosal sites.

Associated abnormalities and visceral organs involvement in this study were predominantly associated with GI abnormalities ($n = 18$, 50.0%), especially transaminitis ($n = 18$, 50.0%) and electrolyte abnormalities ($n = 16$, 44.4%) but this was not significant between both groups (Table 2).

3.4. Treatment. All cases were treated with multidisciplinary team, meticulous wound care with or without dressings (Acticoat™, Biobrane™), hydration, pain control, and isolation at either intensive care unit or a specialised unit as the supportive care. Majority of cases in the SJS group ($n = 16$, 80.0%) and overlap-TEN group ($n = 12$, 75.0%) were treated

TABLE 1: Demographics of patients with Stevens-Johnson syndrome and overlap-toxic epidermal necrolysis.

	SJS, $N = 20$	Overlap-TEN, $N = 16$	Overall, $N = 36$	P value
Male (%)	8 (40.0)	8 (50.0)	16 (44.4)	0.549
Age (yr) (mean ± SD)	8.6 ± 4.2	9.9 ± 3.6	9.2 ± 4.0	0.373
Underlying diseases, N (%)				0.623
None	7 (35.0)	8 (50.0)	15 (41.6)	
Neurological diseases (seizure, MELAS, GBS)	6 (30.0)	6 (37.5)	12 (33.3)	
HIV	2 (10.0)	1 (6.2)	3 (8.3)	
ESRD	1 (5.0)	1 (6.2)	2 (5.6)	
Wilson disease	2 (10.0)	0	2 (5.6)	
SLE	1 (5.0)	0	1 (2.8)	
Cyanotic heart disease	1 (5.0)	0	1 (2.8)	
Probable causative factors (%)				0.185
Unknown	4 (20.0)	2 (12.5)	6 (16.6)	
Infection	1 (5.0)	3 (18.8)	4 (11.1)	
Drug	15 (75.0)	11 (68.7)	26 (72.3)	
Antiepileptics	5 (25.0)	8 (50.0)	13 (36.1)	
Antibiotics	7 (35.0)	2 (12.5)	9 (25.0)	
D-penicillamine	2 (10.0)	0	2 (5.6)	
Antivirus	1 (5.0)	1 (6.2)	1 (2.8)	
NSAIDs	0	0	1 (2.8)	

MELAS, mitochondrial myopathy, encephalopathy, lactic acidosis, and stroke; GBS, Guillain-Barre syndrome; HIV, human immunodeficiency virus; ESRD, end-stage renal disease; SLE, systemic lupus erythematosus.

TABLE 2: Clinical features of patients with Stevens-Johnson syndrome and overlap-toxic epidermal necrolysis.

	SJS, $N = 20$	Overlap-TEN, $N = 16$	Overall, $N = 36$	P value[*]
Prodromal symptoms, N (%)	15 (75.0)	11 (68.8)	26 (72.2)	0.677
Fever	14 (70.0)	11 (68.8)	25 (69.4)	0.352
Stinging eye	4 (20.0)	4 (25.0)	8 (22.2)	0.477
Sore throat	5 (25.0)	1 (6.2)	6 (16.7)	0.274
Cutaneous findings at the presentation, N (%)				
Morbilliform rash	19 (95.0)	11 (68.8)	30 (83.3)	**0.036**
Blister	5 (25.0)	9 (56.3)	14 (38.9)	0.056
Targetoid lesions	6 (30.0)	3 (18.8)	9 (25.0)	0.439
Purpuric macules	1 (5.0)	0	1 (2.8)	0.364
Mucosal involvement, N (%)				
Oral	19 (95.0)	16 (100.0)	35 (97.2)	0.364
Eye	17 (85.0)	13 (81.2)	30 (83.3)	0.764
Genital	15 (75.0)	11 (68.8)	26 (72.2)	0.677
Anus	3 (15.0)	3 (18.8)	6 (16.7)	0.764
Associated abnormalities				
GI abnormalities	9 (45.0)	9 (56.3)	18 (50.0)	0.502
Transaminitis	9 (45.0)	9 (56.3)	18 (50.0)	0.645
Direct hyperbilirubinemia	3 (15.0)	0	3 (8.3)	0.106
Electrolyte abnormalities	8 (40.0)	8 (50.0)	13 (44.4)	0.568
Hyponatremia	5 (25.0)	3 (18.8)	8 (22.2)	0.654
Hypokalemia	3 (15.0)	4 (25.0)	7 (19.4)	0.451
Hypocalcemia, hypophosphatemia	0	1 (6.2)	1 (2.8)	0.257
Renal abnormalities	1 (5.0)	1 (6.2)	2 (5.6)	0.359
Rising creatinine	1 (5.0)	0	1 (2.8)	0.364
Rising creatinine and hematuria	0	1 (6.2)	1 (2.8)	0.257

[*]Significant values are shown in bold.

TABLE 3: Treatment and treatment outcomes of patients with Stevens-Johnson syndrome and overlap-toxic epidermal necrolysis.

	SJS, N = 20	Overlap-TEN, N = 16	Overall, N = 36	P value*
Treatment, N (%)				
Specific treatment	16 (80.0)	75.0	77.8	0.720
Supportive treatment only	4 (20.00)	25.0	22.2	0.720
Duration of hospital stay (d) (mean ± SD)	7.1 ± 4.1	17.7 ± 13.1	11.8 ± 10.6	**<0.001**
Comorbidities/short-term complication, N (%)				
Skin	10 (50.0)	16 (100.00)	26 (72.2)	**0.001**
Dyspigmentation	10 (50.0)	16 (100.00)	26 (72.2)	**0.001**
Nail change	0	4 (25.00)	4 (11.1)	**0.018**
Eye	10 (50.0)	14 (87.5)	24 (66.7)	**0.018**
Conjunctivitis	8 (40.0)	9 (56.3)	17 (47.2)	0.332
Corneal epithelial defects	2 (10.0)	4 (25.0)	6 (16.7)	0.230
Synechiae/symblepharon	2 (10.0)	4 (25.0)	6 (16.7)	0.248
Pseudomembrane	3 (15.0)	3 (18.8)	6 (16.7)	0.764
Superinfection	3 (15.0)	7 (43.8)	10 (27.8)	0.053
Vaginal adhesion	0	3 (18.8)	3 (8.3)	**0.043**
Pneumonia	1 (5.0)	1 (6.2)	2 (5.6)	0.871
Pancreatitis	0	1 (6.2)	1 (2.8)	0.257
Adrenal insufficiency	0	1 (6.2)	1 (2.8)	0.257
Long-term sequel, N (%)				
Skin	5 (25.0)	14 (87.5)	19 (52.8)	**0.001**
Eye	4 (20.0)	9 (56.3)	13 (36.1)	**0.042**
GI (transaminitis)	2 (10.0)	6 (37.5)	8 (22.2)	0.124
Recurrence, N (%)	1 (5.0)	0	1 (2.8)	0.364
Mortality rate, N (%)	0	0	0	

*Significant values are shown in bold.

with systemic treatment (systemic corticosteroids (SCS) at the dose equivalent to prednisolone 1–4 mg/kg/day, intravenous immunoglobulin (IVIG) at the total dose 2–7 mg/kg, or both). All 16 cases from the SJS group, who received systemic treatment, were treated with SCS. The duration of SCS treatment including tapering period varied from 7 to 60 days with the mean (SD) of 22.9 (14.5) days.

In regard to the overlap-TEN group who received systemic treatment (n = 12), 8 cases (66.7%) were treated with SCS alone, 1 case (8.3%) was treated with IVIG only at the dose of 1 mg/kg/day for 4 days, and 3 cases (25.0%) were treated with both SCS and IVIG. Of these 3 cases treated with both SCS and IVIG, 1 case with severe epidermal detachment (>90% BSA) received IVIG 1 mg/kg/day for 3 days and SCS at the dose equivalent to prednisolone 4 mg/kg/day but the degree of skin detachment still progressed so additional IVIG 2 mg/kg/day for 2 days was prescribed. The duration of SCS treatment in this group ranged from 4 to 69 days with the mean (SD) of 39.3 (21.0) days. There was no significant difference between the duration of SCS treatment between the SJS group and the overlap-TEN group (P = 0.171).

3.5. Treatment Outcomes. The duration of hospital stay was significantly different between the SJS (7.1 ± 4.1 days) and overlap-TEN groups (17.7 ± 13.1 days) (P < 0.001). Also, the overall short-term eye complication was significantly

different between the SJS (n = 10, 50.0%) and overlap-TEN groups (n = 14, 87.5%) (P = 0.018). In addition, skin change (dyspigmentation), nail change, and vaginal adhesion were significantly different between the SJS and overlap-TEN groups. Other outcomes such as prevalence of superinfection, pneumonia, pancreatitis, and adrenal insufficiency were comparable between the SJS and overlap-TEN groups (Table 3). No case of the SJS group had pancreatitis or adrenal insufficiency where the overlap-TEN group had 1 case (6.2%, P = 0.257) of each.

The mean duration of follow-up was 13.1 months (SD 19.9, 1–80 months). In regard to long-term skin sequel, dyspigmentation was the most common finding in the SJS (n = 4, 20.0%) and overlap-TEN (n = 14, 87.5%) groups (P < 0.001). One case (5.0%) from the SJS group had xerosis and 1 case (6.2%) from the overlap-TEN group had nail loss. For long-term eye sequel, dry eye was the single long-term complication found in the SJS group (n = 4, 20.0%), while, in the overlap-TEN group, dry eye was the most common long-term sequel (n = 6, 37.5%), followed by corneal scar (n = 4, 25.0%), keratopathy (n = 3, 18.8%), and subconjunctival fibrosis (n = 1, 6.2%). Transaminitis was the long-term GI problem found in the SJS group (n = 2, 10.0%) and overlap-TEN group (n = 6, 37.4%) (Table 4). There was no deceased SJS/TEN case in this study. Recurrence occurred in only 1 case from the SJS group (5.0%).

TABLE 4: Long-term sequel according to diagnosis and treatment.

	Diagnosis			Treatment		
	SJS, $N = 20$	Overlap-TEN, $N = 16$	P value*	Supportive care, $N = 8$	Systemic treatment, $N = 28$	P value*
Long-term skin sequel, N (%)						
Dyspigmentation	4 (20.0)	14 (87.5)	**<0.001**	3 (37.5)	15 (53.6)	0.423
Xerosis	1 (5.0)	0	0.364	1 (12.5)	0	0.058
Nail loss	0	1 (6.2)	0.257	0	1 (3.6)	0.588
Long-term eye sequel, N (%)						
Dry eye	4 (20.0)	6 (37.5)	0.244	4 (50.0)	6 (21.6)	0.112
Corneal scar	0	4 (25.0)	**0.018**	1 (12.5)	3 (10.7)	0.887
Keratopathy	0	3 (18.8)	**0.043**	2 (25.0)	1 (3.6)	0.053
Subconjunctival fibrosis	0	1 (6.2)	0.257	0	1 (3.6)	0.588
Long-term GI sequel, N (%)						
Transaminitis						
Less than 3 m	2 (10.0)	5 (31.2)	0.109	2 (25.0)	5 (17.9)	0.653
More than 3 m	0	1 (6.2)	0.257	0	1 (3.6)	0.588

*Significant values are shown in bold.

TABLE 5: Treatment outcomes according to supportive care alone versus systemic treatment.

	Supportive care only, $N = 8$	Systemic treatment, $N = 28$	P value
Length of hospital stay (d) (mean ± SD)	9.9 ± 7.4	12.3 ± 11.4	0.593
Comorbidities/short-term complication, N (%)			
Skin			
Dyspigmentation	5 (62.5)	21 (75.0)	0.486
Nail change	0	4 (14.3)	0.257
Eye	5 (62.5)	19 (67.9)	0.777
Conjunctivitis	3 (37.5)	14 (50.0)	0.532
Corneal epithelial defects	2 (25.0)	4 (14.3)	0.473
Synechiae/symblepharon	2 (25.0)	4 (14.3)	0.608
Pseudomembrane	1 (12.5)	5 (17.9)	0.720
Superinfection	1 (12.5)	9 (32.1)	0.532
Vaginal adhesion	1 (12.5)	2 (7.1)	0.629
Pneumonia	1 (12.5)	1 (3.6)	0.331
Pancreatitis	0	1 (3.6)	0.588
Adrenal insufficiency	0	1 (3.6)	0.588
Long-term sequel, N (%)			
Skin	4 (50.0)	15 (53.6)	0.261
Eye	5 (62.5)	8 (28.6)	0.302
GI (transaminitis)	2 (25.0)	6 (21.4)	0.795
Recurrence, N (%)	0	1 (3.6)	0.588

Comparing between those receiving only supportive care ($n = 8$, 22.2%) and those receiving systemic treatment ($n = 28$, 77.8%), mean (SD) of duration of hospital stay was 9.9 (7.4) and 12.3 (11.4) ($P = 0.593$). Overall short-term and long-term complications were comparable between both groups without significant differences (Table 5).

Comparisons of clinical features, laboratory findings, and treatment outcomes between children in this study and adults from previous studies were shown in Table 6.

4. Discussion

This study confirms the rarity of SJS/TEN cases. For our institution, a main tertiary referral hospital in Thailand, the prevalence was 1.8 cases/year. This finding is similar to other previous studies; there was a slightly higher risk for girls and a higher number of chronic health conditions associated with SJS cases [20, 21] in contrast to overlap-TEN patients. Drugs were the leading causative factors for both

TABLE 6: Comparison of clinical features and treatment outcomes between children and adults with Stevens-Johnson syndrome and toxic epidermal necrolysis.

	Children	Adult
Sex, %		
Male	44.4	42.1–58.3 [6–13]
Mean age (yr)	9.2	40.1–56.6 [6–13]
Underlying disease, %	58.4	33.3–76.9 [8, 11–14]
Causative factor, %		
Drug-related	72.3	52.4–100.0 [7–9, 11–13]
Non-drug-related	27.7	0–47.6 [7–9, 11–13]
Prodromal symptoms, %		
Fever	69.4	59.8–94.7 [11, 13, 14]
Mucosal involvement, %		
Oral	97.2	38.6–85.4 [7, 8, 11, 13]
Eye	83.3	59.8–64.4 [7, 8, 11, 13]
Genital	72.2	32.9–41.4 [7, 8, 11, 13]
Anus	16.7	n/a
Nose	-	3.6 [11]
Associated abnormalities, %		
GI (Liver) abnormalities	50.0	36.4–48.8 [7, 8, 11]
Renal abnormalities	5.6	9.1–17.1 [7, 8, 11]
Lung abnormalities	-	11.4 [8]
Encephalopathy	-	8.0 [7, 8]
Treatment, %		
Specific treatment	77.8	46.6–97.7 [7–9, 11–13]
Supportive care only	22.2	2.3–53.4 [7–9, 11–13]
Duration of hospital stay (d)	11.8	10.0–37.0 [6–9, 11–14]
Short-term complication, %		
Skin		
Dyspigmentation	72.2	13.7–69.0 [6, 12]
Nail change/loss	11.1	2.9–46.0 [6, 7, 12]
Eye	66.7	0–69.2 [7, 11, 12]
Conjunctivitis	47.2	n/a
Corneal epithelial defects	16.7	Unidentified [11]
Synechiae/symblepharon	16.7	Unidentified [11]
Pseudomembrane	16.7	4.8 [11]
Superinfection	27.8	8.0–56.2 [7, 8, 14]
Vaginal adhesion	8.3	7.7 [12]
Pneumonia	5.6	9.2 [7]
Pancreatitis	2.8	Cases report [15–17]
Adrenal insufficiency	2.8	Case report [18]
Long-term sequel, %		
Skin		
Dyspigmentation	50.0	13.7–69.0 [6, 12]
Xerosis	2.8	n/a
Nail loss	2.8	1.1 [7]
Eye	36.1	9.8–77.0 [6, 11, 12, 19]
Dry eye	27.8	31.0–32.4 [6, 12]
Corneal scar	11.1	4.9–15.4 [6, 12]
Keratopathy	8.3	n/a
Subconjunctival fibrosis	2.8	n/a
Mortality rate, %	0	6.8–34.4 [6–9, 11–14]

n/a, not available.

groups. These results are consistent with prior findings [22–24]. Antiepileptics were the most common culprit drugs for the overlap-TEN group in this study. It is thought that a reactive drug metabolite exerts a direct effect on the keratinocytes [25]. CD8+ T cells, stimulated by the causative drugs or drug metabolites, mediate keratinocyte apoptosis by at least 3 different pathways: (1) Fas/Fas ligand interaction, (2) cytotoxic T-cell, and (3) natural killer- (NK-) cell damage via perforin/granzyme B/granulysin, and tumor necrosis factor-α (TNF-α) [26, 27]. In this study, 2 cases with TEN had mycoplasma infection without the previous history of any drug exposure whereas, in other studies, only SJS cases had mycoplasma infection [23]. We did not assume that these 2 cases had mycoplasma induced rash and mucositis [28] because both of them had severe clinical courses which needed 22 and 55 days of admission and both of them encountered long-term eye sequel. There was no report of herpes simplex virus (HSV) infection in this study which contradicts previous reports that there was 9.0–19.7% of HSV infection among SJS patients [24, 29].

The most common cutaneous findings at the presentation in this study were morbilliform rash, defined as maculopapular rash or exanthematous rash, but excluding atypical targetoid macules or purpuric macules. One-fourth of cases from the SJS group and 56.3% cases ($n = 9$) from the overlap-TEN group had blisters. The difference in the prevalence of blisters in overlap-TEN group was 2.25 times more common than in SJS group but it did not reach statistical significance. The combination of SJS-TEN overlap cases with TEN cases in this study may explain the skewness of the trend. Mucosal involvement was predominant at the oral mucosa (95.0–100.0%), followed by eye (81.2–85.0%), genitalia (68.6–75.0%), and anus (15.0–18.8%). Lesions at more than 2 sites were 50.0–55.0%. The prevalence of ocular involvement, genital involvement, and lesions at more than 2 sites was slightly higher than the previous data [7, 23].

The prevalence of mucosal involvement was comparable between the SJS and over-TEN groups. However, its severity of involvement leading to either short-term complication or long-term sequel was statistically significant in overlap-TEN groups, especially for the eye ($P = 0.018$) and genital involvement ($P = 0.043$).

No case with encephalopathy was observed in the present study in contrast to Yamane's study which found 3.8% in SJS and 14.3% in TEN cases [7].

For treatments, systemic corticosteroids were mainly used in both groups. SCS treatment can decrease the percentage of perforin-positive CD8+ T lymphocytes [30] and decrease excessive immune response [7]. SCS has been suggested to be a valid treatment [31, 32] for the disease but the result of this study did not support the efficacy of SCS treatment over the supportive care alone. The duration of hospital stay, short-term and long-term sequel, and recurrence were comparable between systemic treatment group and the supportive care alone group. Although the prevalence of long-term eye sequel in cases with supportive care alone (62.5%) was 2.18 times higher than in the systemic treatment (28.6%) group, this was not statistically significant ($P = 0.302$). There was no deceased case in this study.

As for the IVIG therapy, only 1 patient in this study was treated with IVIG alone. Additional 3 cases were treated with both IVIG and SCS. Because few were treated with IVIG, therefore we cannot assess the treatment outcome of IVIG to be positive or negative. However, there were studies documenting the favourable outcome of IVIG either alone or combined with SCS in slowing the disease progression among SJS/TEN patients [23, 33, 34].

Ophthalmic complications were found in SJS/TEN with the incidence ranging from 20.0–81.0% [4, 6, 35–37]. In this study, short-term complications were seen in 66.7% of cases and long-term complications were seen in 36.1% of cases. The incidence of these complications was significantly higher in overlap-TEN group than in the SJS group for both short-term ($P = 0.018$) and long-term ($P = 0.042$) complications. In addition, this trend was significantly observed in skin dyspigmentation ($P = 0.001$), nail change ($P = 0.018$), and vaginal adhesion ($P = 0.043$).

Other complications were rare but were present in this study. A case with TEN had adrenal insufficiency and another case with SJS-TEN overlap had pancreatitis. Both of them were previously healthy and had no prior medical exposure to anything that can cause the complication. *Mycoplasma pneumoniae* was presumed to be the cause for the case with adrenal insufficiency by positive IgM serology to *Mycoplasma pneumoniae*. Epstein-Barr virus was the cause for the case with pancreatitis by positive IgM serology to viral capsid antigen. It has been reported that adrenal insufficiency and tuberculosis in an adult were associated with SJS [18]. To our knowledge, there has been no report of TEN associated with adrenal insufficiency in children. In regard to the pancreatitis, there have been only 2 reports associated with TEN and SJS in children [38, 39] and few reports in adults [15–17].

Comparing to adults' data from previous studies [6–14, 19], children tend to have higher frequency of mucosal involvement in all areas including short-term dyspigmentation. However, renal abnormalities were less frequent and there were no lung abnormalities, encephalopathy, or mortality in this study.

The limitation in the present study was that the data was from a single referral centre. Another limitation was its retrospective design. Therefore, we cannot identify the causative factors for all patients. In addition, there were few cases that were treated with IVIG so that we cannot make any assumption toward its treatment outcome. However, it is difficult and unethical to perform a randomized controlled trial for these diseases.

5. Conclusion

SJS/TEN are serious diseases even though they are rare diseases. Compared to the SJS group, the overlap-TEN group had more significant morbidities of the skin, eye, and genital organs. Early and prompt recognition, early withdrawal of suspicious causative factors, meticulous supportive care, and an early admission to a specialised unit are the most essential parts of managing these patients. In this study, the treatment outcomes were comparable between systemic treatment and supportive care only. This indicated that systemic treatment was not superior to supportive care only.

Acknowledgments

The authors would like to gratefully acknowledge the Chulalongkorn University research affairs team for English editing of this manuscript.

References

[1] B. Rzany, M. Mockenhaupt, S. Baur et al., "Epidemiology of erythema exsudativum multiforme majus, Stevens-Johnson syndrome, and toxic epidermal necrolysis in Germany (1990-1992): Structure and results of a population-based registry," *Journal of Clinical Epidemiology*, vol. 49, no. 7, pp. 769–773, 1996.

[2] J. C. Roujeau and R. S. Stern, "Severe adverse cutaneous reactions to drugs," *The New England Journal of Medicine*, vol. 331, no. 19, pp. 1272–1285, 1994.

[3] P. Dilokthornsakul, R. Sawangjit, C. Inprasong et al., "Healthcare utilization and cost of Stevens-Johnson syndrome and toxic epidermal necrolysis management in Thailand," *Journal of Postgraduate Medicine*, vol. 62, no. 2, pp. 109–114, 2016.

[4] R. Gerull, M. Nelle, and T. Schaible, "Toxic epidermal necrolysis and Stevens-Johnson syndrome: A review," *Critical Care Medicine*, vol. 39, no. 6, pp. 1521–1532, 2011.

[5] T. Harr and L. E. French, "Toxic epidermal necrolysis and Stevens-Johnson syndrome," *Orphanet Journal of Rare Diseases*, vol. 5, no. 1, article no. 39, 2010.

[6] C.-W. Yang, Y.-T. Cho, K.-L. Chen, Y.-C. Chen, H.-L. Song, and C.-Y. Chu, "Long-term sequelae of stevens-johnson syndrome/toxic epidermal necrolysis," *Acta Dermato-Venereologica*, vol. 96, no. 4, pp. 525–529, 2016.

[7] Y. Yamane, S. Matsukura, Y. Watanabe et al., "Retrospective analysis of Stevens-Johnson syndrome and toxic epidermal necrolysis in 87 Japanese patients - Treatment and outcome," *Allergology International*, vol. 65, no. 1, pp. 74–81, 2016.

[8] L. Wang and X.-L. Mei, "Retrospective analysis of stevens-johnson syndrome and toxic epidermal necrolysis in 88 Chinese patients," *Chinese Medical Journal*, vol. 130, no. 9, pp. 1062–1068, 2017.

[9] J. Thammakumpee and S. Yongsiri, "Characteristics of toxic epidermal necrolysis and stevens-johnson syndrome: A 5-year retrospective study," *Journal of the Medical Association of Thailand*, vol. 96, no. 4, pp. 399–406, 2013.

[10] M. A. Miliszewski, M. G. Kirchhof, S. Sikora, A. Papp, and J. P. Dutz, "Stevens-Johnson Syndrome and Toxic Epidermal Necrolysis: An Analysis of Triggers and Implications for Improving Prevention," *American Journal of Medicine*, vol. 129, no. 11, pp. 1221–1225, 2016.

[11] H.-I. Kim, S.-W. Kim, G.-Y. Park et al., "Causes and treatment outcomes of Stevens-Johnson syndrome and toxic epidermal necrolysis in 82 adult patients," *Korean Journal of Internal Medicine*, vol. 27, no. 2, pp. 203–210, 2012.

[12] J. Haber, W. Hopman, M. Gomez, and R. Cartotto, "Late outcomes in adult survivors of toxic epidermal necrolysis after treatment in a burn center," *Journal of Burn Care & Rehabilitation*, vol. 26, no. 1, pp. 33–41, 2005.

[13] B. Gerdts, A. F. P. M. Vloemans, and R. W. Kreis, "Toxic epidermal necrolysis; 15.years'experience in a Dutch burns centre," *Journal of the European Academy of Dermatology and Venereology*, vol. 21, no. 6, pp. 781–788, 2007.

[14] G. Gravante, D. Delogu, M. Marianetti, M. Trombetta, G. Esposito, and A. Montone, "Toxic epidermal necrolysis and Steven Johnson syndrome: 11-years experience and outcome," *European Review for Medical and Pharmacological Sciences*, vol. 11, no. 2, pp. 119–127, 2007.

[15] H. Tagami and K. Iwatsuki, "Elevated serum amylase in toxic epidermal necrolysis," *British Journal of Dermatology*, vol. 115, no. 2, pp. 250-250, 1986.

[16] M. Coetzer, A. E. Van Der Merwe, and B. L. Warren, "Toxic epidermal necrolysis in a burn patient complicated by acute pancreatitis," *Burns*, vol. 24, no. 2, pp. 181–183, 1998.

[17] F. M. Tatnall, H. J. Dodd, and I. Sarkany, "Elevated serum amylase in a case of toxic epidermal necrolysis," *British Journal of Dermatology*, vol. 113, no. 5, pp. 629-630, 1985.

[18] W. Wermut and A. Kubasik, "Erythema muldforme, addison's disease; and stevens-johnson syndrome," *British Medical Journal*, vol. 3, no. 5825, p. 531, 1972.

[19] J. Wilkins, L. Morrison, and C. R. White Jr., "Oculocutaneous manifestations of the erythema multiforme/Stevens-Johnson syndrome/toxic epidermal necrolysis spectrum," *Dermatologic Clinics*, vol. 10, no. 3, pp. 571–582, 1992.

[20] D. Y. Hsu, J. Brieva, N. B. Silverberg, A. S. Paller, and J. I. Silverberg, "Pediatric Stevens-Johnson syndrome and toxic epidermal necrolysis in the United States," *Journal of the American Academy of Dermatology*, vol. 76, no. 5, pp. 811–817.e4, 2017.

[21] J. Diphoorn, S. Cazzaniga, C. Gamba et al., "Incidence, causative factors and mortality rates of Stevens-Johnson syndrome (SJS) and toxic epidermal necrolysis (TEN) in northern Italy: Data from the REACT registry," *Pharmacoepidemiology and Drug Safety*, vol. 25, no. 2, pp. 196–203, 2016.

[22] F. Zhang and J. Zhou, "Toxic epidermal necrolysis: 13 years of experience in the management at a Department of Dermatology in China," *Cutaneous and Ocular Toxicology*, vol. 36, no. 1, pp. 19–24, 2017.

[23] M. J.-A. Koh and Y.-K. Tay, "Stevens-Johnson syndrome and toxic epidermal necrolysis in Asian children," *Journal of the American Academy of Dermatology*, vol. 62, no. 1, pp. 54–60, 2010.

[24] Y. Finkelstein, G. S. Soon, P. Acuna et al., "Recurrence and outcomes of Stevens-Johnson syndrome and toxic epidermal necrolysis in children," *Pediatrics*, vol. 128, no. 4, pp. 723–728, 2011.

[25] A. Nassif, A. Bensussan, L. Boumsell et al., "Toxic epidermal necrolysis: Effector cells are drug-specific cytotoxic T cells," *The Journal of Allergy and Clinical Immunology*, vol. 114, no. 5, pp. 1209–1215, 2004.

[26] M. J.-A. Koh and Y.-K. Tay, "An update on Stevens-Johnson syndrome and toxic epidermal necrolysis in children," *Current Opinion in Pediatrics*, vol. 21, no. 4, pp. 505–510, 2009.

[27] R. A. Schwartz, P. H. McDonough, and B. W. Lee, "Toxic epidermal necrolysis: part I. Introduction, history, classification, clinical features, systemic manifestations, etiology, and immunopathogenesis," *Journal of the American Academy of Dermatology*, vol. 69, no. 2, pp. 173.e1-173.e13, 2013.

[28] T. N. Canavan, E. F. Mathes, I. Frieden, and K. Shinkai, "Mycoplasma pneumoniae-induced rash and mucositis as a syndrome distinct from Stevens-Johnson syndrome and erythema multiforme: A systematic review," *Journal of the American Academy of Dermatology*, vol. 72, no. 2, pp. 239–245.e4, 2015.

[29] R. Forman, G. Koren, and N. H. Shear, "Erythema multiforme, Stevens-Johnson syndrome and toxic epidermal necrolysis in children: A review of 10 years' experience," *Drug Safety*, vol. 25, no. 13, pp. 965–972, 2002.

[30] S. J. Posadas, A. Padial, M. J. Torres et al., "Delayed reactions to drugs show levels of perforin, granzyme B, and Fas-L to be related to disease severity," *The Journal of Allergy and Clinical Immunology*, vol. 109, no. 1, pp. 155–161, 2002.

[31] A. Tripathi, A. M. Ditto, L. C. Grammer et al., "Corticosteroid therapy in an additional 13 cases of Stevens-Johnson syndrome: a total series of 67 cases.," *Allergy and asthma proceedings : the official journal of regional and state allergy societies*, vol. 21, no. 2, pp. 101–105, 2000.

[32] K. Hirahara, Y. Kano, Y. Sato et al., "Methylprednisolone pulse therapy for Stevens-Johnson syndrome/toxic epidermal necrolysis: Clinical evaluation and analysis of biomarkers," *Journal of the American Academy of Dermatology*, vol. 69, no. 3, pp. 496–498, 2013.

[33] S. Jagadeesan, K. Sobhanakumari, S. Sadanandan et al., "Low dose intravenous immunoglobulins and steroids in toxic epidermal necrolysis: A prospective comparative open-labelled study of 36 cases," *Indian Journal of Dermatology, Venereology and Leprology*, vol. 79, no. 4, pp. 506–511, 2013.

[34] L.-P. Ye, C. Zhang, and Q.-X. Zhu, "The effect of intravenous immunoglobulin combined with corticosteroid on the progression of stevens-Johnson syndrome and toxic epidermal necrolysis: A meta-Analysis," *PLoS ONE*, vol. 11, no. 11, Article ID e0167120, 2016.

[35] C. J. Catt, G. M. Hamilton, J. Fish, K. Mireskandari, and A. Ali, "Ocular Manifestations of Stevens-Johnson Syndrome and Toxic Epidermal Necrolysis in Children," *American Journal of Ophthalmology*, vol. 166, pp. 68–75, 2016.

[36] R. A. Schwartz, P. H. McDonough, and B. W. Lee, "Toxic epidermal necrolysis: Part II. Prognosis, sequelae, diagnosis, differential diagnosis, prevention, and treatment," *Journal of the American Academy of Dermatology*, vol. 69, no. 2, pp. 187–e16, 2013.

[37] S. Alerhand, C. Cassella, and A. Koyfman, "Stevens-Johnson Syndrome and Toxic Epidermal Necrolysis in the Pediatric Population: A Review," *Pediatric Emergency Care*, vol. 32, no. 7, pp. 472–478, 2016.

[38] M. L. Dylewski, K. Prelack, T. Keaney, and R. L. Sheridan, "Asymptomatic hyperamylasemia and hyperlipasemia in pediatric patients eith toxic epidermal necrolysis," *Journal of Burn Care & Research*, vol. 31, no. 2, pp. 292–296, 2010.

[39] M. Garcia, M. J. Mhanna, M.-J. Chung-Park, P. H. Davis, and M. D. Srivastava, "Efficacy of early immunosuppressive therapy in a child with carbamazepine-associated vanishing bile duct and Stevens-Johnson syndromes," *Digestive Diseases and Sciences*, vol. 47, no. 1, pp. 177–182, 2002.

14

Hidradenitis Suppurativa in Kuala Lumpur, Malaysia: A 7-Year Retrospective Review

Moonyza Akmal Ahmad Kamil ⓘD and Azura Mohd Affandi ⓘD

Department of Dermatology, Kuala Lumpur Hospital, Kuala Lumpur, Malaysia

Correspondence should be addressed to Moonyza Akmal Ahmad Kamil; moonyza@yahoo.com

Academic Editor: Markus Stucker

Introduction. Hidradenitis Suppurativa (HS) is a chronic inflammatory skin condition characterized by inflamed nodules, abscesses, sinus tracts, and scarring, which can occur in any skin containing folliculopilosebaceous units. We aim to identify the demographic and clinical characteristics and treatment modalities in patients with HS. *Methods.* A retrospective analysis involving records of patients diagnosed with HS in Hospital Kuala Lumpur from July 2009 to June 2016. *Results.* Sixty-two patients were identified, with equal cases involving males and females. Majority of patients were Malays (41.9%), followed by Indians (35.5%), Chinese (17.7%), and other ethnicities (4.8%). Median age at diagnosis was 25 (IQR: 14) years. There is a delay in diagnosis with a median of 24 (IQR: 52) months. Most of the patients had lesions on the axilla (85.5%), followed by groin (33.9%) and gluteal region (29%). Gluteal lesions were more common in males. Nodules (67.7%), sinuses (56.5%), and abscesses (33.9%) were the main clinical features, with 43.5% classified under Hurley stage 2. There was no difference in terms of symptoms and types of lesions among different ethnicities and genders. Majority received systemic antibiotics, more than half had retinoid, and third of the patients had surgical intervention. *Conclusions.* A prompt recognition of HS is imperative, to screen for comorbidities and to initiate early treatment to reduce physical and psychological complications.

1. Introduction

Hidradenitis Suppurativa (HS), also known as Verneuil's disease, fox den disease, pyoderma fistulans significa (PFS), or acne inversa, has now been increasingly recognised to be due to a chronic inflammatory recurring skin condition that involves the follicular occlusion of the folliculopilosebaceous units (FPSUs) [1]. HS mainly affects the intertriginous skin areas of the axillary, groin, perianal, perineal, genital, and inframammary skin, as well as other areas of the skin which contains FPSUs. Follicular occlusion, follicular rupture, and the associated innate and adaptive immune dysregulation seem to be the essential events that lead to the development of HS. Bacterial infection and colonization are being regarded as secondary pathogenic factor that may worsen HS. Melnik and Plewig had proposed HS as an autoinflammatory disease characterized by dysregulation of gamma-secretase/Notch pathway [2]. Elevated levels of proinflammatory cytokines such as tumor necrosis factor- (TNF-) α, interleukin- (IL-) 1β, and IL-17 have been reported in HS lesions. Furthermore, there are also reports on genetic susceptibility, mechanical stresses on the skin, obesity, smoking, and hormonal factors which are closely related to HS [3].

The prevalence of HS is varied and not well described. It ranges from 0.05% to 6%, depending on how and where the data were collected [4, 5]. The most recent large population based study involving >48 million patients in United States found a much higher incidence of 11.4 per 100,000 population [6].

HS has a wide spectrum of clinical manifestation. It ranges from the relatively mild cases characterized by recurrent appearance of papules, pustules, and inflammatory nodules, to severe cases of deep fluctuant abscesses, draining sinuses, and keloidal scars. Although HS is not a life-threatening condition, the pain, foul odour, and disfigurement are associated with significant decrease in quality of life [7]. The diagnosis of HS is made clinically but may be misdiagnosed especially by clinicians who are not familiar with this disease. In case of doubt, a skin biopsy may aid in excluding other diagnoses.

Hurley staging is frequently used to classify patients into 3 disease severity groups:

Stage I: abscess formation (single or multiple) without sinus tracts and scaring

Stage II: recurrent abscesses with sinus tracts and scarring, single, or multiple widely separated lesions

Stage III: diffuse or almost diffuse involvement, or multiple interconnected sinus tracts and abscesses across the entire area

HS is notoriously difficult to treat as it has multiple presentation and runs an unpredictable course. Treatment is based on disease severity, presence of comorbidities, patients' tolerance and preferability to the treatment, treatment cost, and the availability of treatment options. Besides the usual topical antibiotics and antiseptics dressings, there are systemic antibiotics, retinoids, and hormonal therapy. Recent evidence has shown that adalimumab and infliximab, 2 different monoclonal antibodies against TNF-α, are effective in the treatment of moderate to severe HS. Adalimumab is the first Food and Drug Administration (FDA) approved treatment for moderate to severe HS in adults. The European Medicine Agency has also recently accepted HS as an indication for adalimumab. In 2015, the Board of the Italian Society of Dermatology and Venereology (SIDeMaST) has also given out guidelines on the role of TNF-α inhibitors in the management of HS [8]. Other trial drugs, such as IL-1 receptor antagonist (anakinra) and Human IgG kappa monoclonal antibody to IL-1β (canakinumab), have also shown improvement in HS [9, 10]. Above all, patient education and psychological support play an important role in managing HS.

This study aims to identify the demographic and clinical characteristics and treatment modalities in patients with HS in Hospital Kuala Lumpur (HKL). We also compare the clinical characteristics of HS patients of different ethnicity and gender group.

2. Materials and Methods

This was a retrospective study involving all patients who had been clinically diagnosed with Hidradenitis Suppurativa from 1 July 2009 to 30 June 2016 in Dermatology Clinic, Kuala Lumpur Hospital. Based on the electronic record from the clinic registration, all of the clinic notes of these patients with the diagnosis of HS were traced and reviewed by 3 doctors from the clinic who had been trained to collect the data. Information such as the demographic information, clinical characteristics, and treatment modalities were extracted from patients' clinic notes and transcribed into the data collection form.

The collected data were analyzed using SPSS 22.0. Descriptive data were performed. All categorical variables such as gender and ethnicity, clinical characteristics, and treatment modalities were summarized as numbers and percentage, while continuous variables such as current age, age at diagnosis, and duration of illness before diagnosis were calculated and expressed in median and interquartile range

TABLE 1: Demographic characteristics of patients with HS.

Characteristics	n (%)	Median (IQR)
Gender		
Male	31 (50)	
Female	31 (50)	
Ethnicity		
Malay	26 (41.9)	
Indian	22 (35.5)	
Chinese	11 (17.7)	
Others	3 (4.8)	
Current age (years old)		31.5 (14)
Age at diagnosis (years old)		25.0 (14)
Duration of illness before diagnosis (months)		24.0 (52)

(IQR). Assumption of normality was based on Kolmogorov-Smirnov statistics, skewness, kurtosis, histograms, and Q-Q plots. The majority of our continuous variables were not normally distributed; therefore, nonparametric tests were used for further data analysis. The tests used were chi-square test for independence, Fisher's exact test, and Mann–Whitney U test. A 2-tailed p value of <0.05 is considered as statistically significant.

3. Results

Of the 47067 records of new cases registered in HKL Dermatology Clinic from 1 July 2009 to 30 June 2016, a total of 62 patients were identified to have the diagnosis of HS. This led to an incidence rate of 0.013 per 100,000 clinic population. An equal number of cases were seen between females and males. HS were seen in patients between 14 and 79 years old. The median age at diagnosis was 25 (IQR: 14) years. Male patients were noted to be diagnosed at an older age (median age: 33, IQR 16 years old) when compared to female patients (median age: 24, IQR: 12 years old, $p = 0.006$). There was no significant difference between both genders in the duration of illness before being diagnosed with HS ($p = 0.101$).

Table 1 shows the demographic characteristics of patients with HS according to gender, ethnicity, age at diagnosis, and duration of illness before diagnosis. HS was more frequently seen in Malay (41.9%), followed by Indian (35.5%), Chinese (17.7%), and other ethnicities (4.8%). There was a delay in making the diagnosis with median duration of illness prior to diagnosis of 24 (IQR: 52) months, with the longest duration of 30 years. There were only 2 patients with similar family history of HS. Nine patients were cigarette smokers. Median BMI of our patients was 34.0 (IQR 20.2), calculated with missing data of up to 90%.

Table 2 shows the clinical characteristics of our study cohort. Majority of the patients had lesions over the axilla (85.5%), followed by groin (33.9%) and gluteal region (29%). Male patients had significant lesions over the gluteal region ($p = 0.002$) (Table 5).

The types of lesions commonly seen were nodules (67.7%), sinuses (56.5%), pustules (37.1%), keloid scar (35.5%),

TABLE 2: Clinical characteristics of patients with HS.

Characteristics	n (%)
Types of lesions	
Nodules	42 (67.7)
Sinus	35 (56.5)
Pustules	23 (37.1)
Keloid scar	22 (35.5)
Abscess	21 (33.9)
Double comedones	2 (3.2)
Fistula	2 (3.2)
Location	
Axilla	53 (85.5)
Groin	21 (33.9)
Gluteal	18 (29)
Chest	10 (16.1)
Back	9 (14.5)
Neck	8 (12.9)
Inframammary	4 (6.5)
Genitalia	2 (3.2)
Postauricular	1 (1.6)
Hurley staging	
1	22 (35.5)
2	27 (43.5)
3	13 (21)
Symptoms	
Pain	35 (56.5)
Pruritus	23 (37.1)
Embarrassment	12 (19.4)

TABLE 3: Cultures taken from patients with HS.

Bacteriological culture (swab or tissue)	Number (%)
Gram-positive	
Staphylococcus	7 (11.3)
MSSA	4 (6.5)
MRSA	3 (4.8)
GBS	4 (6.5)
Streptococcus pyogenes	1 (1.6)
Diphtheroids	4 (6.5)
Enterococcus	1 (1.6)
Gram-negative	
E. coli	6 (9.7)
Proteus sp.	5 (8.1)
Klebsiella pneumonia	4 (6.5)
Acinetobacter	2 (3.2)
Mixed growth	7 (11.3)
Others	
Chrysosporium sp.	1 (1.6)

MSSA: Methicillin Sensitive *Staphylococcus aureus*, MRSA: Methicillin Resistant *Staphylococcus aureus*, and GBS: Group B *Streptococcus*.

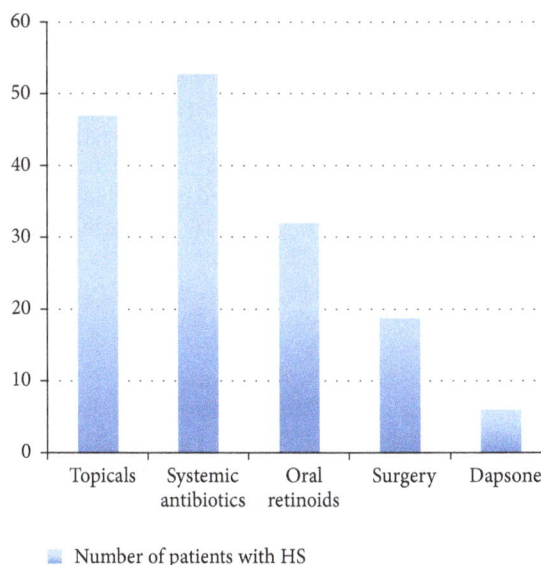

FIGURE 1: Treatment modalities of patients with HS.

and abscesses (33.9%). More than half of them (56.5%) reported symptoms of pain, while a third (37.1%) reported pruritus. There was no significant difference detected in the type of lesions, severity, and symptoms of HS, in between different ethnicities, as well as between male and female patients (Tables 5 and 6)

About 35.5% of patients had positive swab or tissue culture, which grew a mixture of Gram-positive and Gram-negative organisms (Table 3).

In terms of treatment modalities, more than 75% of the patients had topical treatment, which include topical fusidic acid (30.6%), mupirocin (8.1%), clindamycin (4.8%), and antiseptic wash such as chlorhexidine, prontosan, and octenisan wash (66.1%). Fifty-two patients had received systemic antibiotics such as doxycycline (29%), rifampicin (29%), clindamycin (21.1%), tetracycline (8.1%), metronidazole (6.5%), and minocycline (1.6%). Thirty patients had isotretinoin while only 6 patients had acitretin. Six patients had dapsone for the treatment of HS. None of these patients had biologics. A third of these patients had some surgical intervention, which include incision and drainage (14 patients), localised excision (6 patients), and wide local excision and skin graft (3 patients). Figure 1 shows the treatment modalities of patients with HS.

Table 4 shows the comorbidities of the patients with HS. Seventeen patients (27.4%) had Acne Conglobata or Nodulocystic Acne. Pilonidal sinus was diagnosed in 3 patients.

None of these patients fulfilled the criteria of the follicular occlusion triad or tetrad, only 9 patients (14.5%) with obesity, 6 patients (9.7%) with diabetes mellitus, and 4 (6.5%) with hypertension and dyslipidemia. One patient had concurrent HIV and hepatitis C infection. Depression was also detected in 1 patient with HS. In Table 6, HS patients with concurrent hypertension and dyslipidemia are seen more in the Chinese population ($p = 0.039$, $p = 0.031$ consecutively).

4. Discussion

Sixty-two patients had the diagnosis of HS from the review of medical records from 1 July 2009 to 30 June 2016. This has shown an increasing trend when we compare to a similar

TABLE 4: Comorbidities in patients with HS.

Comorbidities	Number (%)
Acne conglobata/nodulocystic	17 (27.4)
Obesity	9 (14.5)
Diabetes	6 (9.7)
Hypertension	4 (6.5)
Dyslipidemia	4 (6.5)
Pilonidal sinus	3 (4.8)
Anemia	3 (4.8)
Neoplasm (SCC)	1 (1.6)
RVD and hepatitis C	1 (1.6)
Depression	1 (1.6)

study done by Leelavathi et al. which reported only 15 patients over 5-year period [11] (Table 7).

Many studies reported that HS is a rarely diagnosed disease [4, 12, 13]. Vazquez et al. reported that only 268 patients were diagnosed with HS in Minnesota between 1968 and 2008, with an overall annual age- and sex-adjusted incidence of 6.0 per 100,000. Cosmatos et al. found a low rate of clinically detected HS where the overall prevalence estimate was 0.053% in a retrospective analysis using health insurance database in the United States (Table 7). We found an incidence rate of 0.013 in 100,000 clinic population, which is much lower than previous studies. This is because Hospital Kuala Lumpur, being a fully subsidized government hospital, is a major tertiary center in Malaysia. Although primarily covering Kuala Lumpur and its surrounding area, it also has patients coming from other parts of the country, including almost the whole of Peninsular Malaysia.

We noted that the ratio of male to female patients was equal, which is inconsistent with previous studies [4, 5, 13–15]. Our number of male to female patients visits to dermatology clinic during this study period was almost equal (1 : 0.94). Shali Alikhan et al. reported that women outnumbered men with HS by nearly 3 to 1, and Garg et al. reported that prevalence of female patients was more than 2-fold greater than in male patients. The only study that reported an obvious male predominant in HS was seen in a study in Tunisia [16].

In our study, the median age at diagnosis was 25 (IQR: 14) years. Male patients with HS were found to be significantly older at the time of diagnosis compared to female patients, with median age of 33, IQR 16 years old for males, compared to median age of 24, IQR 12 years old for females, with $p = 0.006$. This is in line with a study in Minnesota which found that the highest incidence of HS is among young women aged 20–29 (18.4 per 100,000) [4]. Cosmatos et al. [13] found that most patients with HS were aged 30 to 64 years (Table 7).

The diagnosis of HS is often delayed. This is due to the fact that HS has a wide spectrum of manifestation and may mimic other illnesses and commonly treated as skin infections such as recurrent furuncles. This delay may be caused by patient delay in seeking treatment, the clinician not making the correct diagnosis, or both. The longest duration of diagnosis after the onset of symptoms in this study was 30 years. This patient had gone to multiple primary care physicians who

had failed to give the accurate diagnosis. We also had a patient who had underwent several surgical interventions to the abscesses and only later diagnosed with HS. This finding is in line with previous studies, which reported significant delay in the diagnosis of HS [4, 17].

It was also surprising to see that, in our study, the proportion of Indians diagnosed with HS was much higher (35.5%) when compared with the number of new cases of Indian patients during the study period (18.1%). A study by McMillan in 2014 reported that the percentage of visits with HS diagnosis in black patients was significantly higher than the percentage of all visits by black patients in a combined data from the National Ambulatory Medical Care Survey (NAMCS) and National Hospital Ambulatory Medical Care Survey (NHAMCS) in the United States [12]. In another study, the adjusted HS prevalence among African American patients with HS was more than 3-fold than that among white patients [15]. An increased frequency of HS is observed in blacks, possibly because blacks have a greater density of apocrine glands than whites. This same explanation can be postulated in our finding associating HS with the Indian ethnicity in Malaysia, who has darker Fitzpatrick phototype as compared to other ethnicities such as Malay and Chinese.

Although there are emerging data on the association of obesity, metabolic syndrome, and other related comorbidities with HS [18–20], we did not find significant difference statistically between obesity and metabolic syndrome with HS. This is due to the limited documentation in our retrospective study. Missing data were up to 90% in certain categories, as they were not documented in patients' record.

However, with the limited data, we noted that Chinese patients had significantly higher percentage of having concurrent hypertension and dyslipidemia, but there was no difference of comorbidities in between males and females. With the combination of smoking in patients with HS, these contribute to a higher risk of cardiovascular-associated death, as shown in Danish HS patients [21]. None of our patients reported having inflammatory bowel disease or rheumatology condition, as described previously. Previous studies have found that patients with HS have a higher risk of developing depression [22]. In our study, only 1 patient had been diagnosed with depression and currently being treated by the psychiatry team. The low prevalence of depression may be due to the fact that psychiatry illness is still a taboo in our country and therefore patients do not openly express their emotional distress to the clinician.

Majority of the patients had lesions over the axilla, followed by groin and gluteal region, inframammary, chest, back, neck, and postauricular region. The lesions were composed of nodules, sinuses, pustules, keloid scar, and abscesses. At diagnosis, majority of the patients had moderate to severe symptoms (Hurley stages 2 and 3) and more than half of them reported symptoms of pain, while a third reported pruritus. Previous studies had reported that the distribution of lesions in HS is influence by gender. Primary sites of involvement in females are the groin or upper inner thigh, axilla, upper anterior torso (including breast and inframammary regions), and the buttocks or gluteal clefts [4, 23]. In males, the common sites are the groin or thigh, axilla, perineal or

TABLE 5: Comparison of HS clinical characteristics between male and female patients with HS.

Clinical characteristics	Male (n = 31) n (%)	Female (n = 31) n (%)	p value
Severity of HS			
Mild (Hurley stage 1)	8 (25.8)	14 (45.2)	0.111
Moderate to severe (Hurley stage 2-3)	23 (74.2)	17 (54.8)	
Symptoms			
Embarrassment	4 (12.9)	0 (0)	0.113
Pain	18 (58.1)	17 (54.8)	0.798
Pruritus	11 (35.5)	12 (38.7)	0.793
Location of lesion			
Axilla	25 (80.6)	28 (90.3)	0.279
Groin	9 (29.0)	12 (38.7)	0.421
Gluteal	15 (48.4)	3 (9.7)	0.002
Chest	4 (12.9)	6 (19.4)	0.490
Back	7 (22.6)	2 (6.5)	0.071
Neck	2 (6.5)	6 (19.4)	0.130
Inframammary	2 (6.5)	2 (6.5)	1.000
Genitalia	1 (3.2)	1 (3.2)	1.000
Postauricular	1 (3.2)	0 (0)	0.313
Types of lesion			
Papules	8 (25.8)	7 (22.6)	0.767
Nodules	22 (71.0)	20 (64.5)	0.587
Sinus	19 (61.3)	16 (51.6)	0.442
Pustules	12 (38.7)	11 (35.5)	0.793
Keloid scar	13 (41.9)	9 (29.0)	0.288
Abscess	12 (38.7)	9 (29.0)	0.421
Double comedones	1 (3.2)	1 (3.2)	1.000
Fistula	1 (3.2)	1 (3.2)	1.000
Comorbidities			
Nodulocystic acne	9 (29.0)	8 (25.8)	0.776
Obesity	4 (12.9)	5 (16.1)	0.718
Diabetes	4 (12.9)	2 (6.5)	0.671
Hypertension	3 (9.7)	1 (3.2)	0.612
Dyslipidemia	2 (6.5)	2 (6.5)	1.000

perianal regions, and buttocks or gluteal cleft [24]. However, when comparing between males and females in our patients with HS, there was no significant difference between the severity, symptoms of HS, or the location of lesions, except that male patients had more significant lesions over the gluteal region.

Although routine bacterial culture is not indicated, we noted that patients with secondary bacterial infection worsened HS condition. In this study, the swab and/or tissue culture grew mixture of Gram-positive and Gram-negative organism, which can aid in the choice of antibiotics for these patients.

The most common oral tetracycline regime in our clinic is doxycycline, given in the highest percentage of patients, at the dosage of 100 mg once to twice daily. This is the key treatment for mild to moderate HS with favourable adverse effect profile. Combination therapy with clindamycin and rifampicin is the next option, usually to those who have failed oral tetracycline. Our regimen of combination therapy is clindamycin 300 mg twice daily and rifampicin 300 mg twice daily. Previous studies have shown that 35%–70% of patients had at least some improvement in their disease course, with sustained efficacy of more than 40% in 1 year [25–27].

Besides systemic antibiotics, more than half of our cohort received oral retinoid. Most of these patients were on isotretinoin, especially those with concurrent nodulocystic acne. Studies involving acitretin treatment have reported significant improvements in up to 60% of patients [27]. It is also more effective when used as an adjuvant to other systemic medications. Surgical interventions were also treatment choice for those with recurrent and complicated HS.

Table 6: Comparison of clinical characteristics of HS among different ethnicity group.

Clinical characteristics	Malay ($n = 26$) n (%)	Chinese ($n = 11$) n (%)	Indian ($n = 22$) n (%)	Others ($n = 3$) n (%)	Total ($n = 62$)	p value
Severity of HS						
Mild	9 (34.6)	3 (27.3)	9 (40.9)	1 (33.3)	22 (35.5)	0.892
Moderate-severe	17 (65.4)	8 (72.7)	13 (59.1)	2 (66.7)	40 (64.5)	
Symptoms						
Pain	14 (53.8)	4 (36.4)	15 (68.2)	2 (66.7)	35 (56.5)	0.357
Pruritus	8 (30.8)	3 (27.3)	10 (45.5)	2 (66.7)	23 (37.1)	0.443
Embarrassment	1 (3.8)	1 (9.1)	1 (4.5)	1 (33.3)	12 (19.4)	0.246
Location of lesion						
Axilla	23 (88.5)	6 (54.5)	21 (95.5)	3 (100)	53 (85.5)	0.022
Groin	7 (26.9)	6 (54.5)	7 (31.8)	1 (33.3)	21 (33.9)	0.440
Gluteal	6 (23.1)	7 (63.6)	5 (22.7)	0 (0)	18 (29)	0.061
Chest	5 (19.2)	0 (0)	5 (22.7)	0 (0)	10 (16.1)	0.310
Back	4 (15.4)	4 (36.4)	1 (4.5)	0 (0)	9 (14.5)	0.089
Neck	4 (15.4)	2 (18.2)	2 (9.1)	0 (0)	8 (12.9)	0.766
Inframammary	3 (11.5)	0 (0)	0 (0)	1 (33.3)	4 (6.5)	0.072
Genitalia	1 (3.8)	0 (0)	1 (4.5)	0 (0)	2 (3.2)	0.892
Postauricular	1 (3.8)	0 (0)	0 (0)	0 (0)	1 (1.6)	0.704
Types of lesion						
Nodules	18 (69.2)	8 (72.7)	15 (68.2)	1 (33.3)	42 (67.7)	0.620
Sinus	14 (53.8)	8 (72.7)	11 (50.0)	2 (66.7)	35 (56.5)	0.624
Pustules	6 (23.1)	6 (54.5)	9 (40.9)	2 (66.7)	23 (37.1)	0.180
Keloid scar	9 (34.6)	6 (54.5)	7 (31.8)	0 (0)	22 (35.5)	0.316
Abscess	7 (26.9)	4 (36.4)	8 (36.4)	2 (66.7)	21 (33.9)	0.553
Double comedones	0 (0)	0 (0)	1 (4.5)	1 (33.3)	2 (3.2)	0.083
Fistula	2 (7.7)	0 (0)	0 (0)	0 (0)	2 (3.2)	0.413
Comorbidities						
Acne conglobata/nodulocystic	8 (30.8)	3 (27.3)	6 (27.3)	0 (0)	17 (27.4)	0.734
Obesity	5 (19.2)	1 (9.1)	3 (13.6)	0 (0)	9 (14.5)	0.741
Diabetes	3 (11.5)	2 (18.2)	0 (0)	1 (33.3)	6 (9.7)	0.152
Hypertension	1 (3.8)	3 (27.3)	0 (0)	0 (0)	4 (6.5)	0.039
Dyslipidemia	1 (3.8)	2 (18.2)	0 (0)	1 (33.3)	4 (6.5)	0.031

Although recent studies have shown that monoclonal antibodies against TNF-α are effective in moderate to severe HS, none of our patients had yet to receive biologic treatment [28]. This is due to our limited financial resources in this fully funded government clinic. Perhaps when the generic version of biologics or "biosimilars" is widely available, and cost is not an issue anymore, more patients would be on biologic treatment especially those with recalcitrant HS.

We had difficulty in ascertaining the outcome of treatment, as most of them had received multiple treatment modalities in their course of management. Furthermore, we noted that about half of these patients had defaulted on their appointment. This is the limitation that needs to be addressed as this study relied on previous documentations on patients' medical record. In addition, our result may have limited generalizability, as the population size is very small.

Therefore, a larger, prospective cohort study is recommended to look specifically at the treatment modalities and the outcome of each treatment in the near future.

5. Conclusion

In conclusion, there is an equal gender distribution in our HS patients, with higher proportion in Indian population. Most of our patients were young adults, with a median age of diagnosis of 25 years, with long delay in the diagnosis of HS. Thus, it is pertinent that clinicians should be able to make an accurate diagnosis with comprehensive clinical examination, to screen for the associated comorbidities and to initiate treatment early to avoid the physical and emotional complications of this debilitating chronic skin disease.

TABLE 7: Comparison between our study cohort and previous studies.

Variables	Vazquez et al., 2013	Cosmatos et al., 2013	Vinding et al., 2014	Leelavathi et al., 2009	Our study
Country	Minnesota, USA	USA	Copenhagen, Denmark	HKL	HKL
Year	1968–2008	2007	2014	2002–2006	2009–2016
Study type	Retrospective, medical records	Registry, insurers database	Self-administered questionnaires	Retrospective, medical records	Retrospective, medical records
Number of cases	268 cases 6.0/100,000 (incidence)	0.053% (7927/144,000) (prevalence)	2.10%, (Total patients 16404) (prevalence)	15 cases	62 cases 0.013/100,000 hospital population (incidence)
Age at diagnosis	Median 30.6 years (9.9–78.5)	Mean 38.2 (14.73) years		Mean 27.8 years (21–30)	Median 25.0 (12–69) years
Gender F:M	2.2:1	3:1	1.6:1	2.8:1	1:1
Duration between onset of symptom & diagnosis	3.3 years (0 to 30 years)	-	-	-	24 months (1 to 360 months)
Obesity	54.9%		72.9%	13.3% (33% missing data)	9 patients (14.5%) (up to 90% missing data)

Acknowledgments

The authors would like to thank the Director General of Health Malaysia for his permission to publish this article. The authors would also like to express their gratitude to Dr. Ong Sian Yen and Dr. Kanimoli Rathakrishnan for helping in data collection.

References

[1] H. H. van der Zee, J. D. Laman, J. Boer, and E. P. Prens, "Hidradenitis suppurativa: viewpoint on clinical phenotyping, pathogenesis and novel treatments," *Experimental Dermatology*, vol. 21, no. 10, pp. 735–739, 2012.

[2] B. C. Melnik and G. Plewig, "Impaired Notch-MKP-1 signalling in hidradenitis suppurativa: An approach to pathogenesis by evidence from translational biology," *Experimental Dermatology*, vol. 22, no. 3, pp. 172–177, 2013.

[3] M. Napolitano, M. Megna, E. A. Timoshchuk et al., "Hidradenitis suppurativa: From pathogenesis to diagnosis and treatment," *Clinical, Cosmetic and Investigational Dermatology*, vol. 10, pp. 105–115, 2017.

[4] B. G. Vazquez, A. Alikhan, A. L. Weaver, D. A. Wetter, and M. D. Davis, "Incidence of hidradenitis suppurativa and associated factors: a population-based study of Olmsted County, Minnesota," *Journal of Investigative Dermatology*, vol. 133, no. 1, pp. 97–103, 2013.

[5] G. R. Vinding, I. M. Miller, K. Zarchi, K. S. Ibler, C. Ellervik, and G. B. E. Jemec, "The prevalence of inverse recurrent suppuration: A population-based study of possible hidradenitis suppurativa," *British Journal of Dermatology*, vol. 170, no. 4, pp. 884–889, 2014.

[6] A. Garg et al., "Incidence of hidradenitis suppurativa in the United States: A sex- and age-adjusted population analysis," *Journal of the American Academy of Dermatology*, vol. 77, no. 1, pp. 118–122, 2017.

[7] Ł. Matusiak, A. Bieniek, and J. C. Szepietowski, "Psychophysical aspects of hidradenitis suppurativa," *Acta Dermato-Venereologica*, vol. 90, no. 3, pp. 264–268, 2010.

[8] M. Megna et al., "Hidradenitis suppurativa: guidelines of the Italian Society of Dermatology and Venereology (SIDeMaST) for the use of anti-TNF-alpha agents," *Giornale Italiano di Dermatologia e Venereologia*, vol. 150, no. 6, pp. 731–739, 2015.

[9] V. Tzanetakou et al., "Safety and Efficacy of Anakinra in Severe Hidradenitis Suppurativa: A Randomized Clinical Trial," *JAMA Dermatol*, vol. 152, no. 1, pp. 52–59, 2016.

[10] C. Houriet, S. M. Seyed Jafari, R. Thomi et al., "Canakinumab for severe hidradenitis suppurativa: Preliminary experience in 2 cases," *JAMA Dermatology*, vol. 153, no. 11, pp. 1195–1197, 2017.

[11] Leelavathi M. et al., "Hidradenitis Suppurativa: A Review of 15 Patients," *Malaysian Journal of Dermatology*, vol. 23, p. 10, 2009.

[12] K. McMillan, "Hidradenitis suppurativa: Number of diagnosed patients, demographic characteristics, and treatment patterns in the United States," *American Journal of Epidemiology*, vol. 179, no. 12, pp. 1477–1483, 2014.

[13] I. Cosmatos, A. Matcho, R. Weinstein, M. O. Montgomery, and P. Stang, "Analysis of patient claims data to determine the prevalence of hidradenitis suppurativa in the United States," *Journal of the American Academy of Dermatology*, vol. 68, no. 3, pp. 412–419, 2013.

[14] A. Alikhan, P. J. Lynch, and D. B. Eisen, "Hidradenitis suppurativa: a comprehensive review," *Journal of the American Academy of Dermatology*, vol. 60, no. 4, pp. 539–561, 2009.

[15] A. Garg, J. S. Kirby, J. Lavian, G. Lin, and A. Strunk, "Sex- and age-adjusted population analysis of prevalence estimates for hidradenitis suppurativa in the United States," *JAMA Dermatology*, vol. 153, no. 8, pp. 760–764, 2017.

[16] A. Mebazaa et al., "Hidradenitis suppurativa: a disease with male predominance in Tunisia," *Acta Dermatovenerol Alp Pannonica Adriat*, vol. 18, no. 4, pp. 165–172, 2009.

[17] R. Simpson, "Diagnostic delay in hidradenitis suppurativa is a global problem," *British Journal of Dermatology*, vol. 173, no. 6, pp. 1546–1549, 2015.

[18] V. Bettoli, L. Naldi, S. Cazzaniga et al., "Overweight, diabetes and disease duration influence clinical severity in hidradenitis suppurativa-acne inversa: evidence from the national Italian registry," *British Journal of Dermatology*, vol. 174, no. 1, pp. 195–197, 2016.

[19] I. M. Miller, C. Ellervik, G. R. Vinding et al., "Association of metabolic syndrome and hidradenitis suppurativa," *JAMA Dermatology*, vol. 150, no. 12, pp. 1273–1280, 2014.

[20] J. Shlyankevich, A. J. Chen, G. E. Kim, and A. B. Kimball, "Hidradenitis suppurativa is a systemic disease with substantial comorbidity burden: A chart-verified case-control analysis," *Journal of the American Academy of Dermatology*, vol. 71, no. 6, pp. 1144–1150, 2014.

[21] A. Egeberg, G. H. Gislason, and P. R. Hansen, "Risk of major adverse cardiovascular events and all-cause mortality in patients with hidradenitis suppurativa," *JAMA Dermatology*, vol. 152, no. 4, pp. 429–434, 2016.

[22] E. Shavit, J. Dreiher, T. Freud, S. Halevy, S. Vinker, and A. D. Cohen, "Psychiatric comorbidities in 3207 patients with hidradenitis suppurativa," *Journal of the European Academy of Dermatology and Venereology*, vol. 29, no. 2, pp. 371–376, 2015.

[23] J. Revuz, "Hidradenitis suppurativa," *Journal of the European Academy of Dermatology and Venereology*, vol. 23, no. 9, pp. 985–998, 2009.

[24] A. M. R. Schrader, I. E. Deckers, H. H. Van Der Zee, J. Boer, and E. P. Prens, "Hidradenitis suppurativa: A retrospective study of 846 Dutch patients to identify factors associated with disease severity," *Journal of the American Academy of Dermatology*, vol. 71, no. 3, pp. 460–467, 2014.

[25] H. H. Van Der Zee, J. Boer, E. P. Prens, and G. B. E. Jemec, "The effect of combined treatment with oral clindamycin and oral rifampicin in patients with hidradenitis suppurativa," *Dermatology*, vol. 219, no. 2, pp. 143–147, 2009.

[26] V. Bettoli, S. Zauli, A. Borghi et al., "Oral clindamycin and rifampicin in the treatment of hidradenitis suppurativa-acne inversa: A prospective study on 23 patients," *Journal of the European Academy of Dermatology and Venereology*, vol. 28, no. 1, pp. 125-126, 2014.

[27] J. Boer and M. Nazary, "Long-term results of acitretin therapy for hidradenitis suppurativa. Is acne inversa also a misnomer?" *British Journal of Dermatology*, vol. 164, no. 1, pp. 170–175, 2011.

[28] N. Scuderi, A. Monfrecola, L. A. Dessy, G. Fabbrocini, M. Megna, and G. Monfrecola, "Medical and Surgical Treatment of Hidradenitis Suppurativa: A Review," *Skin Appendage Disorders*, vol. 3, no. 2, pp. 95–110, 2017.

15

Epidemiology and Clinical Features of Adult Patients with Psoriasis in Malaysia: 10-Year Review from the Malaysian Psoriasis Registry (2007–2016)

Azura Mohd Affandi ⓘ, Iman Khan, and Nooraishah Ngah Saaya

Department of Dermatology, Hospital Kuala Lumpur, Kuala Lumpur, Malaysia

Correspondence should be addressed to Azura Mohd Affandi; affandi_azura@yahoo.co.uk

Academic Editor: Markus Stucker

Background. Psoriasis is a chronic inflammatory skin disease affecting 2-3% of the general population. *Aim.* To evaluate the epidemiology and clinical characteristics of patients with psoriasis who seek treatment in outpatient dermatology clinics throughout hospitals in Malaysia. *Materials and Methods.* Data were obtained from the Malaysian Psoriasis Registry (MPR). All patients (aged 18 and above) who were notified to the registry from July 2017 to December 2017 were included in this study. *Results.* Among 15,794 patients, Malays were the most common (50.4%), followed by Chinese (21.4%), Indian (17.6%), and others (10.6%). The mean age onset of psoriasis for our study population was 35.14 ± 16.16 years. Male to female ratio was 1.3 : 1. 23.1% of patients had positive family history of psoriasis. The most common clinical presentation was chronic plaque psoriasis (85.1%), followed by guttate psoriasis (2.9%), erythrodermic psoriasis (1.7%), and pustular psoriasis (1.0%). Majority of our patients (76.6%) had a mild disease with BSA < 10%. 57.1% of patients had nail involvement, while arthropathy was seen in 13.7% of patients. Common triggers of the disease include stress (48.3%), sunlight (24.9%), and infection (9.1%). Comorbidities observed include obesity (24.3%), hypertension (25.6%), hyperlipidemia (18%), diabetes mellitus (17.2%), ischaemic heart disease (5.4%), and cerebrovascular disease (1.6%). The mean DLQI (Dermatology Life Quality Index) was 8.5 ± 6.6. One-third (33.1%) of the patients had a DLQI score of more than 10, while 14.2% of patients reported no effect at all. *Conclusion.* Our study on the epidemiological data of adult patients with psoriasis in Malaysia showed a similar clinical profile and outcome when compared to international published studies on the epidemiology of psoriasis.

1. Introduction

Psoriasis is a chronic, immune-mediated inflammatory skin disease that is often associated with systemic manifestations. It is a lifelong disease that can have negative impact on patients' quality of life. Psoriasis has a strong genetic component but environmental factors play an important role in the presentation of this disease [1, 2].

Psoriasis affects approximately 2.0% to 3.0% of the world's population [3–5]. To date, epidemiological studies have demonstrated variable prevalence among different population and ethnic groups worldwide. Higher prevalence rates were found in western countries; the distribution ranges from 2.2% in the U.K [6] to as high as 4.5% in Norway [7]. The prevalence of psoriasis among patients in the United States was 2.2% to 3.15% [8], while lower rates were observed in Latin Americans, Indians, Africans (Egypt and Tanzania) [9], and in Asia at less than 0.5% [10–12]. The wide variation in estimates of prevalence between regions may be attributed to the differences in ethnic or racial composition, genetics, and environmental and climate conditions [13, 14].

Although the number of studies conducted locally is increasing, there is still limited information concerning the epidemiological and clinical data pertaining to psoriasis. Informed data prevalence may contribute to a better understanding of the disease burden, updating population research, and advancement of health policies. Thus, this study aims to define the epidemiology, clinical profile, and the impact on quality of life among adult patients with psoriasis in Malaysia.

2. Materials and Methods

This was a multicenter study involving adult patients with psoriasis (aged 18 and above) attending 25 dermatology outpatient clinics throughout Malaysia from July 2007 to December 2016. Data collection was based on the Malaysian Psoriasis Registry (MPR). The MPR is a prospective, ongoing, systematic collection of data on patients with psoriasis in Malaysia. Data was collected at baseline and every 6 months. However, follow-up data was not available for all patients, as some were notified only once. The diagnosis of psoriasis is made based on clinical evaluation. Confirmation of diagnosis by histopathology examination is optional. Data were analyzed using descriptive analyses for sociodemographic characteristics of the patients, aggravating factors, comorbidities, types of psoriasis, and treatment modalities.

The disease severity was assessed using the body surface area (BSA) involvement and presence of nail and joint involvement. The impact of skin symptoms on quality of patient's life was evaluated using the Dermatology Life Quality Index (DLQI). The score ranges from 0 to 30 and severe impact on health-related quality of life (HRQoL) by psoriasis is defined as a DLQI score ≥ 10 [15].

2.1. Statistical Analysis. Descriptive statistics were presented as number and percentages for categorical variables. Mean with standard deviation (SD) was used for normally distributed data, while median with interquartile range (IQR) was used for data that were not normally distributed. Collected data was tabulated using SPSS.

3. Results

There were a total of 15,794 patients (aged 18 years and above) notified to the MPR between July 2007 and December 2016. 56.6% of the patients were male and 43.4% were female patients. The racial distributions of patients were Malay (50.5%), Chinese (21.4%), Indian (17.6%), and others (10.6%) (Table 1).

Psoriasis can present at any time of life. Female patients had an earlier age of onset of psoriasis, with a mean age of 32.59 ± 16.64, compared to male, with a mean age of 37.09 ± 15.51. Positive family history was reported in 23.1% of patients, and female patients had a higher percentage of family members with psoriasis, compared to male patients (Table 1).

Psoriasis can have several presentations. The most common type of psoriasis in our study was plaque psoriasis (85.1%), followed by guttate psoriasis (2.9%), erythrodermic psoriasis (1.7%), and pustular psoriasis (1.0%). Other less common types include flexural psoriasis and palmoplantar nonpustular psoriasis, each with 0.4% (Figure 1).

In terms of disease severity, 25.2% of patients had a body surface area (BSA) of less than 5%, while 51.4% of our patients had BSA involvement of 5–10%, and 21.7% of patients had a BSA of >10–90%. Only 1.8% were reported to be erythrodermic (BSA > 90%). Male patients had more severe disease (BSA > 10%), compared to female patients (26.7% and 19.6%, resp.) (Table 1).

Of 15,794 patients, 57.1% of patients had nail involvement, and the percentage is higher in male patients, compared to

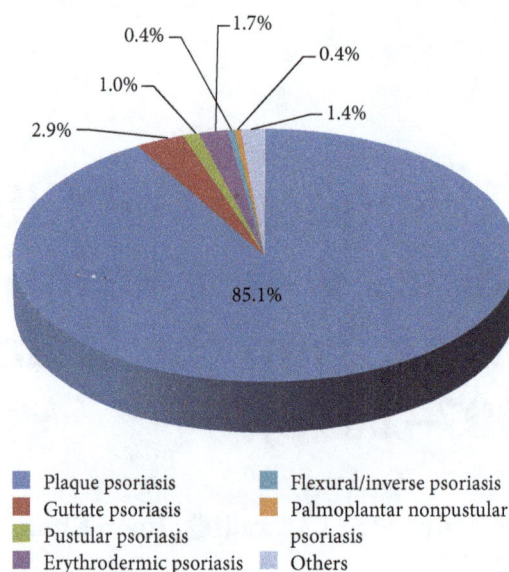

FIGURE 1: Type of psoriasis.

Legend:
- Plaque psoriasis
- Guttate psoriasis
- Pustular psoriasis
- Erythrodermic psoriasis
- Flexural/inverse psoriasis
- Palmoplantar nonpustular psoriasis
- Others

female ones (62.0% and 50.6%, resp.). Nail pitting was the most common form (72.3%) followed by onycholysis (48.3%), nail discolouration (29.4%), subungual hyperkeratosis (12.6%), and total nail dystrophy (4.8%) (Table 1).

Psoriatic arthropathy was reported in 2,168 (13.7%) patients. Psoriatic arthropathy was more commonly reported in female compared to male patients (16.3% and 11.8%, resp.).

Oligo/monoarthropathy (37.9%) was the most common type, followed by symmetrical polyarthropathy (30.6%), distal hand joint arthropathy (29.6%), spondylitis/sacroiliitis (7.4%), and arthritis mutilans (2.8%) (Table 1).

52% of patients in our study had identifiable aggravating factors. Most of the patients confirmed stress as an aggravating factor (48.3%), followed by sunlight (24.9%) and infection (9.1%). Other less common aggravating factors include smoking, trauma, drugs, alcohol, and pregnancy.

3,377 (24.3%) of our patients were obese (BMI >= 30). Other common comorbidities associated with psoriasis in patients in this study were hypertension (25.6%), hyperlipidemia (18%), diabetes mellitus (17.2%), ischaemic heart disease (5.4%), and cerebrovascular disease (1.6%) (Table 1).

4. Treatment

Data on types of therapy was available for 15,635 patients at baseline/first visit. However, only 5,701 patients have complete data on types of therapy at last follow-up (6 months and above). Between 93.6% and 95.4% were prescribed topical treatment at baseline and at follow-up. There were not many differences in the types of topical treatment prescribed at baseline and at follow-up. Topical steroid was the most common treatment prescribed, followed by emollients and tar preparation. Other types of topical treatments include keratolytics, calcipotriol, calcipotriol with betamethasone dipropionate, and dithranol (Table 2).

TABLE 1: Patients' characteristics at baseline.

Variable	Male		Female		Total
	n	%	n	%	
Number of patients	8,947	56.6	6,847	43.4	15,794
Ethnicity					
Malay	4,083	45.6	3,885	56.7	7,968 (50.5%)
Chinese	2,164	24.2	1,215	17.7	3,379 (21.4%)
Indian	1,779	19.9	994	14.6	2,773 (17.6%)
Others	922	10.3	753	11.0	1,669 (10.6%)
Mean age of onset of psoriasis	37.09 ± 15.51		32.59 ± 16.64		35.14 ± 16.16
Positive family history	1,926	21.5	1,737	25.4	3,663 (23.1%)
Types of psoriasis					
Plaque psoriasis	7,696	86.0	5,752	84.0	13,448 (85.1%)
Guttate psoriasis	240	2.7	216	3.2	456 (2.9%)
Erythrodermic psoriasis	182	2.0	85	1.2	267 (1.7%)
Pustular psoriasis	50	0.6	105	1.5	155 (1.0%)
Flexural psoriasis	24	0.3	43	0.6	67 (0.4%)
Palmoplantar nonpustular psoriasis	36	0.4	23	0.3	59 (0.4%)
Severity of psoriasis					
BSA < 5%	1,029	25.9	801	24.4	1,826 (25.2%)
BSA 5–10%	1,882	47.5	1,843	56.0	3,725 (51.4%)
BSA > 10–90%	972	24.5	600	18.2	1,572 (21.7%)
BSA > 90%	86	2.2	45	1.4	131 (1.8%)
Nail involvement					
Yes	5,549	62.0	3,463	50.6	9,012 (57.1%)
Pitting	4,025	72.5	2,429	70.1	6,519 (72.3%)
Onycholysis	2,792	50.3	1,561	45.1	4,353 (48.3%)
Nail discolouration	1,783	32.1	870	25.1	2,653 (29.4%)
Subungual hyperkeratosis	816	14.7	316	9.1	1,132 (12.6%)
Total nail dystrophy	333	6.0	102	2.9	435 (4.8%)
No	3,091	34.5	3,135	45.8	6,226 (39.4%)
Joint involvement					
Yes	1,053	11.8	1,115	16.3	2,168 (13.7%)
Oligo/monoarthropathy	407	38.7	414	37.1	821 (37.9%)
Symmetrical polyarthropathy	286	27.2	378	33.9	664 (30.6%)
Distal hand joint arthropathy	301	28.6	340	30.5	641 (29.6%)
Spondylitis/sacroiliitis	89	8.5	71	6.4	160 (7.4%)
Arthritis mutilans	39	3.7	22	2.0	61 (2.8%)
No	7,573	84.6	5,503	80.4	13,076 (82.8%)
Comorbidities					
Obese (BMI > 30)	1,642	20.8	1,735	28.9	3,377 (24.3%)
Hypertension	2,535	28.3	1,750	25.6	4,285 (25.6%)
Hyperlipidemia	1,817	20.3	1,195	17.5	3,012 (18.0%)
Diabetes mellitus	1,713	19.1	1,179	17.2	2,892 (17.2%)
Ischaemic heart disease	698	7.8	203	3.0	901 (5.4%)
Cerebrovascular disease	192	2.1	78	1.1	270 (1.6%)
Mean DLQI	8.8 ± 6.6		8.2 ± 6.6		8.5 ± 6.6

A total of 449 (2.9%) patients received phototherapy at baseline and the number reduced to 1.2% at last follow-up. Since phototherapy was given for 3-4 months only, this could be an explanation as to why the number of patients receiving phototherapy during last visit was less, since notification to the registry was made at 6 months and above. Most of the patients received Narrow Band UVB (NBUVB). Not many patients had oral/topical/bath PUVA (Table 2).

Systemic therapy was required in 2,910 (18.5%) patients at baseline. During last follow-up (6 months and above),

TABLE 2: Types of treatment and outcome.

Type of therapy	Baseline/first visit (n = 15,635)		Last follow-up (6 months and above) (n = 5,701)	
	n	%	n	%
Topical	14,741	93.6	5,441	95.4
Topical steroids	13,079	89.4	5,022	92.3
Emollient	11,526	78.8	4,360	80.1
Tar preparation	10,546	72.1	3,789	69.6
Keratolytics	8,089	55.3	3,069	56.4
Calcipotriol	2,410	16.5	968	17.8
Calcipotriol with betamethasone dipropionate	2,202	15.1	818	15.0
Dithranol	242	1.7	100	1.8
Others	208	1.4	60	1.1
Phototherapy	449	2.9	184	1.2
NB-UVB	391	87.1	169	91.8
BB-UVB	28	6.2	7	3.8
Oral PUVA	12	2.7	4	2.2
Topical PUVA	7	1.6	2	1.1
Bath PUVA	4	0.9	3	1.6
Excimer laser	1	0.2	0	0.0
Others	14	3.1	5	2.7
Systemic therapy	2,910	18.5	1,405	8.9
Methotrexate	2,154	78.0	1,012	72.0
Acitretin	515	18.7	276	19.6
Sulphasalazine	176	6.4	67	4.8
Cyclosporin	120	4.3	56	4.0
Systemic corticosteroids	108	3.9	24	1.7
Hydroxyurea	18	0.7	3	0.2
Biologics	90	3.3	34	2.4
Ustekinumab	31	36.5	11	32.4
Adalimumab	25	29.4	8	23.5
Etanercept	14	16.5	7	20.6
Infliximab	3	3.5	2	5.9
Golimumab	4	4.7	1	2.9
Efalizumab	1	1.2	0	0.0
Secukinumab	2	2.4	0	0.0
Severity of psoriasis				
BSA < 5%	1,826	25.2	666	25.7
BSA 5–10%	3,725	51.4	1,284	49.6
BSA > 10–90%	1,572	21.7	598	23.1
BSA > 90%	131	1.8	43	1.7
Mean DLQI	8.51 ± 6.58		8.29 ± 6.56	

the percentage of patients on systemic therapy reduced to 8.9% only. This might be explained by missing data, as data for follow-up was only available for 5,701 patients. The most common systemic agents given were methotrexate, followed by acitretin, sulphasalazine, and cyclosporine. Biologics therapy was given in 3.3% of patients at baseline and 2.4% of patients continued the treatment at last follow-up (6 months and above). The three most common biologics given were ustekinumab, adalimumab, and etanercept (Table 2).

Despite the treatments instituted, there was not much difference in the outcomes of the patients as measured by BSA affected during follow-up (6 months and above). However, the amount of data available during follow-up was a lot less than baseline (15,635 patients at baseline and 5,701 patients during last follow-up). Even though there was not much difference in terms of BSA affected, there was a reduction in mean DLQI at baseline and follow-up (8.51 ± 6.58 and 8.29 ± 6.56, resp.) (Table 2).

5. Quality of Life

Psoriasis can impose major psychological impact on patients and affect their quality of life. The mean DLQI for our patients was 8.5 ± 6.6. There was not much difference in mean DLQI between males and females (Table 1). One-third (33.1%) of patients scored more than 10, which indicates severe impairment of quality of life, while 14.2% of patients reported no effect at all. Patients who reported small effect and moderate effect were 25.2% and 27.2%, respectively (Figure 2).

6. Discussion

6.1. Demography. Psoriasis occurs worldwide, affecting men and women of all ages and ethnic origins. It can present at any age and usually persists for life. Several large studies have found that the age of onset for psoriasis has a bimodal distribution (early and late onset) [16–18]. It is suggested that the bimodal distribution of psoriasis incidence represents two clinical presentations of the disease, type I (early onset) presenting at <40 years of age and type II (late onset) at >40 years of age [16]. This bimodality, however, was not observed in our study. The mean age of onset of psoriasis in our population was 35.14 ± 16.16, which is consistent with other studies that reported that psoriasis generally appears in the third decade [19, 20]. The male to female ratio in our study revealed a slightly higher incidence in men than in women at 1.3 : 1, which was similar to a study by Ejaz et al. [19] who reported a male to female ratio of 1.2 : 1. Although most studies that reported prevalence by sex showed no significant difference in the frequency of psoriasis between genders [9, 11, 12, 21, 22], there are some studies that showed a higher incidence in women than in men [9].

6.2. Clinical Features. Plaque psoriasis was the most common type of psoriasis, accounting for 85.1% of patients, followed by guttate psoriasis (2.9%), erythrodermic psoriasis (1.7%), and pustular psoriasis (1.0%).

Nail involvement is common in patients with psoriasis. The prevalence of psoriasis-related nail disease was observed in 57.1% of our patients. The most common nail changes seen were pitting, seen in 72.3% of our patients, followed by onycholysis (48.3%), nail discolouration (29.4%), subungual hyperkeratosis (12.6%), and total nail dystrophy (4.8%). In contrast, a cross-sectional study by Brazzelli et al. [23] in Italy reported onycholysis as the most common nail change. However, the exact prevalence of specific nail patterns in psoriatic patients is still relatively underreported.

6.3. Obesity and Psoriasis. In the present study, we found 24.3% of psoriasis patients with obesity. Numerous studies have implicated a close association between obesity and psoriasis. In a systematic review and meta-analysis by Armstrong et al. [24], it was reported that psoriasis patients have >50%

likelihood for obesity compared to those without psoriasis. Similarly, in a recent study, Helmick et al. [25] found that the prevalence of obesity in patients with psoriasis was also reported to be higher than the general population.

So far, the role of weight loss as treatment for psoriasis in obese patients is unclear; however, it is reasonable to assume that weight loss in such patients may reduce the obesity-induced inflammation, which may in turn improve the skin disease [26].

6.4. Comorbidities. Epidemiological studies revealed that patients with psoriasis have an increased risk of developing comorbidities related to the metabolic syndrome which include arterial hypertension and abnormalities in lipid and glucose metabolism [27].

In this study, our patients were shown to have hypertension (25.6%), hyperlipidemia (18%), diabetes mellitus (17.2%), ischaemic heart disease (5.4%), and cerebrovascular disease (1.6%). Similar findings were also reported in a study by Cohen et al. [27], which involved 16,851 patients with psoriasis and 48,681 controls. The study reported hypertension in 27.5% of the patients with psoriasis and 14.4% of the controls ($p < 0.001$), while diabetes mellitus occurred in 13.8% of psoriasis patients as compared to 7.3% of the controls ($p < 0.001$). In a cross-sectional study by Shapiro et al. [28] on 46,095 patients with psoriasis (case patients) and 1,579,037 subjects without psoriasis (control patients), it was revealed that diabetes was significantly higher in psoriasis patients as compared with the control group (odds ratio [OR]: 1.27, 95% confidence interval [CI]: 1.1–1.48). Atherosclerosis was also found to be significantly higher in psoriasis patients as compared to the control group (OR: 1.28, 95% CI: 1.04–1.59).

Numerous studies have shown a great correlation between the prevalence of metabolic syndrome and individuals with psoriasis. Given the serious complications, screening for metabolic syndrome should be included in the long-term management of individuals with psoriasis.

6.5. Stress and Psoriasis. Up to 48.3% patients in our study described stress as the main triggering factor for their disease. Psoriasis exacerbations have been frequently related to acute stressful events. The normal physiological response to stress involves activation of the hypothalamus-pituitary-adrenal (HPA) axis and sympathetic adrenomedullary (SAM) axis, both of which interact with immune functions [29]. In normal individuals, stress usually elevates stress hormones (i.e., raised cortisol levels). However, there are available studies to suggest that HPA responses are reduced, while SAM responses are upregulated in psoriasis patients exposed to stress [29–31]. A study by Evers et al. [32] found that psoriasis patients had significantly lower cortisol levels at moments when daily stressors are at peak levels. The study also reported that psoriasis patients with high levels of daily stressors exhibited lower mean cortisol levels, as compared to psoriasis patients with low levels of daily stressors [32].

Other exacerbating factors include sunlight (24.9%) and infection (9.1%). Smoking, trauma, drugs, alcohol, and pregnancy were reportedly less common. Although our study did

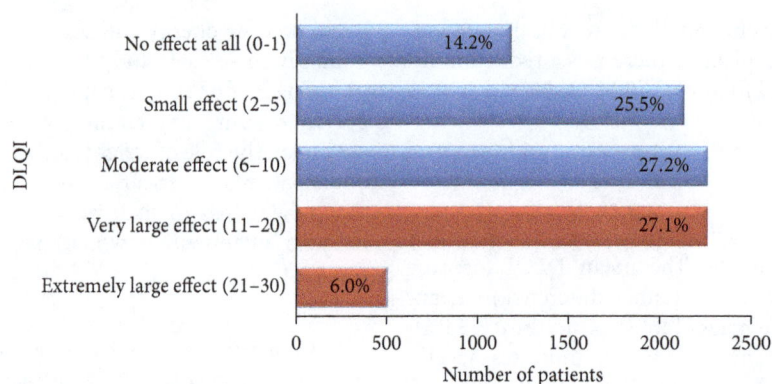

FIGURE 2: Quality of life in adult patients with psoriasis.

not show any strong relationship of smoking with psoriasis, there are several studies that have shown a significant association of smoking being a predisposing environmental factor for the development of psoriasis [3]. The severity of psoriasis seems to be correlated with the intensity of smoking [12].

6.6. DLQI and Psoriasis. The Dermatology Life Quality Index (DLQI), despite methodological limitations, is currently the most commonly used method for evaluating quality of life for patients with skin conditions. The term quality of life, or health-related quality of life (HRQoL), refers to a quantitative estimation of the global impact of a disease on physical, social, and psychological well-being of a patient [3]. Factors such as disease severity, gender, age, anatomical sites of lesion, presence of comorbidities, and psychological distress can all be associated with reduced HRQoL in people with psoriasis [33].

Patients in our study had a mean DLQI score of 8.5 ± 6.6. One-third (33.1%) of our patients had a DLQI score of more than 10, which indicates severe impairment. This was similar to a local study on 223 patients, evaluating the HRQoL using DLQI [34]. The study reported 67 patients (30%) with severe impairment (DLQI score = 11–30) and a median DLQI score of 7. A study conducted in Germany reported marked impairment of health-related life quality, with a mean DLQI of 8.6. The study also reported 32% patients with QoL score of more than 10, while 15.2% had no effect on their QoL [35].

6.7. Psoriatic Arthropathy. Psoriatic arthritis (PsA) is a seronegative arthritis that is associated with psoriasis. PsA affects the quality of life of patients and has a considerable impact on annual healthcare expenditure and results in increased risk of mortality. Several researches have reported the prevalence of psoriatic arthropathy (PsA) in psoriasis patients, varying from 6.25% to 48% in western countries and from 1% to 9% in Asian countries [36, 37]. The differences in the prevalence can possibly be explained by geographical and ethnic differences and the differences in the applied diagnostic criteria of PsA [38]. Joint involvement was reported in 13.7% of our patients. Our prevalence was higher than that in reported studies from other Asian countries. However, our data was mainly based on history and clinical examination. The other studies

focused more on psoriatic arthropathy and more stringent inclusion criteria were employed.

Moll and Wright first described five clinical patterns among patients with PsA: distal hand joint arthropathy, asymmetrical oligo/monoarthritis, symmetrical polyarthritis, spondylitis/sacroiliitis, and arthritis mutilans [39]. The exact frequency of the patterns is variable but oligoarthritis was the most commonly reported pattern [39]. Comparably, in our study, oligo/monoarthritis (37.3%) was the most common pattern, followed by symmetrical polyarthritis (30.6%), distal hand joint arthropathy (29.6%), spondylitis/sacroiliitis (7.4%), and arthritis mutilans (2.8%).

A very recent study by Mishra et al. [38] used four different types of screening tools to diagnose PsA and found that the most common pattern of PsA was symmetrical polyarthritis (46%) followed by oligoarthritis (44%). Regardless of the differences in prevalence of PsA, early screening for PsA is necessary for prevention of joint damage. In patients who were diagnosed with PsA early in arthritis clinics, up to 47% have been shown to develop erosions within the first 2 years [40]. However, patients treated within 2 years of diagnosis have less progression of joint damage than those treated 2 years after diagnosis [41]. Thus, early diagnosis has the potential to prevent joint damage and improve patient outcomes.

6.8. Treatment in Psoriasis. Treatment of psoriasis is based on controlling the symptoms. Topical therapies such as corticosteroids, vitamin D analogs, keratolytics, and tar preparation are useful for treating mild-to-moderate psoriasis. More severe psoriasis may be treated with phototherapy or may require systemic therapy.

A large majority of our patients were prescribed with topical treatments as first-line therapy, the most common being topical corticosteroid (75.3%). 2.8% of patients received phototherapy, while 18.4% of patients received systemic therapy. Our data was closely similar to other published studies. A retrospective study by Gillard and Finlay, based on data from a primary-care medical record database of psoriasis patients from 2002 to 2003 in the UK, demonstrated that only 4% of 6120 patients with psoriasis received either phototherapy or systemic therapy [42]. Majority of their patients (93.6%) received topical treatment only.

7. Conclusion

This study describes the sociodemographic characteristics, clinical features, and the impact of disease in patients with psoriasis in Malaysia. Our findings are similar to other published epidemiological studies on psoriasis. In the future, there is a need for more epidemiological studies, as they are an important contributor to a better understanding of the disease burden, updating population research, and advancement of health policies.

Acknowledgments

The authors would like to thank all doctors and allied health personnel from the participating centres of the Malaysian Psoriasis Registry. The authors would also like to thank Nurakmal Baharum from Clinical Research Malaysia for statistical support. They acknowledge the support of Ministry of Health, Malaysia, and the Dermatological Society of Malaysia.

References

[1] R. G. B. Langley, G. G. Krueger, and C. E. M. Griffiths, "Psoriasis: epidemiology, clinical features, and quality of life," *Annals of the Rheumatic Diseases*, vol. 64, Suppl 2, no. 2, pp. ii18–ii23, 2005.

[2] A. S. Lønnberg, L. Skov, A. Skytthe, K. O. Kyvik, O. B. Pedersen, and S. F. Thomsen, "Smoking and risk for psoriasis: A population-based twin study," *International Journal of Dermatology*, vol. 55, no. 2, pp. 72–78, 2016.

[3] J. Hayes and J. Koo, "Psoriasis: Depression, anxiety, smoking, and drinking habits," *Dermatologic Therapy*, vol. 23, no. 2, pp. 174–180, 2010.

[4] G. K. Perera, P. Di Meglio, and F. O. Nestle, "Psoriasis," *Annual Review of Pathology: Mechanisms of Disease*, vol. 7, pp. 385–422, 2012.

[5] D. A. Springate, R. Parisi, E. Kontopantelis, D. Reeves, C. E. M. Griffiths, and D. M. Ashcroft, "Incidence, prevalence and mortality of patients with psoriasis: a U.K. population-based cohort study," *British Journal of Dermatology*, vol. 176, no. 3, pp. 650–658, 2017.

[6] N. M. Seminara, K. Abuabara, D. B. Shin et al., "Validity of the Health Improvement Network (THIN) for the study of psoriasis," *British Journal of Dermatology*, vol. 164, no. 3, pp. 602–609, 2011.

[7] A. O. Olsen, A. Grjibovski, P. Magnus, K. Tambs, and J. R. Harris, "Psoriasis in Norway as observed in a population-based Norwegian twin panel," *British Journal of Dermatology*, vol. 153, no. 2, pp. 346–351, 2005.

[8] S. K. Kurd and J. M. Gelfand, "The prevalence of previously diagnosed and undiagnosed psoriasis in US adults: results from NHANES 2003-2004," *Journal of the American Academy of Dermatology*, vol. 60, no. 2, pp. 218–224, 2009.

[9] R. Parisi, D. P. M. Symmons, C. E. M. Griffiths, and D. M. Ashcroft, "Global epidemiology of psoriasis: a systematic review of incidence and prevalence," *Journal of Investigative Dermatology*, vol. 133, no. 2, pp. 377–385, 2013.

[10] T. D. Rachakonda, C. W. Schupp, and A. W. Armstrong, "Psoriasis prevalence among adults in the United States," *Journal of the American Academy of Dermatology*, vol. 70, no. 3, pp. 512–516, 2014.

[11] X. Ding, T. Wang, Y. Shen, X. Wang, C. Zhou, and S. Tian, "Prevalence of psoriasis in China: a population-based study in six cities," *European Journal of Dermatology*, vol. 22, no. 5, pp. 663–667, 2012.

[12] K. Bo, M. Thoresen, and F. Dalgard, "Smokers report more psoriasis, but not atopic dermatitis or hand eczema: Results from a Norwegian population survey among adults," *Dermatology*, vol. 216, pp. 40–45, 2008.

[13] C. E. Griffiths and J. N. Barker, "Pathogenesis and clinical features of psoriasis," *The Lancet*, vol. 370, no. 9583, pp. 263–271, 2007.

[14] A. F. Alexis and P. Blackcloud, "Psoriasis in Skin of Color: Epidemiology, Genetics, Clinical Presentation, and Treatment Nuances. Desai SR, Alexis A," *Journal of Clinical and Aesthetic Dermatology*, vol. 7, no. 11, pp. 16–24, 2014.

[15] A. Y. Finlay and G. K. Khan, "Dermatology Life Quality Index (DLQI)—a simple practical measure for routine clinical use," *Clinical and Experimental Dermatology*, vol. 19, no. 3, pp. 210–216, 1994.

[16] T. Henseler and E. Christophers, "Psoriasis of early and late onset: characterization of two types of psoriasis vulgaris," *Journal of the American Academy of Dermatology*, vol. 13, no. 3, pp. 450–456, 1985.

[17] C. Huerta, E. Rivero, and L. A. García Rodríguez, "Incidence and risk factors for psoriasis in the general population," *Archives of Dermatology*, vol. 143, no. 12, pp. 1559–1565, 2007.

[18] M. Icen, C. S. Crowson, M. T. McEvoy, F. J. Dann, S. E. Gabriel, and H. Maradit Kremers, "Trends in incidence of adult-onset psoriasis over three decades: a population-based study," *Journal of the American Academy of Dermatology*, vol. 60, no. 3, pp. 394–401, 2009.

[19] A. Ejaz, N. Raza, N. Iftikhar, A. Iftikhar, and M. Farooq, "Presentation of early onset psoriasis in comparison with late onset psoriasis: A clinical study from Pakistan," *Indian Journal of Dermatology, Venereology and Leprology*, vol. 75, no. 1, pp. 36–40, 2009.

[20] Y. T. Chang, T. J. Chen, P. C. Liu et al., "Epidemiological study of psoriasis in the national health insurance database in Taiwan," *Acta Dermato-Venereologica*, vol. 89, no. 3, pp. 262–266, 2009.

[21] J. M. Gelfand, D. D. Gladman, P. J. Mease et al., "Epidemiology of psoriatic arthritis in the population of the United States," *Journal of the American Academy of Dermatology*, vol. 53, no. 4, pp. 573–577, 2005.

[22] B. Sinniah, P. S. Saraswathy Devi, and B. S. Prasant, "Epidemiology of psoriasis in Malaysia: A hospital based study," *Medical Journal of Malaysia*, vol. 65, no. 2, pp. 112–114, 2010.

[23] V. Brazzelli, A. Carugno, A. Alborghetti et al., "Prevalence, severity and clinical features of psoriasis in fingernails and toenails in adult patients: Italian experience," *Journal of the*

European Academy of Dermatology and Venereology, vol. 26, no. 11, pp. 1354–1359, 2012.

[24] A. W. Armstrong, C. T. Harskamp, and E. J. Armstrong, "The association between psoriasis and obesity: a systematic review and meta-analysis of observational studies," *Nutrition & Diabetes*, vol. 2, no. 12, p. e54, 2012.

[25] C. G. Helmick, H. Lee-Han, S. C. Hirsch, T. L. Baird, and C. L. Bartlett, "Prevalence of psoriasis among adults in the U.S.: 2003-2006 and 2009-2010 National Health and Nutrition Examination Surveys," *American Journal of Preventive Medicine*, vol. 47, no. 1, pp. 37–45, 2014.

[26] F. O. Nestle, P. Di Meglio, J.-Z. Qin, and B. J. Nickoloff, "Skin immune sentinels in health and disease," *Nature Reviews Immunology*, vol. 9, no. 10, pp. 679–691, 2009.

[27] A. D. Cohen, M. Sherf, L. Vidavsky, D. A. Vardy, J. Shapiro, and J. Meyerovitch, "Association between psoriasis and the metabolic syndrome: A cross-sectional study," *Dermatology*, vol. 216, no. 2, pp. 152–155, 2008.

[28] J. Shapiro, A. D. Cohen, M. David et al., "The association between psoriasis, diabetes mellitus, and atherosclerosis in Israel: A case-control study," *Journal of the American Academy of Dermatology*, vol. 56, no. 4, pp. 629–634, 2007.

[29] A. Buske-Kirschbaum, M. Ebrecht, S. Kern, and D. H. Hellhammer, "Endocrine stress responses in TH1-mediated chronic inflammatory skin disease (psoriasis vulgaris)—do they parallel stress-induced endocrine changes in TH2-mediated inflammatory dermatoses (atopic dermatitis)?" *Psychoneuroendocrinology*, vol. 31, no. 4, pp. 439–446, 2006.

[30] A. W. M. Evers, Y. Lu, P. Duller, P. G. M. Van Der Valk, F. W. Kraaimaat, and P. C. M. Van De Kerkhoft, "Common burden of chronic skin diseases? Contributors to psychological distress in adults with psoriasis and atopic dermatitis," *British Journal of Dermatology*, vol. 152, no. 6, pp. 1275–1281, 2005.

[31] H. L. Richards, D. G. Fortune, T. M. O'Sullivan, C. J. Main, and C. E. M. Griffiths, "Patients with psoriasis and their compliance with medication," *Journal of the American Academy of Dermatology*, vol. 41, no. 4, pp. 581–583, 1999.

[32] A. W. M. Evers, E. W. M. Verhoeven, F. W. Kraaimaat et al., "How stress gets under the skin: Cortisol and stress reactivity in psoriasis," *British Journal of Dermatology*, vol. 163, no. 5, pp. 986–991, 2010.

[33] World Health Organization, *Global Report on Psoriasis*, World Health Organization, 2016.

[34] W. W. T. Nyunt, W. Y. Low, R. Ismail, S. Sockalingam, and A. K. K. Min, "Determinants of health-related quality of life in psoriasis patients in Malaysia," *Asia-Pacific Journal of Public Health*, vol. 27, no. 2, pp. NP662–NP673, 2015.

[35] M. Augustin, K. Reich, G. Glaeske, I. Schaefer, and M. Radtke, "Co-morbidity and age-related prevalence of psoriasis: Analysis of health insurance data in Germany," *Acta Dermato-Venereologica*, vol. 90, no. 2, pp. 147–151, 2010.

[36] F. C. Wilson, M. Icen, C. S. Crowson, M. T. McEvoy, S. E. Gabriel, and H. M. Kremers, "Incidence and clinical predictors of psoriatic arthritis in patients with psoriasis: A population-based study," *Arthritis Care & Research*, vol. 61, no. 2, pp. 233–239, 2009.

[37] L. S. Tam, Y. Y. Leung, and E. K. Li, "Psoriatic arthritis in Asia," *Rheumatology*, vol. 48, no. 12, pp. 1473–1477, 2009.

[38] S. Mishra, H. Kancharla, S. Dogra, and A. Sharma, "Comparison of four validated psoriatic arthritis screening tools in diagnosing psoriatic arthritis in patients with psoriasis (COMPAQ

Study)," *British Journal of Dermatology*, vol. 176, no. 3, pp. 765–770, 2017.

[39] J. M. Moll and V. Wright, "Psoriatic arthritis," in *Seminars in Arthritis and Rheumatism*, vol. 3, pp. 55–78, WB Saunders, 1973.

[40] D. Kane, L. Stafford, B. Bresniham, and O. FitzGerald, "A prospective, clinical and radiological study of early psoriatic arthritis: An early synovitis clinic experience," *Rheumatology*, vol. 42, no. 12, pp. 1460–1468, 2003.

[41] D. D. Gladman, P. J. Mease, V. Strand et al., "Consensus on a core set of domains for psoriatic arthritis," *The Journal of Rheumatology*, vol. 34, no. 5, pp. 1167–1170, 2007.

[42] S. E. Gillard and A. Y. Finlay, "Current management of psoriasis in the United Kingdom: Patterns of prescribing and resource use in primary care," *International Journal of Clinical Practice*, vol. 59, no. 11, pp. 1260–1267, 2005.

16

Career Choices and Career Progression of Junior Doctors in Dermatology: Surveys of UK Medical Graduates

Atena Barat, Michael J. Goldacre, and Trevor W. Lambert ⓘ

UK Medical Careers Research Group, Unit of Health-Care Epidemiology, Nuffield Department of Population Health, University of Oxford, Old Road Campus, Oxford OX3 7LF, UK

Correspondence should be addressed to Trevor W. Lambert; trevor.lambert@dph.ox.ac.uk

Academic Editor: Craig G. Burkhart

Objective. To report UK-trained doctors' career choices for dermatology, career destinations, and factors influencing career pathways. *Methods.* Multicohort multipurpose longitudinal surveys of UK-trained doctors who graduated between 1974 and 2015. *Results.* In all, 40,412 doctors (58% of graduates) responded in year 1, 31,466 (64%) in year 3, and 24,970 (67%) in year 5. One year after graduation, 1.7% of women and 0.6% of men made dermatology their first choice but by five years after graduation the respective figures were 1.0% and 0.7%. Compared to their predecessors, its popularity fell more substantially from years 1 to 5 among recent graduates (2005–15), particularly for women (from 2.1% in year 1 to 0.8% in year 5) compared with a fall from 0.8% to 0.5% among men. The most important factor influencing dermatology choice was "hours/working conditions": in year one, 69% regarded this as important compared with 31% of those choosing other hospital physician specialties. Only 18% of respondents who chose dermatology at year 1 eventually worked in it; however, almost all practising dermatologists (94%), 10 years after qualifying, had made their future career decision by year 5. *Conclusion.* Dermatology is popular among female UK graduates. Most dermatologists made their career decision late but decisively.

1. Introduction

Dermatology is a highly competitive specialty to enter both globally and within the UK [1–3]. In the UK, all aspiring dermatologists begin their training by becoming fully registered with the General Medical Council (GMC). This is achieved by completing a two-year Foundation Programme which follows their medical degree and is common to all specialties. Trainees then spend two to three years in one of three core training programmes: Core Medical Training (CMT), which is the first stage of postgraduate training for many physician specialties; Acute Care Common Stem (ACCS) training, which is a training pathway parallel to CMT for those particularly interested in acute specialties; or Paediatrics. All intending dermatologists must attain, at the end of that period of training, membership of the Royal College of Physicians (MRCP) or membership of the Royal College of Paediatrics and Child Health (MRCPCH) before commencing specialty training in dermatology which takes at least four years. Finally, successful trainees are awarded

their certificate of completion of training (CCT) and can apply for consultant dermatologist positions [4, 5]. In 2017, dermatology recorded the highest level of competition for training posts among all specialties in the UK, with 5.58 applicants for each available post [3].

Dermatology has some characteristics that make it appealing for medical graduates. It is considered a rewarding specialty due to recent advances in medicine which have rendered chronic diseases curable or controllable [5, 6]. Dermatologists interact with a variety of patients from all ages but they are rarely life threateningly unwell [5]. Since dermatology is mainly an outpatient-based specialty with a relatively low on-call commitment, flexible training is available and many of its consultants work less than full time [7, 8]. The controllable lifestyle features, including control of working hours, of dermatology make it popular among female doctors [2, 9, 10]: in the UK in 2016, 57% of consultants and 75% of higher specialty trainees in dermatology were women [11].

Dermatological conditions are extremely prevalent, accounting for around 13 million patients annually presenting to GPs in England and Wales; and nearly 6.1% (0.8 m) are referred for specialist consultation. In 2005, approximately 4000 deaths in the UK were ascribed to skin disease [12]. In the UK, multidisciplinary teams led by consultants provide specialist care services. The team may include specialist registrars (StR) in Dermatology, Staff and Associate Specialist (SAS) doctors, specialist dermatology nurses, general practitioners with a special interest (GPwSI) in dermatology, and specialist trainees [4, 12]. In 2016, 538 consultant and 259 medical registrars, in terms of full-time equivalents, were working in dermatology in England [13]. Ideally, 1.6 consultants per 100,000 population are recommended by the Royal College of Physicians [14], indicating a shortage of approximately 100 dermatology consultant posts [15], with particular shortages in rural or remote areas [16]; however, no region in the UK has sufficient dermatology consultants [14]. The reported shortfall and uneven distribution of dermatology professionals has resulted in unmet patient needs [16].

The distribution of physicians in different specialties across a country is affected by the career choices of medical graduates [2]. Thus, understanding their preferences for a career specialty can help to improve the educational programmes, plan for a balanced distribution of workforce, and evolve the health system to better suit the needs of specialties and the choices of doctors [17]. The goal of this paper is to report trends in choosing dermatology as a career over various cohorts, to identify factors which principally motivate medical graduates choosing dermatology, and to compare their early career intention with their eventual destination. The information should be helpful to workforce planners, providers of care, and educational commissioners in supporting the provision of an effective and sustainable health system. It should also help medical graduates to understand important issues related to dermatology careers.

2. Methods

2.1. Data Collection. We analysed a large national database generated during the multicohort surveys conducted by the UK Medical Careers Research Group. Detailed information about study design, methods, and participants has been reported previously [18]. Briefly, the target population was all UK-trained doctors, registered by the General Medical Council (GMC), since 1974, in particular years of graduation. Participants have been followed up with questionnaire surveys at the first, third, and fifth years after graduation and longer intervals thereafter. To enhance the reliability of the study and increase the response rate [19], up to four follow-up reminders were sent to those who were initially nonrespondents.

Our data related to 15 cohorts: the UK medical graduates of 1974, 1977, 1980, 1983, 1993, 1996, 1999, 2000, 2002, 2005, 2008, 2009, 2011, 2012, and 2015. The analysis focused on three main concepts: early career preferences, influencing factors on career choices, and eventual career destinations.

Information on the first two measures was obtained from 15 cohorts (1974–2015), 12 cohorts (1974–2008 and 2012), and 10 cohorts (1974–1980 and 1993–2008) at the first, third, and fifth year after qualification, respectively. Information on the last measure, career destination, was obtained from 5 cohorts (1993–2002) at 10 years after graduation.

2.2. Research Instrument. A self-administered, postal or electronic, questionnaire containing sections on demographic information, career choices and plans, and employment history was completed by each respondent. The content and construct of the questionnaire were checked and revised over many years [20].

The questionnaire asked participants about their specialty preferences using the question "What is your choice of long-term career specialty?," enabling up to three specialty choices to be specified in order of preference. The questionnaire also asked about certainty of choices. Participants could rate their level of certainty about their career choice as "definite," "probable," or "uncertain." A three-point scale covering "not at all," "a little," and "a great deal" was used to explore participants' views regarding each of 13 influencing factors on career choices.

2.3. Data Analysis. To increase statistical power, we combined the individual cohort data into three groups: graduates of 1974–1983, 1993–2002, and 2005–2015. This classification corresponds to pivotal periods when changes happened in medical education in the UK.

In analysing specialty choices, we used the term "tied choices" to refer to choices of equal priority for a respondent. Similarly, "untied choices" refers to a solo choice that a participant explicitly named it as his/her preferred specialty. Moreover, hospital medical specialties other than dermatology, whose training is managed by the Joint Royal Colleges of Physicians Training Board (JRCPTB), were grouped together and named in this paper as "other hospital physician specialties" as a comparative group to compare with dermatologists. This group included the following: general medicine, cardiology, endocrinology, geriatrics, nephrology, neurology, chest medicine, rheumatology/rehabilitation, genitourinary medicine, gastroenterology, vascular medicine, tropical medicine, clinical pharmacology, infectious diseases, and occupational medicine. These trainees complete a similar core medical training (CMT) stage prior to their specialty training programme as dermatologists, and like dermatologists their working environment is mainly in hospital rather than in the community [21].

The statistical analyses were carried out with IBM SPSS Statistics for Windows, V22 [22], and Microsoft Excel (2010). Heterogeneity of cohort group was examined through the χ^2 statistic test. Bivariate cross-tabulation and Chi-square test with the appropriate number of degrees of freedom were applied for comparison of proportions and the Mantel–Haenszel linear-by-linear χ^2 test was performed to identify linear trends over cohorts. The corresponding 95% confidence interval was calculated and statistical significance inferred at a 2-tailed probability value < 0.05. All analysis was

TABLE 1: Trends in early first choices for eventual career in dermatology: percentages of doctors who specified dermatology at years 1, 3, and 5 after graduation.

Year after graduation	Cohorts (years of graduation)				Statistical tests	
	1974–83 N (%)	1993–2002 N (%)	2005–15 N (%)	All cohorts N (%)	Linear trend $(\chi^2 1, p)$	Heterogeneity $(\chi^2 2, p)$
Men and women						
Year 1	88 (0.8)	133 (0.9)	263 (1.7)	484 (1.2)	41.8, <0.001	48.7, <0.001
Year 3	98 (1.0)	169 (1.2)	90 (1.1)	357 (1.1)	0.64, 0.42	2.41, 0.29
Year 5	65 (0.9)	121 (0.9)	34 (0.7)	220 (0.9)	1.06, 0.3	1.76, 0.41
Men						
Year 1	32 (0.5)	35 (0.6)	49 (0.8)	116 (0.6)	7.4, 0.006	8.07, 0.018
Year 3	47 (0.8)	54 (0.9)	18 (0.6)	119 (0.8)	0.23, 0.62	2.11, 0.34
Year 5	33 (0.7)	44 (0.8)	10 (0.6)	87 (0.7)	0.09, 0.75	0.61, 0.73
Women						
Year 1	56 (1.5)	98 (1.3)	214 (2.1)	368 (1.7)	12.3, <0.001	21.06, <0.001
Year 3	51 (1.5)	115 (1.5)	72 (1.4)	238 (1.5)	0.03, 0.85	0.09, 0.95
Year 5	32 (1.4)	77 (1.1)	24 (0.8)	133 (1.0)	3.85, 0.05	3.87, 0.14

reported stratified by sex and cohort group and all results are also presented as sex-combined.

3. Results

3.1. Response Rate. In the first year after graduation, we contacted 69,670 registered doctors covering all 15 cohorts: 40,412 (58.0%) replied. The questionnaire was sent to 48,899 subjects in year 3 covering all 12 cohorts and 31,466 (64.3%) responded. For five years after qualification, covering 10 cohorts, 24,970 from a possible 37,424 doctors (66.7%) replied.

3.2. Early Career Choices for Dermatology: One, Three, and Five Years after Graduation. In total, the percentage of doctors who specified dermatology as their first choice showed a gradual fall from 1.2% in year 1 to 0.9% in year 5 (Table 1). Testing for trend across the three cohort groups defined by the graduates of 1974–1983, 1993–2002, and 2005–2015, in each row of Table 1, no trend was found for years 3 and 5, but a linear upward trend was found for year 1 ($\chi^2 = 41.8$, df = 1).

Examination of individual groups of cohorts (Table 1) showed no evident trend in the popularity of dermatology as a first choice of long-term career, moving from year 1 to year 5, for the two earlier groups (1974–83 and 1993–2002), but a downward trend for the recent group (2005–15), with only 0.7% of the cohorts of 2005 and 2008 choosing dermatology in year 5 compared to 1.4% (92/6430 from Table 2) of those cohorts in year 1.

Results for individual cohorts are shown in Table 2.

3.3. Certainty of Career Choice. Doctors who chose dermatology were surer of their choice than doctors who chose other hospital specialties (Table 3). Their level of certainty rose from 18% in year 1 to 72.6% in year 5. Similar increases in certainty applied to both genders. Male doctors regardless of their chosen specialty were more certain of their choice than female doctors.

3.4. Choices by Gender. Over all cohort groups and all years of graduation, higher percentages of women than men chose dermatology as their first choice of future career (Table 1, Figure 1). Nevertheless, its popularity for both genders varied across cohorts and survey years. Comparing year 1 with year 5 across all cohorts, choices for dermatology for men remained roughly constant at 0.6% and 0.7%, respectively, while for women choices fell from 1.7% to 1.0%.

Comparing cohort groups in year 1, we identified an upward trend in choosing dermatology from 1974 to 2015 for both genders but the statistical evidence for the trend was weaker for men (men: $\chi^2 = 8.07$, $p = 0.018$; women: $\chi^2 = 21.06$, $p < 0.001$, any first choice). Gender differences continued in years 3 and 5 but showed a downward trend across cohorts in the percentages of both male and female doctors choosing dermatology as a first choice, with nonsignificant results. Generally, the difference between men and women who chose dermatology increased from 1974 to 2015 in years 1 and 3 but narrowed in year 5.

Gender variation was reduced at all three cohort groups, moving from years 1 to 5. The most recent cohort group (2005–15) showed the largest gender gap in year 1 (1.29%) and the smallest in year 5 (0.23%). Among women, choices for dermatology fell from 2.1% to 0.8%, while among men the fall was only from 0.8% to 0.5%, comparing year 1 with year 5.

The gender balance in choices for dermatology was similar whether for the specialty as first choice or as any choice (Figure 2).

3.5. Factors Influencing Choice for Dermatology. Table 4 shows the percentages of dermatologists and of those working in other hospital physician specialties who specified, for each factor, whether it influenced their career choice a great deal.

TABLE 2: Choices for dermatology in individual cohorts: percentages and numbers of respondents.

Graduation year	Year 1 % (N)	Year 3 % (N)	Year 5 % (N)	Year 1 % (N)	Year 3 % (N)	Year 5 % (N)
	Dermatology as any first choice			Dermatology as any choice		
1974	0.9 (18/1940)	1.2 (18/1486)	1.0 (18/1755)	2.1 (41/1940)	2.0 (29/1486)	1.4 (25/1755)
1977	0.8 (20/2637)	1.3 (31/2336)	1.2 (30/2602)	2.5 (66/2637)	2.5 (59/2336)	2.0 (52/2602)
1980	1.0 (29/2853)	1.0 (28/2843)	0.6 (17/2716)	2.9 (84/2853)	1.9 (54/2843)	1.0 (27/2716)
1983	0.7 (21/3166)	0.7 (21/3037)	0.0	1.8 (56/3166)	1.1 (33/3037)	0.0
1993	1.0 (26/2621)	1.0 (27/2777)	0.9 (24/2729)	1.9 (49/2621)	1.4 (39/2777)	1.1 (31/2729)
1996	0.7 (21/2926)	0.7 (20/2721)	0.7 (28/2521)	1.7 (51/2926)	1.4 (39/2721)	1.0 (24/2521)
1999	0.8 (21/2727)	1.5 (39/2549)	1.4 (38/2661)	1.7 (45/2727)	2.3 (59/2549)	1.8 (47/2661)
2000	1.2 (35/2978)	1.7 (51/2968)	1.0 (27/2703)	2.0 (59/2978)	2.7 (80/2968)	1.4 (38/2703)
2002	1.1 (30/2778)	1.2 (32/2748)	0.5 (14/2552)	2.8 (78/2778)	2.2 (60/2748)	0.6 (15/2552)
2005	1.2 (36/3128)	0.7 (20/2710)	0.6 (13/2362)	3.1 (96/3128)	1.3 (34/2710)	1.0 (24/2362)
2008	1.7 (56/3302)	1.2 (39/3228)	0.9 (21/2369)	3.8 (124/3302)	1.8 (58/3228)	1.4 (34/2369)
2009	1.7 (51/2917)	0.0	0.0	3.8 (110/2917)	0.0	0.0
2011	1.6 (16/1001)	0.0	0.0	3.1 (31/1001)	0.0	0.0
2012	1.9 (45/2398)	1.5 (31/2063)	0.0	3.6 (86/2398)	1.9 (39/2063)	0.0
2015	1.9 (59/3040)	0.0	0.0	3.2 (97/3040)	0.0	0.0

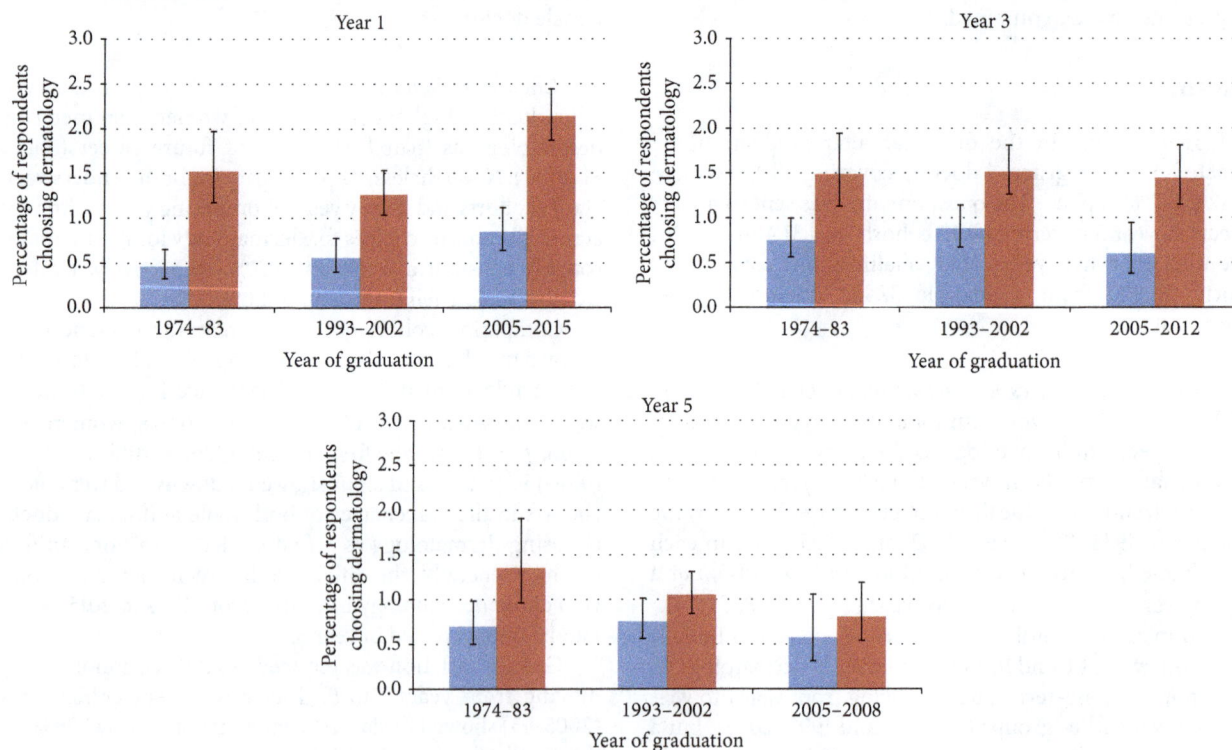

FIGURE 1: Percentages of men (blue) and women (red) doctors who chose dermatology as a first choice of eventual career one, three, and five years after graduation.

Hours and working conditions were the most important factor for doctors who chose dermatology, the importance increasing as time passed from qualification. The factor scoring the second highest percentage for aspiring dermatologists was enthusiasm and commitment. Other important factors for aspiring dermatologists were domestic circumstances, self-appraisal, and student experience of the subject. In contrast, financial circumstances while training, inclinations before medical school, and advice from others were unimportant.

Compared with doctors who chose other hospital physician specialties, dermatologists scored consistently higher on

TABLE 3: Comparison of the firmness of choice between doctors who expressed a first preference for each specialty group at 1, 3, and 5 years after graduation.

Gender	Level of certainty of career choice	Year 1		Year 3		Year 5	
		Dermatology N (%)	Other hospital physician specialties N (%)	Dermatology N (%)	Other hospital physician specialties N (%)	Dermatology N (%)	Other hospital physician specialties N (%)
Male	Definite	22 (19.6)	664 (15.0)	37 (31.1)	707 (28.1)	68 (79.1)	1101 (61.1)
	Probable	54 (48.2)	2356 (53.2)	62 (52.1)	1276 (50.7)	14 (16.3)	570 (31.6)
	Uncertain	36 (32.1)	1407 (31.8)	20 (16.8)	533 (21.2)	4 (4.7)	131 (7.3)
	Total	112 (100.0)	4427 (100.0)	119 (100.0)	2516 (100.0)	86 (100.0)	1802 (100.0)
Female	Definite	64 (17.5)	522 (10.7)	62 (26.4)	507 (22.7)	91 (68.4)	968 (59.6)
	Probable	195 (53.4)	2294 (47.2)	104 (44.3)	1054 (47.3)	34 (25.6)	515 (31.7)
	Uncertain	106 (29.0)	2043 (42.0)	69 (29.4)	668 (30.0)	8 (6.0)	140 (8.6)
	Total	365 (100.0)	4859 (100.0)	235 (100.0)	2229 (100.0)	133 (100.0)	1623 (100.0)
All (men & women)	Definite	86 (18.0)	1186 (12.8)	99 (28.0)	1214 (25.6)	159 (72.6)	2069 (60.4)
	Probable	249 (52.2)	4650 (50.1)	166 (46.9)	2330 (49.1)	48 (21.9)	1085 (31.7)
	Uncertain	142 (29.8)	3450 (37.2)	89 (25.1)	1201 (25.3)	12 (5.5)	271 (7.9)
	Total	477 (100.0)	9286 (100.0)	354 (100.0)	4745 (100.0)	219 (100.0)	3425 (100.0)

For details of specialties included as "other hospital physician" specialties, see Methods.

TABLE 4: Numbers and percentages of doctors who specified each factor affecting their career choice "a great deal."

Factor	Year 1		Year 3		Year 5	
	Dermatology % (N)	Other hospital physician specialty % (N)	Dermatology % (N)	Other hospital physician specialty % (N)	Dermatology % (N)	Other hospital physician specialty % (N)
Hours/working conditions	69% (211***)	31% (1793)	75% (105***)	35% (769)	82% (115***)	38% (981)
Domestic circumstances	54% (195***)	23% (1605)	45% (106***)	22% (731)	44% (90***)	27% (884)
Future financial prospects	25% (59***)	9% (410)	25% (34***)	7% (166)	17% (24***)	7% (193)
Career and promotion prospects	29% (80**)	22% (1250)	48% (96***)	27% (785)	36% (75***)	25% (834)
Experience of jobs so far	34% (79***)	54% (2792)	41% (97***)	59% (1989)	51% (106***)	66% (2197)
Self-appraisal	43% (120*)	49% (2939)	51% (122)	55% (1852)	54% (112)	57% (1894)
Student experience of subject	38% (131)	40% (2620)	33% (71*)	26% (814)	31% (59**)	23% (718)
A particular teacher/department	33% (89)	29% (1680)	30% (59*)	37% (987)	30% (49*)	39% (1045)
Inclinations before medical school	5% (14*)	9% (531)	6% (14)	8% (245)	7% (14)	7% (211)
Enthusiasm/commitment	54% (164)	60% (3492)	65% (90)	70% (1550)	80% (113)	80% (2094)
Advice from others	17% (48)	17% (974)	21% (42)	20% (571)	17% (36)	16% (548)
Other reasons	11% (11)	13% (260)	16% (17)	18% (260)	26% (19)	24% (273)
Financial circumstances while training	6% (3)	3% (31)	5% (6)	5% (82)	3% (3)	6% (71)

* indicates $p < 0.05$; ** indicates $p < 0.01$; *** indicates $p < 0.001$, comparing dermatology with other hospital physician specialties, within each year, for each factor. For details of specialties included as "other hospital physician" specialties, see Methods.

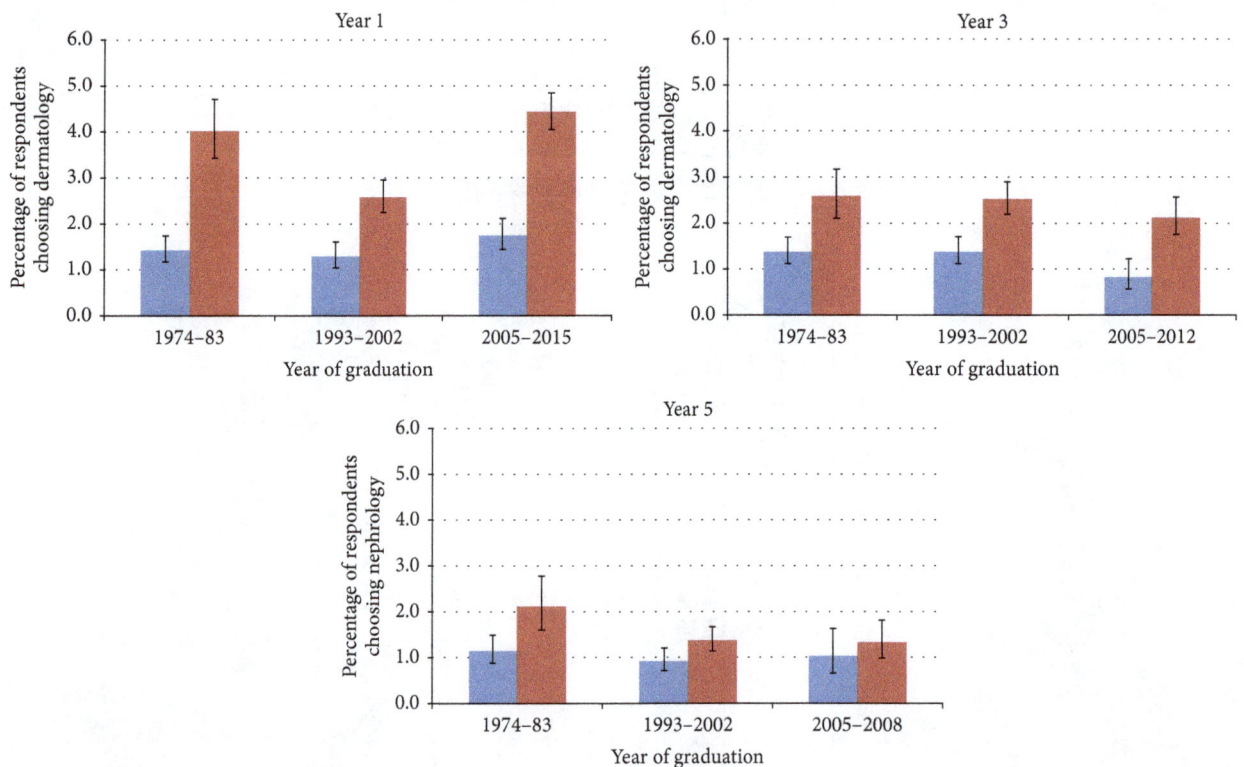

FIGURE 2: Percentages of men (blue) and women (red) doctors who chose dermatology as a first, second, or third choice of eventual career one, three, and five years after graduation.

TABLE 5: Numbers and percentages of medical graduates whose original choice was dermatology and eventually practised at four different destinations in year 10 (looking forwards).

	Four final destinations after 10 years				
	Dermatology % (N)	Other hospital physician specialties % (N)	Other clinical specialties % (N)	GP % (N)	Total % (N)
Year 1 first choice					
Male choosing dermatology	17% (5)	31% (9)	42% (12)	10% (3)	100% (29)
Female choosing dermatology	20% (15)	16% (12)	32% (24)	32% (24)	100% (75)
Total choosing dermatology	19% (20)	20% (21)	35% (36)	26% (27)	100% (104)
Year 3 first choice					
Male choosing dermatology	48% (21)	18% (8)	18% (8)	16% (7)	100% (44)
Female choosing dermatology	41% (36)	14% (12)	24% (21)	21% (18)	100% (87)
Total choosing dermatology	44% (57)	15% (20)	22% (29)	19% (25)	100% (131)
Year 5 first choice					
Male choosing dermatology	89% (33)	5% (2)	3% (1)	3% (1)	100% (37)
Female choosing dermatology	82% (46)	7% (4)	9% (5)	2% (1)	100% (56)
Total choosing dermatology	85% (79)	6% (6)	6% (6)	3% (2)	100% (93)

For details of specialties included as "other hospital physician" specialties, see Methods. "Other clinical specialties" includes the following: emergency medicine, anaesthesia, clinical oncology, surgery, paediatrics, pathology, psychiatry, and radiology.

the importance of hours and working conditions, domestic circumstances, future financial prospects, and career and promotion prospects, but less highly on experience of jobs so far.

3.6. Comparing Early Choice with Eventual Destination

3.6.1. Looking Forward to Eventual Destination. Early career choices for dermatology in years 1, 3, and 5 were matched with four career destination groups in year 10 after qualification (Table 5). Only 19% of respondents who chose dermatology in year 1 were working as dermatologists in year 10. This percentage increased substantially when year 3 and 5 choices were considered, reaching 44% and 85%, respectively. More than half of the respondents who specified dermatology as their first choice in year 1 did not become hospital physicians and more than a quarter of them were in general practice in year 10 including 32% of the women who had chosen dermatology (Table 5). Only very small numbers of those who chose dermatology in year 5 were not working in the specialty at year 10.

3.6.2. Looking Backwards to Early Choices. Looking backwards, 30% of practising dermatologists in year 10 had considered dermatology as a future career in year 1, whether as first, second, or third choice (Table 6). Looking back from year 10 destinations to year 3 and 5 choices in the same way indicated much higher percentages which reached 70.3% and 94%, respectively.

4. Discussion

4.1. Main Findings. Considering choices for dermatology one year after graduation, there was an upward trend across the year of graduation cohorts. However, interest fell in years

three and five, and the percentage of doctors in their fifth postqualification year who chose dermatology was much lower, particularly among women and particularly in the most recent year of graduation cohorts. Research into the causes of this loss of initial interest is suggested. Nevertheless, throughout this study dermatology was more popular among female than male doctors, though this gender difference gradually diminished as time passed from graduation. A third of women who chose dermatology one year after graduation were later working in general practice.

Across all cohorts, three life style and income related factors (i.e., "hours/working conditions," "domestic situation," and "future financial prospects") were more important to intending dermatologists than doctors opting for other hospital medical specialties. The first two factors were more important for female than male doctors while the latter was more influential for male respondents. Aspiring dermatologists scored lower on "experience of jobs so far" than those choosing other hospital specialties. This may reflect low exposure to dermatology in medical school or in the early years after graduation.

Dermatologists were late decision-makers regarding their future career. Over two-thirds of practising dermatologists had not chosen dermatology in their first year after graduation, whereas, in year 5, 94% of them had given dermatology as their first choice. Less than one-fifth of intending dermatologists in year 1 eventually became dermatologists; but the corresponding figure exceeded four-fifths in year 5. Confidence in dermatology choices increased with time for both female and male participants. Considering our data on influencing factors, their relatively late but assured decisions to commit to a career in dermatology could be attributed in part to the field experiences or self-awareness which had been built up over time.

TABLE 6: Numbers and percentages of practicing dermatologists in year 10, based on their original any first career choices in years 1, 3, and 5 (looking backwards).

Career choices	Male % (N)	Female % (N)	Total % (N)
Year 1			
Dermatology as untied first choice	15% (5)	22% (11)	19% (16)
Dermatology as tied 1st choice	0% (0)	8% (4)	5% (4)
Dermatology as 2nd or 3rd choice	9% (3)	4% (2)	6% (5)
Other hospital physician specialties	58% (19)	43% (21)	49% (40)
Others	18% (6)	22% (11)	21% (17)
Total	100% (33)	100% (49)	100% (82)
Year 3			
Dermatology as untied first choice	62% (21)	47% (27)	53% (48)
Dermatology as tied 1st choice	0% (0)	16% (9)	10% (9)
Dermatology as 2nd or 3rd choice	0% (0)	12% (7)	8% (7)
Other hospital physician specialties	15% (5)	10% (6)	12% (11)
Others	23% (8)	14% (8)	18% (16)
Total	100% (34)	100% (57)	100% (91)
Year 5			
Dermatology as untied first choice	100% (33)	88% (45)	93% (78)
Dermatology as tied 1st choice	0% (0)	2% (1)	1% (1)
Dermatology as 2nd or 3rd choice	0% (0)	0% (0)	0% (0)
Other hospital physician specialties	0% (0)	0% (0)	0% (0)
Others	0% (0)	10% (5)	6% (5)
Total	100% (33)	100% (51)	100% (84)

For details of specialties included as "other hospital physician" specialties, see Methods.

4.2. Comparison with Other Research. In this longitudinal study, recent medical graduates were gradually losing their interest in pursuing dermatology as their future career between years 1 and 5. This downward trend was not unique for dermatology and also observed in other specialties such as nephrology [23].

The gender differences in specialty preference in our results were highlighted in studies from other countries, for example, Japan [24] and the US [10]. The reported high rate of women in dermatology in our study corresponds with previous research. For instance, in Japan, dermatology was mentioned as a popular career choice among female physicians [24]. A study of over 11,000 medical students from 11 countries in Latin America indicated female gender was associated with the choice of dermatology [25].

Additionally, life style and income related factors are valued as determinants of motivation for choosing dermatology by our respondents. The "work–life balance" benefit of dermatology was emphasized by not only the UK-trained doctors, but also medical graduates from both developed and underdeveloped countries [2]. In a study of fourth-year medical students in the US, dermatology was rated the highest scoring specialty for lifestyle. Controllable lifestyle in the US study comprised four items: predictable working hours, having extra time for activities outside of work, leisure, and being with family [10]. Further, a cross-sectional study

on 200 Saudi medical students found that the majority of respondents were attracted to dermatology by having roots in life-work balance as well as financial and occupational satisfaction, including how dermatologists lead a satisfying family life, the appeal of being a dermatologist, opportunities for researches, and the reliance on clinical skills for diagnosis. It is notable that 66% of intending dermatologists in that study were females.

Although, in recent years, specialties with controllable lifestyle and work–life balance are highlighted by both male and female doctors [9, 26], their importance is higher for many women [27] which may be due to women's traditional roles in supporting family and competing demands for the time of family and career [28]. Considering dermatology as a career with controllable lifestyle [29] and the tendency of females towards professions compatible with their family life [2], the higher proportion of women in dermatology is understandable. In this respect, for many doctors dermatology will compare well with other specialties such as surgery [30].

Late career decisions among aspiring dermatologists were also reported in other research among those intending other hospital specialties such as cardiology [31]. As time passes from qualification, medical graduates will gain a better assessment of their abilities and a realistic vision of expected career roles through their first-hand experiences and contact with more experienced and informed colleagues [32]. Literature suggests that later preferences encompass factors beyond job values, work–family, and encouragement and mentoring from others [33].

4.3. Implications. The greater influx of female than male doctors in dermatology field, particularly in recent years, may raise concern regarding workforce gender imbalance. Although, in some countries, training and practice in dermatology are combined with venereology [34], in the United Kingdom, genitourinary medicine is a separate specialty [5]. Hence concerns which may be expressed, for example, by a male patient hesitating to discuss their complaint with a female dermatologist would not normally apply in the UK. However, an increasingly female gender balance in the specialty may lead to an increase in part-time working and a consequent reduction in capacity. Further research is needed to elucidate the working status of dermatologists and provide a comprehensive picture of the workforce in this specialty.

Late decisions to commit to a future career are mainly related to applicants' lack of information about their desired specialty, which can be tackled through preparing both clinical and research mentorship programmes [35], offering specialty-specific electives during medical schools [36], and providing career-support services [36]. Late career choice is difficult for applicants and risks wasting societies' resources and talents. Thus, it is crucial to recognise the aptitudes of medical students as early as possible and lead them towards a proper career path tailored to their needs and talents. In doing so, constant and concerted support from all stakeholders particularly educational providers and workforce planners is required.

4.4. Strengths and Limitations. This, the longest multicohort national study, provides an insight into the views of UK medical graduates on dermatology choices and provides an initial point of investigation to start more specific evaluation of their training and experiences. The relatively large sample size and the prospective design over 10 years enable comparison of choices, career outcomes, and motivations. However, some limitations exist. We do not include physicians working in the UK who graduated abroad and, as in any survey work, there is a possibility of responder bias.

5. Conclusions

In summary, the popularity of dermatology was evidently higher among female than male participants across all cohorts. Intending dermatologists significantly valued lifestyle and income related factors higher than those intending to work in other hospital specialties. Furthermore, dermatology choices were relatively stable in the later stages in the career course and changes regarding career decisions tend to occur in the first few years after medical school. Thought should be given to future administrative strategies that can improve the work–life balance in other specialties and support medical students regarding their career choice.

Acknowledgments

The authors thank Janet Justice and Alison Stockford for data entry. They are very grateful to all the doctors who participated in the surveys.

References

[1] F. Gorouhi, A. Alikhan, A. Rezaei, and N. Fazel, "Dermatology residency selection criteria with an emphasis on program characteristics: a national program director survey," *Dermatology Research and Practice*, vol. 2014, Article ID 692760, 8 pages, 2014.

[2] R. A. Aldahash, G. M. Alqahtani, A. K. Alkahtani, H. A. Alnuaim, O. A. Alhathlol, and N. S. Alshahrani, "Reasons for choosing Dermatology as a career choice," *Journal of Health Specialties*, vol. 4, no. 4, pp. 288–293, 2016.

[3] Health Education England, *Competition Ratios*, 2017.

[4] Health Careers, "Training and development," Dermatology, 2017.

[5] I. Yusuf, R. Turner, and S. M. Burge, "A career in dermatology," *BMJ Career*, 2010.

[6] British Association of Dermatologists, "A career in dermatology," *Healthcare Professionals*, 2017.

[7] British Association of Dermatologists, "Flexible training," *Healthcare Professionals*, 2017.

[8] British Association of Dermatologists, "Less than full-time training," *Healthcare Professionals*, 2017, British Association of Dermatologists. Less than Full-Time Training. HealthcareProfessionals.

[9] R. Kawamoto, D. Ninomiya, Y. Kasai et al., "Gender difference in preference of specialty as a career choice among Japanese medical students," *BMC Medical Education*, vol. 16, no. 1, 2016.

[10] K. J. DeZee, L. A. Byars, C. D. Magee, G. Rickards, S. J. Durning, and D. Maurer, "The R.O.A.D. confirmed: ratings of specialties' lifestyles by fourth-year US medical students with a military service obligation," *Family Medicine*, vol. 45, pp. 240–246, 2013.

[11] Royal College of Physicians of Edinburgh, Royal College of Physicians and Surgeons of Glasgow, and Royal College of Physicians of London, *Focus on Physicians. Census of Consultant Physicians and Higher Specialty Trainees in the UK 2016-17*, Royal College of Physicians, 2017.

[12] J. K. Schofield, D. Grindlay, and H. C. William, *Skin Conditions in the UK: A Health Needs Assessment*, Centre of Evidence Based Dermatology, University of Nottingham, Nottingham, UK, 2009.

[13] Workforce and Facilities Team and NHS Digital, *HCHS Doctors by Grade and Specialty in Trusts and CCGs—Full Time Equivalent. NHS Workforce Statistics—September 2016, Provisional Statistics*, NHS Digital part of the Government Statistical Service, Surrey, UK, 2016.

[14] D. Eedy, "The crisis in dermatology," *BMJ Careers*, vol. 350, Article ID h2765, 2015.

[15] S. A. Chan, G. A. Fremlin, and T. M. Finch, "How to succeed in the ST3 dermatology application," *BMJ Careers*, vol. 351, Article ID h5574, 2015.

[16] N. Edwards and C. Imison, "How can dermatology services meet current and future patient needs, while ensuring quality of care is not compromised and access is equitable across the UK?" *King's Fund*, 2015.

[17] K. Van Der Horst, M. Siegrist, P. Orlow, and M. Giger, "Residents' reasons for specialty choice: Influence of gender, time, patient and career," *Medical Education*, vol. 44, no. 6, pp. 595–602, 2010.

[18] M. J. Goldacre and T. W. Lambert, "Participation in medicine by graduates of medical schools in the United Kingdom up to 25 years post graduation: National cohort surveys," *Academic Medicine*, vol. 88, no. 5, pp. 699–709, 2013.

[19] A. I. Christensen, O. Ekholm, P. L. Kristensen et al., "The effect of multiple reminders on response patterns in a Danish health survey," *European Journal of Public Health*, vol. 25, no. 1, pp. 156–161, 2015.

[20] K. E. A. Burns, M. Duffett, M. E. Kho et al., "A guide for the design and conduct of self-administered surveys of clinicians," *Canadian Medical Association Journal*, vol. 179, no. 3, pp. 245–252, 2008.

[21] Royal College of Physicians of Edinburgh, Royal College of Physician and Surgeons of Glasgow, and Royal College of Physician, *Training and Certification*, Joint Royal Colleges of Physicians Training Board (JRCPTB), 2017.

[22] IBM Corp, *IBM SPSS Statistics for Windows. 22.0*, IBM Corp, Armonk, NY, USA, 2013.

[23] A. Barat, M. Glodacre, and T. Lambert, "Career choices for nephrology and factors influencing them: surveys of UK medical graduates," *Medical Teacher*, 2017.

[24] Y. Fukuda and T. Harada, "Gender differences in specialty preference and mismatch with real needs in Japanese medical students," *BMC Medical Education*, vol. 10, no. 1, article 15, 2010.

[25] L. F. Ng-Sueng, I. Vargas-Matos, P. Mayta-Tristán et al., "Gender associated with the intention to choose a medical specialty in medical students: a cross-sectional study in 11 countries in Latin America," *PLoS ONE*, vol. 11, no. 8, Article ID e0161000, 2016.

[26] F. Smith, T. W. Lambert, and M. J. Goldacre, "Factors influencing junior doctors' choices of future specialty: trends over time and demographics based on results from UK national surveys," *Journal of the Royal Society of Medicine*, vol. 108, no. 10, pp. 396–405, 2015.

[27] J. Bickel, *Women in Medicine: Getting in, Growing, and Advancing*, Sage Publications, Thousand Oaks, Calif, USA, 2000.

[28] G. Verlander, "Female physicians: Balancing career and family," *Academic Psychiatry*, vol. 28, no. 4, pp. 331–336, 2004.

[29] L. Enoch, J. T. Chibnall, D. L. Schindler, and S. J. Slavin, "Association of medical student burnout with residency specialty choice," *Medical Education*, vol. 47, no. 2, pp. 173–181, 2013.

[30] M. J. Goldacre, L. Laxton, E. M. Harrison, J. M. J. Richards, T. W. Lambert, and R. W. Parks, "Early career choices and successful career progression in surgery in the UK: prospective cohort studies," *BMC Surgery*, vol. 2, no. 10, article 32, 2010.

[31] F. Smith, T. W. Lambert, A. Pitcher, and M. J. Goldacre, "Career choices for cardiology: Cohort studies of UK medical graduates," *BMC Medical Education*, vol. 13, no. 1, article 10, 2013.

[32] L. K. G. Hsu and M. Hersen, *Research in Psychiatry: Issues, Strategies, and Methods*, Springer, Boston, Mass, USA, 1992.

[33] M. C. Ku, "When does gender matter? Gender differences in specialty choice among physicians," *Work and Occupations*, vol. 38, no. 2, pp. 221–262, 2011.

[34] L. Mahmood Malik and N. Ali Azfar, "Gender shift in dermatology: implications for the profession," *Journal of Pakistan Association of Dermatologists*, vol. 15, pp. 79-80, 2015.

[35] D. E. Girard, D. Choi, J. Dickey, D. Dickerson, and J. D. Bloom, "A comparison study of career satisfaction and emotional states between primary care and speciality residents," *Medical Education*, vol. 40, no. 1, pp. 79–86, 2006.

[36] O. A. Aboshady, M. S. Zenhom, and A. A. Nasr, "What should medical students do to choose their specialty?" *Pan African Medical Journal*, vol. 22, article 282, 2015.

17

Autologous Fat Grafting in the Treatment of Facial Scleroderma

Mehdi Gheisari,[1] **Arman Ahmadzadeh ⓘ,**[2] **Nilofar Nobari,**[1]
Behzad Iranmanesh,[1] **and Nikoo Mozafari ⓘ**[1,3]

[1] *Skin Research Center, Shahid Beheshti University of Medical Sciences, Tehran, Iran*
[2] *Department of Rheumatology, Shahid Beheshti University of Medical Sciences, Tehran, Iran*
[3] *Department of Dermatology, Loghmen-e-Hakim Hospital, Shahid Beheshti University of Medical Sciences, Tehran, Iran*

Correspondence should be addressed to Nikoo Mozafari; nikoo_md@yahoo.com

Academic Editor: Gavin P. Robertson

Systemic sclerosis (SSc) is a rare systemic autoimmune disease, characterized by progressive cutaneous and internal organ fibrosis. Orofacial manifestations of systemic sclerosis are extremely disabling and treatment options are limited. In this study, we aimed to assess the safety and efficacy of autologous fat grafting in the face of patients with systemic sclerosis. We enrolled 16 SSc patients suffering from facial sclerosis and limited mouth opening capacity. Autologous fat injection ranging from 15 to 40 ml was administered per patient, based on their face morphology. The patients were evaluated at baseline and 3 months after fat injection. Evaluations included mouth opening capacity, mouth handicap in systemic sclerosis (MHISS), Rodnan skin sclerosis score, skin biophysical properties using a sensitive biometrologic device with the assessment of cutaneous resonance running time (CRRT), volumizing and aesthetic effects based on pre- and posttreatment photographs, possible side effects, and global patient satisfaction. Clinical assessment showed autologous fat transfer significantly improved mouth opening capacity and the MHISS and Rodnan score of patients with facial scleroderma (p value <.001). The aesthetic and/or functional results of fat injection were satisfying to about 80% of the patients. The changes in CRRT values were not significant. Our findings support the possible therapeutic role of autologous fat grafting in improving facial scleroderma both in aesthetic and in functional aspects. This trial is registered with IRCT20180209038677N1.

1. Introduction

Systemic sclerosis (SSc) is a rare systemic autoimmune connective tissue disease of unknown etiology, characterized by cutaneous and visceral fibrosis [1]. Key pathogenic abnormality in the skin and internal organs are immunologically overactivated fibroblasts which, with the secretion of extraordinary amounts of collagen and extracellular matrix, lead to progressive cutaneous and internal organ fibrosis [1].

Systemic sclerosis is a heterogeneous disease, but two major clinical subtypes based on the extent of skin involvement are typically recognized, namely, limited cutaneous SSc with skin involvement from the distal to the elbows and knees and diffused cutaneous SSc with skin involvement extending to the proximal limbs and/or trunk [2]. The face is frequently involved in both subtypes of this disease. Patients with facial scleroderma often complain of aesthetic and functional concerns [3]. Facial involvement is associated with disfigurement and limited expression with a mask-like stiffness of the face. The loss of elasticity and the thickening of the skin in the perioral area and lips form perioral radial furrowing and narrowing of the oral aperture, leading to mouth opening reduction that interferes considerably with life's basic functions such as eating, speaking, oral hygiene, and professional dental care [3]. Furthermore, dry mouth or xerostomia because of salivary gland fibrosis and reduced saliva production is also a frequent symptom in these patients that increase the risk of periodontal diseases and caries [4]. The orofacial manifestations of systemic sclerosis are extremely disabling and severely impair the patients' self-image and compromise their quality of life [4].

Autologous fat tissue grafting, in addition to a filling effect, seems to have regenerative potentials presumably due to their adipose-derived stem cells (ASCs) content [5]. Currently, lipotransfer has been used for reversing fibrosis in various conditions such as scars, radio dermatitis, and

TABLE 1: The mouth handicap in systemic sclerosis scale (MHISS).

		Never	rarely	occasionally	often	always
1	I have difficulties opening my mouth	0	1	2	3	4
2	I have to avoid certain drinks (sparkling, alcohol, acidic)	0	1	2	3	4
3	I have difficulties chewing	0	1	2	3	4
4	My dentist has difficulties taking care of my teeth	0	1	2	3	4
5	My dentition has become altered	0	1	2	3	4
6	My lips are retracted and/or my cheeks are sunken	0	1	2	3	4
7	My mouth is dry	0	1	2	3	4
8	I must drink often	0	1	2	3	4
9	My meals consist of what I can eat and not what I would like to eat	0	1	2	3	4
10	I have difficulties speaking clearly	0	1	2	3	4
11	The appearance of my face is modified	0	1	2	3	4
12	I have trouble with the way my face looks	0	1	2	3	4

localized forms of scleroderma such as "en coup de sabre" [6, 7]. More recently, some reports have shown the efficacy of autologous fat grafting in patients with SSc to improve mouth opening and fibrosis reduction in the treated skin [5, 8].

In this study, we aimed to assess the safety and efficacy of autologous fat grafting in the face of patients with systemic sclerosis.

2. Material and Methods

This was an open-label study performed at the dermatology operative unit of our center. The study was approved by the ethics committee of the "skin research center". A written informed consent was obtained from all the participants. All procedures were done free of charge.

We enrolled 16 patients by fulfilling the "American College of Rheumatology" criteria for systemic sclerosis with facial involvement. Exclusion criteria were as follows: (1) pregnant or breastfeeding; (2) patients with diffused skin sclerosis who had insufficient fat for harvest; (3) recently diagnosed patients with SSc who had no clear face and oral involvement; (4) patients with a history of neoplasia in the last 5 years; (5) those who were taking prednisolone of more than 10 mg/d.

2.1. Autologous Fat Grafting Procedure. Given an easier access to a sufficient amount of adipose tissues, the trochanteric, the flank, and the periumbilical, or the buttock areas were chosen as the donor sites. The entry points for the infiltration cannula were anesthetized with 1 ml of pure lidocaine with a 30-gauge needle. Then 500 ml of tumescent solution containing normal saline, 25 ml of lidocaine 2%, and .5 ml of epinephrine 1:1000 was infiltrated in the selected donor area with a 1.5 mm cannula. After twenty minutes, the adipose tissue was harvested using a 3 mm blunt tipped cannula connected with a Luer-lock 10 ml syringe, using low vacuum pressure. The collected adipose tissue in each 10 ml syringe was left to sediment by gravity for 10 minutes. Oil and blood excess were eliminated and the remaining fat was transferred to the 1 ml syringe and was directly injected into the face using disposable 18-gauge cannulas.

In this study, 3 of the 4 essential parts of autologous fat transfer technique (donor site preparation, fat harvest, and reinjection) were based on the Coleman method [9]. For adipose tissue processing, the gravity separation technique was used instead of the centrifugation method.

The quantity of injected fat ranged from 15 to 40 ml per patient, based on the morphology of the patients' faces. Subcutaneous injections were administered to different locations: perioral, upper lip, and lower lip, mouth corners, buccal, malar, and periorbital regions. All patients were visited two weeks after AFT to record any possible side effects. During this time, they were asked to contact a physician if any of the following developed: progressive pain, warmness, swelling, and erythema of the face.

2.2. Clinical Outcome Evaluations. All patients were evaluated at baseline and 3 months after the procedure. Patient assessment was based on the following:

(1) Mouth opening capacity: maximal distance in cm between the upper and lower incisors.

(2) Mouth handicap in the systemic sclerosis (MHISS) scale, a 12-item questionnaire that specifically quantifies the mouth disability in SSc, is organized in 3 subclasses representing handicap induced by reduced mouth opening (5 items—1, 3, 4, 5, and 6), handicap induced by the sicca syndrome (5 items—2, 7, 8, 9, and 10), and aesthetic concerns (2 items—11 and 12) (Table 1) [10].

(3) Skin sclerosis based on the Rodnan skin score on face (0: uninvolved, 1: mild thickness, 2: moderate thickness, and 3: sever thickness)

(4) Skin biophysical properties: we used a Reviscometer (MPA9; Courage & Khazaka Electronic GmbH, Koln, Germany) to measure the possible changes in the collagen pattern and content. The measurement was based on cutaneous resonance running time (CRRT): the time that acoustical shock waves take to propagate between two sensors (emitter and receiver) on the skin surface. Two sensors are applied to the skin surface in a supine position. The mean CRRT over the four axes (0, 90, 180, and 270) was calculated for the perioral region.

TABLE 2: Baseline demographic, clinical, and therapeutic characteristics of patients.

Case	Age/sex	Disease duration (year)	Systemic sclerosis type	Liposuction area	Injected fat volume (ml)
1	41/f	8	limited	trochanteric	40
2	54/f	9	diffuse	Buttock	20
3	31/f	5	diffuse	flank	15
4	38/f	6	limited	periumbilical	30
5	37/f	7	diffuse	Buttock	20
6	32/f	5	diffuse	periumbilical	30
7	51/f	8	limited	trochanteric	25
8	49/f	10	limited	periumbilical	30
9	31/f	5	diffuse	trochanteric	20
10	34/f	8	diffuse	trochanteric	30
11	52/f	6	diffuse	Buttock	35
12	34/f	4	limited	trochanteric	40
13	29/f	5	diffuse	trochanteric	25
14	43/f	4	limited	periumbilical	30
15	39/f	7	diffuse	Buttock	15
16	32/f	7	diffuse	Buttock	30

(5) Aesthetic effect: improvement of the patients' appearance was evaluated with the help of pre- and posttreatment photographs. An outside dermatologist was asked to fill out a 4-point scale (-1: worsening, 0: no improvement, 1: some improvement, and 2: much improvement).

(6) Global patients' satisfaction: patients were asked to fill out a 3-point scale to quantify the degree of improvement both from the aesthetic and from the functional points of view (0: unsatisfied, 1: somewhat satisfied, and 2: very satisfied).

2.3. Statistical Analysis. All descriptive data are expressed as mean ± standard deviation (SD) or frequency (%). Comparison between values at the baseline and those at 3 months after treatment was performed by paired t-test and Wilcoxon's test for continuous and noncontinuous variables respectively. Data analysis was carried out using an SPSS software package version 20 (SPSS Inc., Chicago, IL, USA) and significant levels were considered as P value <0.05.

3. Results

3.1. Patient Characteristics. Sixteen patients with SSc, all women with a mean age of 39.18 ± 8.32 years, and mean disease duration of 6.5 ± 1.8 years, were enrolled. Six patients were diagnosed with limited SSc and 10 with the diffused form of SSc. The main characteristics of the patients are shown in Table 2.

3.2. Side Effects. No serious or persistent complications such as a vascular occlusion phenomenon, fat cyst, facial ecchymosis, or edema developed in the participants. Short lasting adverse effects such as bruising at the zone of fat harvest reported by 10 patients were spontaneously resolved within two weeks. No local or systemic infectious complications related to the procedure were recorded.

3.3. Clinical Evaluation of Treatment (Figure 1). (1) Mouth opening capacity (MOC): in all patients, an improvement in MOC was observed in the 3-month follow-up with a mean gain of .78 cm (range 0.5 to 1.5 cm) (p=<0.001) (Figure 2).

(2) MHISS score: at the baseline, the mean MHISS score was 29.37 ± 4.36 and significantly decreased to 23.25 ± 3.13 after 3 months (mean variation: 6.12 ± 2.3, p=<0.001).

(3) The mean face Rodnan score significantly improved with a reduction from 2.06 ± .57 at baseline to 1.56 ± .51 after 3 months (mean variation: .5 ±. 52, p = 0.001).

(4) The mean CRRT did not significantly change from the baseline (1001.12 ± 369.30) to 3 months after fat transfer (1132.75 ± 315.02) (mean variation: 131.62 ± 150.65, p = 0.39).

(5) Aesthetic effect: 13 of the 16 (81%) patients showed an improvement in their appearance (fuller and softer face with less wrinkles)—no improvement was seen in 3, some improvement in 4, and much improvement in 9 of them (Figure 3).

(6) Global patients' satisfaction: three months after fat grafting, 10 (62.5%) patients said they were very satisfied, 2 (12.5%) patients were somewhat satisfied, and 3 (18.75%) patient were unsatisfied.

4. Discussion

The present study demonstrated that autologous fat transfer (AFT) in the face of patients with scleroderma not only improves facial aesthetic aspects but significantly enhances the mouth opening capacity and reduces skin wrinkles and facial sclerosis. Our study showed that AFT was safe for patients with scleroderma and resulted in the reduction of mouth handicap as assessed by the MHISS score.

In 3 of the 16 patients who were unsatisfied with the aesthetic results, nearly the total volume of injected fat had been absorbed after 3 months, but the improvements in mouth opening and function were retained. There is

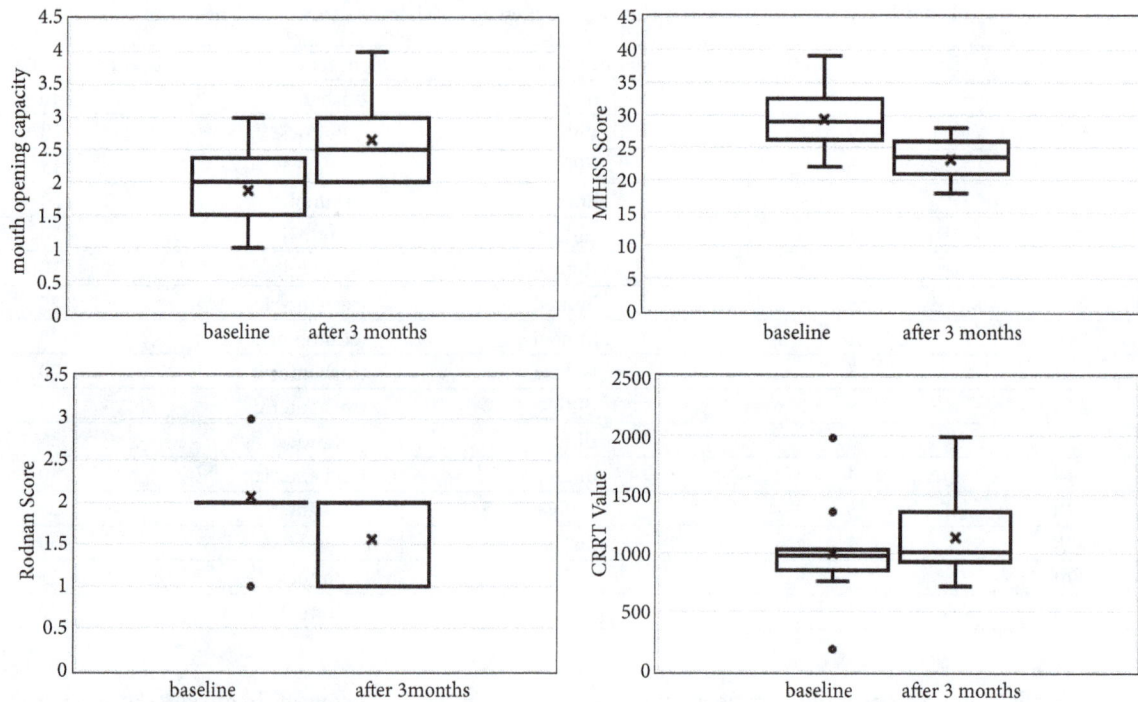

FIGURE 1: Pre- and postoperative changes of several parameters related to oral opening, mouth handicap in systemic sclerosis (MIHSS), sclerosis (Rodnan score), and cutaneous resonance running time (CRRT).

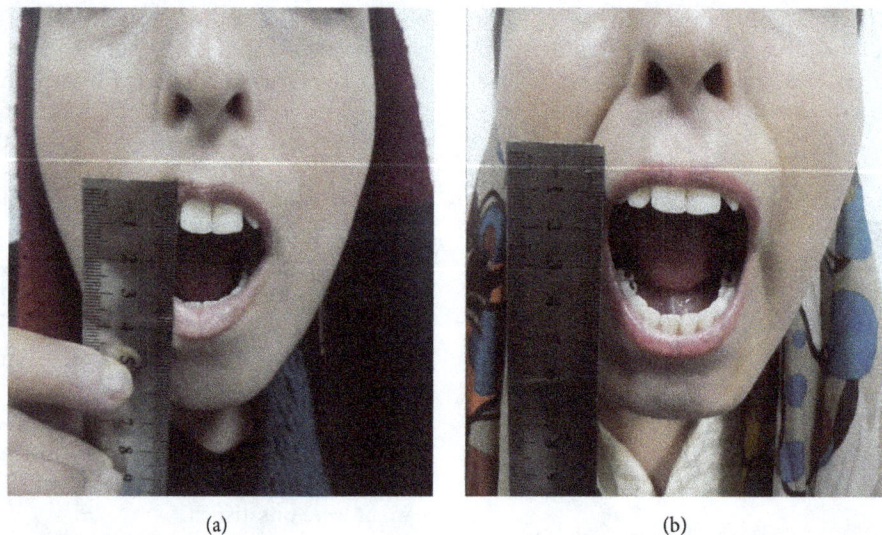

FIGURE 2: Mouth opening capacity at baseline (a) and significant improvement in mouth opening capacity 3 months after autologous fat transfer (b).

some evidence to show functional improvement in scleroderma patients following AFT cannot be ascribed only to the filling effects but rather to the activation of various biological mechanisms that could induce tissue regeneration [11, 12].

Recent studies have demonstrated that a fatty tissue has the highest percentage of adult stem cells compared to any other tissue in the body [12]. Adipose-derived stem cells (ASCs), similar to bone-marrow-derived stem cells, are capable of differentiating into multiple mesodermal tissue types, but, in contrast to bone-marrow-derived stem cells, they can be easily harvested by liposuction, and the abundance of these cells (in comparison to bone-marrow-derived stem cells) avoids the need for expansion in culture. Because of these practical aspects, the adipose tissue is considered an innovative source of mesenchymal stem cells suitable for cell-based therapy in regenerative medicine [12]. The regenerative features of ASCs are attributable to their ability to secrete

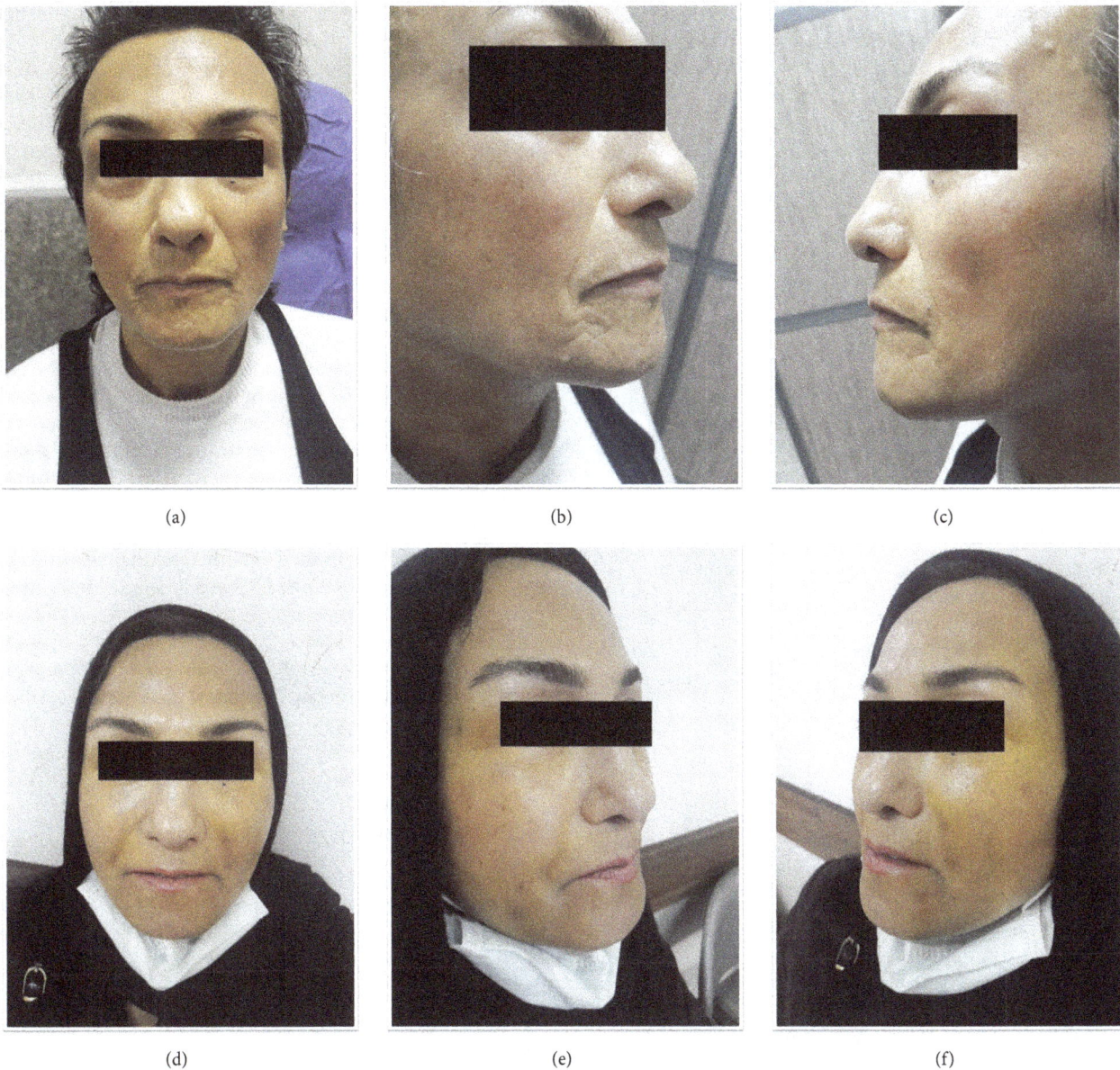

FIGURE 3: Aesthetic improvement after autologous fat transfer, baseline (a, b, c) and 3 months after autologous fat transfer (d, e, f).

angiogenetic factors and immunomodulatory properties that facilitate tissue repair [5].

Increasing evidence shows that lipotransfer in sclerotic tissues may decrease collagen deposition and increase elasticity and vascularization [13]. To measure these changes, we used cutaneous resonance running time (CRRT), which is a noninvasive apparatus to assess skin biophysical properties [14]. CRRT can be influenced by the collagen content, skin elasticity, and hydration. CRRT is negatively correlated with skin stiffness or firmness. For instance, it has been demonstrated that CRRT is decreased in aged skin. In the aging process, defragmentation of the elastin network and configuration change in the dermal collagen network could increase skin stiffness and decrease skin elasticity and CRRT [14]. In our study, mean CRRT values increased after AFT, although the changes were not significant. Indeed, changes

of cutaneous biophysical properties after fat transfer have not been well documented. It would be better if we could perform skin biopsy before and 3 months after the procedure to assess the possible histopathological changes in the pattern and content of collagen and elastic fibers. Unfortunately, none of the participants agreed to undergo skin biopsy. Following AFT in patients with scleroderma, a partial restoration of skin structures has been demonstrated by histological evaluation of the biopsies sections [11]. Del Papa et al. showed, by comparing with the baseline, a reduction in the dermoepidermal junction flattening with the reconstruction of the normal rete ridges and dermal papillae pattern in posttreatment samples [11].

In recent decades, autologous fat tissue grafting has been successfully used to regenerate atrophic or fibrotic skin for a large number of clinical conditions such as radio dermatitis, burning scars, linear scleroderma, and different types of morphea [8]. In most of these cases, a significant increase in skin elasticity and thickening with both aesthetic and functional improvement has been reported [8].

Moreover, the use of lipotransfer to reverse fibrosis is currently being explored in the treatment of the face and hands of patients with SSc [5, 15]. Del papa et al. treated perioral thickening in 20 female patients with the diffused type of SSc with autologous fat. After 3 months of the treatment, a significant increase was observed in the patients' maximum interincisive distance with respect to the baseline value (mean increase: 2.63 mm) [11]. Furthermore, they showed an increase in the neovascularization of the treated perioral skin after AFT [11]. Similarly, Sautereau et al. demonstrated improvements in mouth opening, facial pain, and MHISS scores in all the 14 SSc patients who were treated with autologous micro fat grafting at 3 and 6 months after surgery [16].

There are many ways to process fat after its collection; Del Papa et al. used Coleman's technique. They centrifuged lipoaspirate at $700 \times g$ for 3 minutes before injection [11]. Whereas Sautereau et al. used the pure graft filtration technique to purify the lipoaspirate from blood cells and free lipid content [16]. There is no agreement among authors regarding the best method for processing fat transfer. Similar to our study, Onseti et al. used sedimentation by gravity as a method to eliminate nonviable components of the lipoaspirate. They compared the effects of lipotransfer and expanded 8×10^5 cells/ml of the adipose stem cell injection in 10 patients with SSc. At the one-year follow-up, they noticed that both procedures provided a significant improvement in the mouth opening capacity and MHISS scores; but neither technique offered superior results [17].

In a recent trial, Virzi et al. demonstrated the beneficial effects of the combined use of autologous lipoaspirate and platelet-rich plasma (PRP) in the improvement of the buccal rhyme, skin elasticity, and vascularization of the perioral and malar areas of patients with SSc [18]. Whether this combination is superior to the standard fat transfer or other processing techniques in terms of clinical efficacy or durability needs to be addressed by prospective randomized clinical trials.

One limitation of the current and previous studies is the lack of quantified measurement of fat graft survivability. The actual mechanism on how fat graft survives is not completely understood [19]. According to previous studies, there was no significant difference in the survival of grafted fat obtained from different harvests and implantation techniques [20, 21]. Not any one technique is clearly superior to other techniques. There is no linear relation between the fat graft volume and survival rates [21]. Differences in underlying disease processes or patient variability may significantly impact engraftment. Significant differences in the number of stromal adipose stem cells in lipoaspirates between patients, and underlying conditions associated with poor revascularization, may account for the differences observed between patients in volume retention from fat grafts [20]. To determine if the injected fat in patients with scleroderma can

be expected to survive as long as in the normal population, larger and controlled studies are required.

In the current study, all our participants were women because systemic sclerosis affects women three to four times as often as men [2], orofacial manifestations of scleroderma are four times more common in women [22], and men are generally poor consumers of aesthetic care and dermatology services. Autologous fat transfer has been successfully applied to men and even children [23] in different indications. Apart from fat availability which may be a limit in these groups, the aesthetic and functional results are comparable to women. In recently published articles [11, 15–18] on AFT for scleroderma, among a total of 57 cases, 4 cases were men, and the clinical outcomes were satisfactory, indicating the utility of the AFT in treatment of facial sclerosis in both females and males.

There are limited treatment options for scleroderma microstomia. The recommended treatment for limited mouth opening is based on stretching exercise for 3 months that need to be continued in the long term [4]. Intense pulsed dye light [24] and Co2 laser [25] have been advocated for the treatment of limited mouth opening; however, the reported efficacy was limited. There is a growing body of evidence that suggests autologous fat transfer can be an effective therapeutic alternative in patients with SSc. Our findings support the possible therapeutic role of autologous fat grafting in improving facial scleroderma both in aesthetic and functional aspects.

Acknowledgments

The authors would like to thank the Clinical Research Development Unit (CRDU) of Loghman Hakim Hospital, Shahid Beheshti University of Medical Sciences, Tehran, Iran, for their support, cooperation, and assistance throughout the period of study. The present study was funded by the Skin Research Center, Shahid Beheshti University of Medical Sciences.

References

[1] G. Kumánovics, M. Péntek, S. Bae et al., "Assessment of skin involvement in systemic sclerosis," *Rheumatology*, vol. 56, no. 5, pp. v53–v66, 2017.

[2] H. Alhajeri, M. Hudson, M. Fritzler et al., "2013 American College of Rheumatology/European League against rheumatism classification criteria for systemic sclerosis outperform the 1980 criteria: data from the Canadian Scleroderma Research Group," *Arthritis Care & Research*, vol. 67, no. 4, pp. 582–587, 2015.

[3] A. Panchbhai, S. Pawar, A. Barad, and Z. Kazi, "Review of orofacial considerations of systemic sclerosis or scleroderma with report of analysis of 3 cases," *Indian Journal of Dentistry*, vol. 7, no. 3, p. 134, 2016.

[4] J. B. Albilia, D. K. Lam, N. Blanas, C. M. L. Clokie, and G. K. B. Sándor, "Small mouths··· big problems? A review of scleroderma and its oral health implications," *Journal of the Canadian Dental Association*, vol. 73, no. 9, pp. 831–836, 2007.

[5] G. Magalon, A. Daumas, N. Sautereau, J. Magalon, F. Sabatier, and B. Granel, "Regenerative Approach to Scleroderma with Fat Grafting," *Clinics in Plastic Surgery*, vol. 42, no. 3, pp. 64–353, 2015.

[6] E. Z. Barin, H. Cinal, M. A. Cakmak, and O. Tan, "Treatment of linear scleroderma (en Coup de Sabre) with dermal fat grafting," *Journal of Cutaneous Medicine and Surgery*, vol. 20, no. 3, pp. 269–271, 2016.

[7] T. P. Zanelato, R. F. Magalhães, G. Marquesini, A. M. de Moraes, and P. T. Colpas, "Implantation of autologous fat globules in localized scleroderma and idiopathic lipoatrophy - Report of five patients," *Anais Brasileiros de Dermatologia*, vol. 88, no. 6, pp. 120–123, 2013.

[8] M. F. Griffin, A. Almadori, and P. E. Butler, "Use of Lipotransfer in Scleroderma," *Aesthetic Surgery Journal*, vol. 37, no. suppl_3, pp. S33–S37, 2017.

[9] S. R. Coleman, "Structural fat grafting: more than a permanent filler," *Plastic and Reconstructive Surgery*, vol. 118, no. 3, supplement, pp. 108S–120S, 2006.

[10] L. Mouthon, F. Rannou, A. Bérezné et al., "Development and validation of a scale for mouth handicap in systemic sclerosis: The Mouth Handicap in Systemic Sclerosis scale," *Annals of the Rheumatic Diseases*, vol. 66, no. 12, pp. 1651–1655, 2007.

[11] N. Del Papa, F. Caviggioli, D. Sambataro et al., "Autologous fat grafting in the treatment of fibrotic perioral changes in patients with systemic sclerosis," *Cell Transplantation*, vol. 24, no. 1, pp. 63–72, 2015.

[12] E. Bellini, M. P. Grieco, and E. Raposio, "The science behind autologous fat grafting," *Annals of Medicine and Surgery*, vol. 24, pp. 65–73, 2017.

[13] W. Chen, Z.-K. Xia, M.-H. Zhang et al., "Adipose tissue-derived stem cells ameliorates dermal fibrosis in a mouse model of scleroderma," *Asian Pacific Journal of Tropical Medicine*, vol. 10, no. 1, pp. 52–56, 2017.

[14] S. Xin, W. Man, J. W. Fluhr, S. Song, P. M. Elias, and M.-Q. Man, "Cutaneous resonance running time varies with age, body site and gender in a normal Chinese population," *Skin Research and Technology*, vol. 16, no. 4, pp. 413–421, 2010.

[15] O. Blezien, F. D'Andrea, G. F. Nicoletti, and G. A. Ferraro, "Effects of Fat Grafting Containing Stem Cells in Microstomia and Microcheilia Derived from Systemic Sclerosis," *Aesthetic Plastic Surgery*, vol. 41, no. 4, pp. 839–844, 2017.

[16] N. Sautereau, A. Daumas, R. Truillet et al., "Efficacy of Autologous Microfat Graft on Facial Handicap in Systemic Sclerosis Patients," *Plastic and Reconstructive Surgery Global Open*, vol. 4, no. 3, article no. e660, 2016.

[17] M. G. Onesti, P. Fioramonti, S. Carella, P. Fino, C. Marchese, and N. Scuderi, "Improvement of Mouth Functional Disability in Systemic Sclerosis Patients over One Year in a Trial of Fat Transplantation versus Adipose-Derived Stromal Cells," *Stem Cells International*, vol. 2016, 2016.

[18] F. Virzì, P. Bianca, A. Giammona et al., "Combined platelet-rich plasma and lipofilling treatment provides great improvement in facial skin-induced lesion regeneration for scleroderma patients," *Stem Cell Research & Therapy*, vol. 8, no. 1, 2017.

[19] L. L. Q. Pu, "Mechanisms of fat graft survival," *Annals of Plastic Surgery*, vol. 77, pp. S84–S86, 2016.

[20] A. L. Strong, P. S. Cederna, J. P. Rubin, S. R. Coleman, and B. Levi, "The Current state of fat grafting: A review of harvesting, processing, and injection techniques," *Plastic and Reconstructive Surgery*, vol. 136, no. 4, pp. 897–912, 2015.

[21] N.-Z. Yu, J.-Z. Huang, H. Zhang et al., "A systemic review of autologous fat grafting survival rate and related severe complications," *Chinese Medical Journal*, vol. 128, no. 9, pp. 1245–1251, 2015.

[22] M. Hadj Said, J. M. Foletti, N. Graillon, L. Guyot, and C. Chossegros, "Orofacial manifestations of scleroderma. A literature review," *Revue de Stomatologie, de Chirurgie Maxillo-faciale et de Chirurgie Orale*, vol. 117, no. 5, pp. 322–326, 2016.

[23] M. Guibert, G. Franchi, and E. Ansari, "Fat graft transfer in children's facial malformations: a prospective three-dimensional evaluation," *Journal of Plastic, Reconstructive & Aesthetic Surgery*, vol. 66, no. 6, pp. 799–804, 2013.

[24] L. R. Comstedt, Å. Svensson, and A. Troilius, "Improvement of microstomia in scleroderma after intense pulsed light: A case series of four patients," *Journal of Cosmetic and Laser Therapy*, vol. 14, no. 2, pp. 102–106, 2012.

[25] I. Bennani, R. Lopez, D. Bonnet et al., "Improvement of Microstomia in Scleroderma after Carbon Dioxide Laser Treatment," *Case Reports in Dermatology*, vol. 8, no. 2, pp. 142–150, 2016.

18

Investigation of Interleukin-27 in the Sera of Nonmelanoma Skin Cancer Patients

Mehdi Ghahartars,[1] Shiva Najafzadeh,[2] Shabnam Abtahi,[2]
Mohammad Javad Fattahi,[2] and Abbas Ghaderi ⓘ[2]

[1]*Department of Dermatology, School of Medicine, Shiraz University of Medical Sciences, Shiraz, Iran*
[2]*Shiraz Institute for Cancer Research, School of medicine, Shiraz University of Medical Sciences, Shiraz, Iran*

Correspondence should be addressed to Abbas Ghaderi; ghaderia@sums.ac.ir

Academic Editor: Gavin Robertson

IL-27 has been shown to have both tumor promoting and suppressing functions. IL-27, with its diverse influences on immune responses, has not been studied extensively in nonmelanoma skin cancers (NMSC), including Squamous and Basal Cell Carcinomas (SCC and BCC), and its roles in tumor initiation, progression, and its probable use in NMSC treatment have yet to be unveiled. A cross-sectional analytical study was designed to investigate the serum levels of IL-27 in NMSC patients in comparison to normal individuals. Levels of IL-27 in the sera of 60 NMSC patients along with 28 healthy controls were measured by means of quantitative enzyme-linked immunosorbent assay (ELISA). In this study we observed that IL-27 serum levels were significantly higher in NMSC patients in comparison to healthy individuals (0.0134 *versus* 0.0008 ng/ml; P<0.001). Furthermore, when subcategorized based on pathological diagnosis, both BCC and SCC patients had higher levels of IL-27 in their sera compared to controls (P=0.002 and P=0.033; respectively). However, these levels were not different among SCC and BCC patients. According to our results, it seems that IL-27 is involved in antitumor immune responses in NMSCs. On the other hand, these observations might be indicative of this cytokine involvement in NMSC tumorigenesis and progression. Therefore, administration of this cytokine for therapeutic purposes in patients with such conditions should be erred on the side of caution.

1. Introduction

Attempts for identifying mechanisms underlying carcinogenesis have resulted in discovery of many aspects of tumor immune responses, many of which are already being used in therapeutic protocols for different malignancies [1]. However, there are still aspects in need of being discovered and further clarified. Use of cytokines such as IL-2 and IFN-alpha for cancer immunotherapy is prominent milestones in the history of medical oncology [2], and attempts to identify other cytokines for this purpose have been continuing ever since. Several cytokines, such as IL-12, IL-15, IL-21, and granulocyte macrophage colony-stimulating factor (GM-CSF) have shown promising results for cancer therapy in both murine models and clinical trials [3].

Among cytokines being investigated for probable therapeutic applications, IL-27 has been shown to have both tumor promoting and suppressing functions, depending on the characteristics of the target neoplasm [4–6]. IL-27 is a member of the IL-6/IL-12 family and is considered to be a multifunctional cytokine with both pro- and anti-inflammatory properties [7]. This cytokine is a heterodimer composed of an IL-12 p40-related protein subunit, EBV-induced gene 3 (EBI3) and a unique IL-12p35-like protein, IL-27p28. This cytokine is mainly produced by activated antigen presenting cells (APCs) including dendritic cells (DCs) and macrophages [6, 7].

Several reports have demonstrated IL-27 exerting direct and indirect inhibitory effects on neoplastic cells. Studies have shown the tumor restricting effects of this cytokine on pediatric leukemias [8, 9], lymphomas [10], multiple myeloma (MM) [11], neuroblastoma [12], prostate cancer [13], non-small-cell lung cancer (NSCLC) [14], ovarian cancer (SKOV3 cell line) [15], colon cancer [16], esophageal cancer

[17], head and neck squamous cell carcinoma (SCC) [18], and melanoma [19]. These studies have suggested direct inhibition of cell growth/proliferation, migration, tumor angiogenesis, and IL-17 production, alongside with enhancement of NK cell responses, antibody-dependent cell-mediated cytotoxicity (ADCC), generation of myeloid progenitor cells, promoting M1 macrophage differentiation, and most importantly activation and promotion of tumor specific cytotoxic T cell responses as means of antitumor mechanisms by IL-27 [5–7, 20].

In spite of well-documented antitumor activities for IL-27, tumor promoting effects have been reported for this cytokine, as well. In contrast to pediatric leukemias, a study has shown that IL-27 improves survival of adult Acute Myeloid Leukemia (AML) cells and decreases their responsiveness to chemotherapeutic agents [21]. Other studies have suggested that IL-27 exerts some of its tumor promoting effects through induction of immune regulatory phenotypes, such as increasing the expression of molecules like IL-18BP [22], PD-L1/2 [23, 24], IDO [23], CD39 [25], Tim3 [26], and IL-10 [26].

The significance of the immune system in nonmelanoma skin cancers (NMSC), including Squamous and Basal Cell Carcinomas (SCC and BCC), has been long recognized, mainly based on the increased incidence of these neoplasms in organ transplant patients receiving immune-suppressants and immunomodulation due to ultraviolet light [27]. IL-27, with its diverse influences on immune responses, has not been studied extensively in NMSCs and its roles in cancer initiation, progression, and its probable use in NMSC treatment have yet to be revealed. In an attempt to further clarify the roles of this cytokine in NMSC, we designed a cross-sectional study in order to compare serum levels of IL-27 in NMSC patients and healthy individuals.

2. Materials and Methods

A cross-sectional analytical study was designed to investigate the serum levels of IL-27 in NMSC patients in comparison to normal individuals. A total of 60 patients with histopathologic diagnosis of SCC or BCC, who consented to be involved in the study, were enrolled from a dermatology clinic affiliated with Shiraz University of Medical Sciences. Their demographics, past medical history, and family history were gathered from clinical documents. Patients with previous history of any neoplastic or autoimmune diseases, and those with metastatic NMSC were excluded from the study. The comparison group consisted of 28 age-sex matched nonaffected individuals from the same geographic area with no history of malignant or autoimmune diseases and signs of infection at the time of sampling. The Medical Ethics Committee of Shiraz University of Medical Sciences approved that this study was in agreement with the Declaration of Helsinki principles [28].

5 ml of venous blood was collected from each participant. The blood samples were centrifuged and the obtained sera were stored at −80°C until analysis. Levels of IL-27 in the sera were measured by a quantitative enzyme-linked immunosorbent assay (ELISA) kit (Sigma-Aldrich; USA) according to the protocols described by the manufacturer.

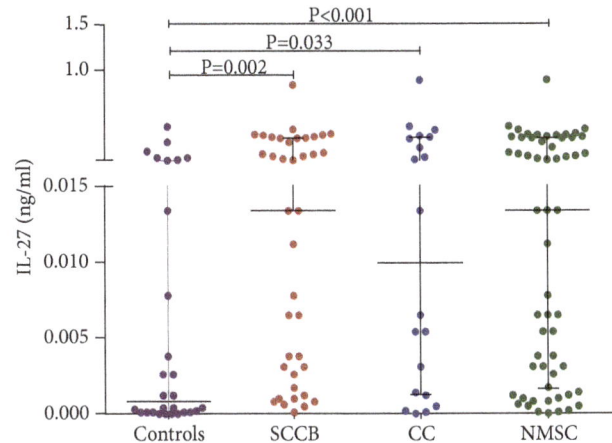

FIGURE 1: Scatter dot plot diagram of IL-27 serum levels; the middle line represents the median levels of serum IL-27. The ends of the whiskers represent 10-90 percentile; outliers are plotted as individual points; SCC: Squamous Cell Carcinoma; BCC: Basal Cell Carcinoma; NMSC: nonmelanoma skin cancer (SCC+BCC); IL-27 serum levels were significantly higher in NMSC, SCC, and BCC patients in comparison to controls (0.0134, 0.0134, and 0.0100 ng/ml respectively *versus* 0.0008 ng/ml).

Statistical Package for Social Sciences (SPSS, version 22; SPSS Inc., Chicago, IL, USA) was used for data analysis. Variables with normal distribution are presented as mean ± standard deviation (SD), otherwise as median. Frequencies are presented as percentages. Mann–Whitney U-test, Kruskal-Wallis, and Dunn's post hoc test were used to analyze the differences among groups. $P < 0.05$ was considered statistically significant.

3. Results

A total number of 60 NMSC patients and 28 healthy age-sex matched individuals, as controls, were involved in the study. The mean age of NMSC patients was 67.60±12.82 years, and male to female ratio was 3:1 (45:15). The most frequent diagnosis was SCC (n=40, 66.67%). Other clinicopathological features of the NMSC patients are presented in Table 1.

When comparing NMSC patients and controls, we observed that IL-27 serum levels were significantly higher in NMSC patients (Figure 1; 0.0134 *versus* 0.0008 ng/ml; P<0.001). In subgroup analysis according to pathologic diagnosis, serum levels of IL-27 were not different between SCC and BCC patients (P=1.000). However, we observed that SCC patients had higher levels of IL-27 in their serum in comparison to controls (Figure 1; 0.0134 *versus* 0.0008 ng/ml; P=0.002). The same was true when comparing IL-27 serum levels of BCC patients with controls (Figure 1; 0.0100 *versus* 0.0008 ng/ml; P=0.033). No other significant difference in IL-27 circulating levels was observed among different subgroups of patients (Table 1).

4. Discussion

Soon after its discovery by Pflanz in 2002 [29], IL-27 became a trendy subject in oncology-immunology, scientists started

TABLE 1: Clinicopathologic characteristics of nonmelanoma skin cancer patients and their respective IL-27 serum levels in each subgroup.

Variables		N(valid percent)	IL-27 serum level(ng/ml)	P-value[1]
Gender	Male	45(75.0%)	0.00715	0.070
	Female	15(25.0%)	0.0989	
Pathology	SCC	40(66.7%)	0.01615	0.621
	BCC	20(33.3%)	0.00995	
Tumor Site	Sun-exposed	54(93.10%)	0.0134	0.091
	Not Sun-exposed	4(6.90%)	0.2812	
Multiple lesions	Yes	8(16.67%)	0.0589	0.778
	No	40(83.33%)	0.0134	

[1] Mann-whitney U-test.

investigating its roles in carcinogenesis, use as a cancer biomarker, and designing novel immune therapies [5]. However the results of the conducted studies were controversial mostly depending on the type of neoplasm, its stage and many other known and unknown factors [4–6]. In this study we observed that IL-27 serum levels were significantly higher in NMSC patients in comparison to healthy individuals. Furthermore, when subcategorized based on pathological diagnosis, both BCC and SCC patients had higher levels of IL-27 in their sera compared to controls.

Studies investigating IL-27 roles in NMSC pathogenesis are scarce. In a study investigating IL-27 roles in skin tumorigenesis, Dibra et al. observed that increased levels of IL-27 enhance papilloma formation in the skin, help proliferation of mutated stem cells, sustain premalignant niche, increase angiogenesis, and augment vessel density, all of which lead to increased tumorigenesis [30]. However, in a survey on potential roles of IL-27 in head and neck SCC, Matsui et al. observed that this cytokine effects on murine NK cells resulted in longer survival, boosted cytotoxic activity, and probably ADCC of these cells, consequently leading to better antitumor responses [18].

Regarding Melanomas, Gonin et al. observed that IL-27 expression in melanomas was associated with tumor progression rather than regression [31]. They found that IL-27 might induce suppressive molecules such as PD-L1 and IL-10 and thus immunosuppressive responses and melanoma progression [31]. However, older studies on the melanomas have had converse results. These studies have shown that IL-27 exerts an antitumor effect on poorly immunogenic B16F10 melanoma by means of antiproliferative, antiangiogenic, Cytotoxic T lymphocyte (CTL), and NK cells activity [19, 32, 33].

NSCLCs are among the carcinomas that have been widely studied in this regard. In all studies, it has been proposed that IL-27 has tumor suppressing effects on NSCLCs [5]. The same seems to be true in cases of esophageal [17] and prostate [13] carcinomas and neuroblastomas [12, 34], and according to published studies IL-27 shows antitumor activity in these neoplasms. In case of hematologic malignancies, studies have shown the opposite roles for this cytokine. IL-27 seems to promote proliferation of human leukemic cell lines, suppresses sensitivity to chemotherapeutic agents [21],

and induces the expression of immunosuppressive molecules like PDL-1/2 [24].

Regarding ovarian carcinomas, study results have been paradoxical. While Zhang et al. have observed that IL-27 expression by plasmid transfected SKOV3 cells leads to suppression of ovarian cancer cells' proliferation and enhanced cytotoxicity [15], other studies have shown that IL-27 helps ovarian tumors' progression by escalating production of IDO, PDL-1 [23], and CD39 [25] and thus induction of immunosuppressive environment in favor of ovarian cancer progression.

The observations of this study are indicative of IL-27 association with NMSC and the results could be both the cause and effect (following host immune responses) of NMSC presence.

5. Conclusion

Although many studies suggested IL-27 administration for cancer immunotherapy [6], its therapeutic use as an anti-cancer agent may not be effective and potentially even detrimental (in certain tumors where IL-27 has been associated with a protumor effect). To draw any definitive conclusion there is a need for studies with larger sample sizes, considering the amount of sun exposure, other skin cancer risk factors, and participants' type of skin. Furthermore, correlating IL-27 levels to NMSC progression and prognosis requires longitudinal studies.

Acknowledgments

This work was supported by a grant from Shiraz University of Medical Sciences (Grant no. 1396-01-01-16171).

References

[1] S. Farkona, E. P. Diamandis, and I. M. Blasutig, "Cancer immunotherapy: the beginning of the end of cancer?" *BMC Medicine*, vol. 14, no. 1, article 73, 2016.

[2] W. K. Decker, R. F. da Silva, M. H. Sanabria et al., "Cancer immunotherapy: historical perspective of a clinical revolution and emerging preclinical animal models," *Frontiers in Immunology*, vol. 8, article 829, 2017.

[3] T. A. Waldmann, "Cytokines in Cancer Immunotherapy," *Cold Spring Harbor Perspectives in Biology*, vol. 10, no. 11, Article ID a028472, 2017.

[4] M.-S. Li, Z. Liu, J.-Q. Liu, X. Zhu, Z. Liu, and X.-F. Bai, "The Yin and Yang aspects of IL-27 in induction of cancer-specific T-cell responses and immunotherapy," *Immunotherapy*, vol. 7, no. 2, pp. 191–200, 2015.

[5] M. Fabbi, G. Carbotti, and S. Ferrini, "Dual roles of IL-27 in cancer biology and immunotherapy," *Mediators of Inflammation*, vol. 2017, Article ID 3958069, 14 pages, 2017.

[6] G. Murugaiyan and B. Saha, "IL-27 in tumor immunity and immunotherapy," *Trends in Molecular Medicine*, vol. 19, no. 2, pp. 108–116, 2013.

[7] N. Orii, I. Mizoguchi, Y. Chiba et al., "Protective effects against tumors and infection by interleukin-27 through promotion of expansion and differentiation of hematopoietic stem cells into myeloid progenitors," *OncoImmunology*, vol. 7, no. 5, Article ID e1421892, 2018.

[8] A. Zorzoli, E. Di Carlo, and C. Cocco, "Interleukin-27 inhibits the growth of pediatric acute myeloid leukemia in NOD/SCID/Il2rg-/- mice," *Clinical Cancer Research*, vol. 18, no. 6, pp. 1630–1640, 2012.

[9] S. Canale, C. Cocco, C. Frasson et al., "Interleukin-27 inhibits pediatric B-acute lymphoblastic leukemia cell spreading in a preclinical model," *Leukemia*, vol. 25, no. 12, pp. 1815–1824, 2011.

[10] C. Cocco, E. Di Carlo, S. Zupo et al., "Complementary IL-23 and IL-27 anti-tumor activities cause strong inhibition of human follicular and diffuse large B-cell lymphoma growth in vivo," *Leukemia*, vol. 26, no. 6, pp. 1365–1374, 2012.

[11] C. Cocco, N. Giuliani, E. Di Carlo et al., "Interleukin-27 acts as multifunctional antitumor agent in multiple myeloma," *Clinical Cancer Research*, vol. 16, no. 16, pp. 4188–4197, 2010.

[12] R. Salcedo, J. K. Stauffer, E. Lincoln et al., "IL-27 mediates complete regression of orthotopic primary and metastatic murine neuroblastoma tumors: role for CD8$^+$ T cells," *The Journal of Immunology*, vol. 173, no. 12, pp. 7170–7182, 2004.

[13] E. Di Carlo, C. Sorrentino, A. Zorzoli et al., "The antitumor potential of Interleukin-27 in prostate cancer," *Oncotarget*, vol. 5, no. 21, pp. 10332–10341, 2014.

[14] I. Airoldi, M. G. Tupone, S. Esposito et al., "Interleukin-27 re-educates intratumoral myeloid cells and down-regulates stemness genes in non-small cell lung cancer," *Oncotarget*, vol. 6, no. 6, pp. 3694–3708, 2015.

[15] Z. Zhang, B. Zhou, K. Zhang, Y. Song, L. Zhang, and M. Xi, "IL-27 suppresses SKOV3 cells proliferation by enhancing STAT3 and inhibiting the Akt signal pathway," *Molecular Immunology*, vol. 78, pp. 155–163, 2016.

[16] M. Hisada, S. Kamiya, K. Fujita et al., "Potent antitumor activity of interleukin-27," *Cancer Research*, vol. 64, no. 3, pp. 1152–1156, 2004.

[17] L. Liu, S. Wang, B. Shan et al., "IL-27-mediated activation of natural killer cells and inflammation produced antitumour effects for human oesophageal carcinoma cells," *Scandinavian Journal of Immunology*, vol. 68, no. 1, pp. 22–29, 2008.

[18] M. Matsui, T. Kishida, H. Nakano et al., "Interleukin-27 activates natural killer cells and suppresses NK-resistant head and neck squamous cell carcinoma through inducing antibody-dependent cellular cytotoxicity," *Cancer Research*, vol. 69, no. 6, pp. 2523–2530, 2009.

[19] T. Yoshimoto, N. Morishima, I. Mizoguchi et al., "Antiproliferative activity of IL-27 on melanoma," *The Journal of Immunology*, vol. 180, no. 10, pp. 6527–6535, 2008.

[20] Y. Chiba, I. Mizoguchi, J. Furusawa et al., "Interleukin-27 exerts its antitumor effects by promoting differentiation of hematopoietic stem cells to M1 macrophages," *Cancer Research*, vol. 78, no. 1, pp. 182–194, 2018.

[21] H. Jia, P. Dilger, C. Bird, and M. Wadhwa, "IL-27 promotes proliferation of human leukemic cell lines through the MAPK/ERK signaling pathway and suppresses sensitivity to chemotherapeutic drugs," *Journal of Interferon & Cytokine Research*, vol. 36, no. 5, pp. 302–316, 2016.

[22] G. Carbotti, G. Barisione, A. M. Orengo et al., "The IL-18 antagonist IL-18-binding protein is produced in the human ovarian cancer microenvironment," *Clinical Cancer Research*, vol. 19, no. 17, pp. 4611–4620, 2013.

[23] G. Carbotti, G. Barisione, I. Airoldi et al., "IL-27 induces the expression of IDO and PD-L1 in human cancer cells," *Oncotarget*, vol. 6, no. 41, pp. 43267–43280, 2015.

[24] H. Horlad, C. Ma, H. Yano et al., "An IL-27/Stat3 axis induces expression of programmed cell death 1 ligands (PD-L1/2) on infiltrating macrophages in lymphoma," *Cancer Science*, vol. 107, no. 11, pp. 1696–1704, 2016.

[25] S. M. d'Almeida, G. Kauffenstein, C. Roy et al., "The ecto-ATPDase CD39 is involved in the acquisition of the immunoregulatory phenotype by M-CSF-macrophages and ovarian cancer tumor-associated macrophages: regulatory role of IL-27," *OncoImmunology*, vol. 5, no. 7, Article ID e1178025, 2016.

[26] C. Zhu, K. Sakuishi, S. Xiao et al., "An IL-27/NFIL3 signalling axis drives Tim-3 and IL-10 expression and T-cell dysfunction," *Nature Communications*, vol. 6, article 6072, 2015.

[27] S. Rangwala and K. Y. Tsai, "Roles of the immune system in skin cancer," *British Journal of Dermatology*, vol. 165, no. 5, pp. 953–965, 2011.

[28] World Medical Association, "World Medical Association declaration of Helsinki ethical principles for medical research involving human subjects," *Journal of the American Medical Association*, vol. 310, no. 20, pp. 2191–2194, 2013.

[29] S. Pflanz, J. C. Timans, J. Cheung et al., "IL-27, a heterodimeric cytokine composed of EBI3 and p28 protein, induces proliferation of naive CD4$^+$ T cells," *Immunity*, vol. 16, no. 6, pp. 779–790, 2002.

[30] D. Dibra, A. Mitra, M. Newman et al., "IL27 controls skin tumorigenesis via accumulation of ETAR-positive CD11b cells in the pre-malignant skin," *Oncotarget*, vol. 7, no. 47, pp. 77138–77151, 2016.

[31] J. Gonin, A. Carlotti, and C. Dietrich, "Expression of IL-27 by tumor cells in invasive cutaneous and metastatic melanomas," *PLoS ONE*, vol. 8, no. 10, Article ID e75694, 2013.

[32] S. Oniki, H. Nagai, T. Horikawa et al., "Interleukin-23 and interleukin-27 exert quite different antitumor and vaccine effects on poorly immunogenic melanoma," *Cancer Research*, vol. 66, no. 12, pp. 6395–6404, 2006.

[33] Y. Chiba, I. Mizoguchi, K. Mitobe et al., "IL-27 enhances the expression of TRAIL and TLR3 in human melanomas and inhibits their tumor growth in cooperation with a TLR3 agonist Poly(I:C) partly in a TRAIL-dependent manner," *PLoS ONE*, vol. 8, no. 10, Article ID e76159, 2013.

[34] R. Salcedo, J. A. Hixon, J. K. Stauffer et al., "Immunologic and therapeutic synergy of IL-27 and IL-2: enhancement of T cell sensitization, tumor-specific CTL reactivity and complete regression of disseminated neuroblastoma metastases in the liver and bone marrow," *The Journal of Immunology*, vol. 182, no. 7, pp. 4328–4338, 2009.

19

Is Oral Omega-3 Effective in Reducing Mucocutaneous Side Effects of Isotretinoin in Patients with Acne Vulgaris?

Mina Mirnezami[1] and Hoda Rahimi ⓘ[2]

[1]*Department of Dermatology, Faculty of Medicine, Arak University of Medical Sciences, Arak, Iran*
[2]*Skin Research Center, Shahid Beheshti University of Medical Sciences, Tehran, Iran*

Correspondence should be addressed to Hoda Rahimi; hoda_rahimi@yahoo.com

Academic Editor: Bruno A. Bernard

Background. Acne vulgaris is an inflammatory disease of pilosebaceous units which may cause permanent dyspigmentation and/or scars if not treated. Isotretinoin is recommended in the treatment of recalcitrant or severe acne, but it is associated with common adverse effects that frequently result in patients incompliance and discontinuation of the drug. The present study was designed to assess the efficacy of oral omega-3 in decreasing the adverse effects of isotretinoin. *Materials and Methods.* In this randomized double-blind clinical trial, a total of 118 patients with moderate or severe acne were randomly divided into two (case and control) groups. The control group was treated with isotretinoin 0.5 mg/kg, and the case group was treated with the same dose of isotretinoin combined with oral omega-3 (1 g/day). The treatment was lasted for 16 weeks and mucocutaneous side effects of isotretinoin were recorded and compared between the two groups in weeks 4, 8, 12, and 16. *Results.* Cheilitis (at weeks 4, 8, and 12), xerosis, dryness of nose at all weeks, and dryness of eyes (at week 4) were less frequent in the group that received isotretinoin combined with oral omega-3 compared to the group that received isotretinoin alone. *Conclusion.* Administration of oral omega-3 in acne patients who are receiving isotretinoin decreases the mucocutaneous side effects of isotretinoin. *This trial is registered with* IRCT201306238241N2.

1. Introduction

Acne vulgaris is a common disease of the pilosebaceous units that affects both sexes during puberty. Although, severity and duration of acne vary in different people [1], its severe types are more common in males and its long-term forms are more common in women. Some studies have reported prevalence rate of 85% among people aged 12 to 25 [2, 3]. Mild acne resolves without scars, but the severe types may cause permanent scars [2–4]. Lesions are more common and severe in areas of the skin rich in sebaceous glands [5]. During puberty, following sebum production, *Propionibacterium* acne proliferates in the skin and some alterations occur in the follicular epithelial membrane, resulting in closed comedones which are the origin of the subsequent lesions. Effective medications for acne include benzoyl peroxide, topical/systemic retinoids, and topical/systemic antibiotics [6].

Isotretinoin is an oral retinoid and a derivative of vitamin A which has revolutionized the treatment of severe acne in recent years. However, it has significant mucocutaneous and systemic side effects such as teratogenicity and hepatotoxicity [7, 8]. Dryness of lips and nasal mucosa, conjunctivitis, and xerosis are the most common side effects [9–11]. In some cases, these side effects are so severe and annoying for the patient, which results in patient being incompliant and urging the physician to taper or discontinue the medication.

Omega-3 fatty acids (n-3 FAs) are a group of long-chain and very-long-chain polyunsaturated fatty acids (PUFAs) [12]. Since they cannot be produced by human body, their dietary intake is essential [13]. The main sources of omega-3 PUFAs are fish oils [14] and plants [15]. According to the 2012 National Health Interview Survey, omega-3 is a safe supplement without any major side effect. Omega-3 not only does not have any adverse effect on liver, but also can improve serum lipid profile by decreasing serum triglyceride and total cholesterol levels and increasing HDL cholesterol concentration [16]. Furthermore, several clinical trials have confirmed the efficacy of omega-3 in treatment of depression [17]. Lipid mediators derived from omega-3 fatty acids are anti-inflammatory molecules and play a major role in resolution of inflammation [18]. Some studies have reported their effectiveness in resolution of eczematous lesions [19] and prevention of allergic diseases [20]. Kangari et al. observed the effects of omega-3 in alleviating symptoms of dry eye syndrome [21]. In a study by Bhargava and Kumar on patients with contact lens-related dryness of eye, omega-3 significantly reduced this complication [22]. Creuzot et al. also proved the improvement of dry eye symptoms following administration of omega-3 [9]. In a study by Barcelos et al., administration of omega-3 reduced epidermal water loss and thus reduced xerosis symptoms in rats [23].

The impact of oral omega-3 on mucocutaneous side effects of isotretinoin in patients with acne vulgaris has not been evaluated yet. Since omega-3 is an inexpensive and available oral supplement with no adverse effect, if it proved to be effective in controlling mucocutaneous side effects of isotretinoin, it can be prescribed for patients receiving oral isotretinoin, resulting in more satisfaction and compliance of patients.

2. Materials and Methods

This case-control study included 118 patients with acne vulgaris, presenting to our dermatology clinic between May 2014 and May 2015. Patients with moderate or severe acne who did not respond to conventional therapy were enrolled after obtaining their written consent. The study was approved by our institutional ethics committee. Patients with hyperlipidemia, hepatitis, seafood allergy, or bleeding disorders; pregnant or lactating women; those who did not intend to use long-term contraception; and those who were receiving anticoagulant drugs, omega-3, or vitamin A derivates were excluded from the study.

Patients were randomly divided into two groups. The case group received oral isotretinoin (0.5 mg/kg) plus omega-3 soft gel capsules (1 g/day; Nature Made Company, CA, USA) and the control group received only oral isotretinoin with the same dose for 16 weeks. Mucocutaneous side effects of isotretinoin, including scaling/dryness of skin, cheilitis, crust formation in the nose, epistaxis, and conjunctivitis, were assessed in both groups by a dermatologist who was blind to the study at baseline and weeks 4, 8, 12, and 16.

Finally, these side effects were compared in two groups using chi-square test and t-test. All statistical analyses were performed using SPSS 16.0 (SPSS Inc., Chicago, IL, USA). $P < 0.05$ was considered as statistically significant.

3. Results

A total of 104 patients completed the study. Fourteen patients did not agree to complete the study because of remission of their lesions after the first prescription of isotretinoin. The case group included 50 patients and the control group included 54. The subjects were 67 females (64.4%) and 37

Table 1: Comparison of the frequency of sex and location of acne in case and control group.

	Isotretinoin group N (%)	Isotretinoin + omega-3 group N (%)	P value
Sex			
Male	19 (35)	18 (36)	0.931
Female	35 (65)	32 (64)	
Acne location			
Face	37 (68.5)	40 (80)	0.182
Face and trunk	17 (31.5)	10 (20)	

males (35.6%). Acne lesions in 77 cases (74%) were limited to the face and in 27 cases (36%) were located on both face and trunk. Eighty patients (77%) had severe (nodulocystic) acne and 24 patients (23%) had moderate (papulopustular) acne. The mean age of patients was 22.8 ± 4.9 years and the mean duration of the disease was 4.9 ± 3.6 years.

The two groups had no significant differences in age and mean duration of the disease. The two groups were also matched for the frequency of sex and location of acne lesions. (Table 1).

Table 2 summarizes mucocutaneous side effects of isotretinoin in case and control groups. Dry lips were significantly less frequent in case group in weeks 4, 8, and 12. Dry nose was found to be less frequent in the group treated with isotretinoin and omega-3 in comparison to the group treated with isotretinoin alone in weeks 4, 8, 12, and 16. Also, the dryness of skin in weeks 4, 8, 12, and 16 was significantly less frequent in the group treated with isotretinoin and omega-3 in comparison to the group treated with isotretinoin alone. Dry eyes were significantly less frequent in case group only in week 4, but it did not show significant difference between two groups in weeks 8, 12, and 16.

4. Discussion

In recent years, retinoids have been administered in a wide range of clinical conditions. Besides their several indications and well-established efficacy in dermatology, they are under investigation for their possible role in treatment and prevention of different kinds of malignancies [24, 25]. However, retinoid therapy may be complicated by some side effects, especially mucocutaneous toxicity, which can reduce patient compliance and result in tapering or even discontinuation of the treatment.

Currently, omega-3 PUFAs are in extensive research, particularly for their preventing and treating effects in organ-specific inflammation. They have also been shown to play a protective role in some degenerative diseases such as rheumatoid arthritis [25], type 2 diabetes mellitus [26], autoimmune disorders, cardiovascular diseases [12, 27], and malignancies [28, 29].

TABLE 2: Comparison of the frequency of mucocutaneous side effects of isotretinoin between case and control groups.

	Isotretinoin group (%)	Isotretinoin + omega-3 group (%)	P value
Dry lips			
Baseline	0	0	
Week 4	78.7	58	0.030*
Week 8	64.8	50	0.041*
Week 12	44.4	26	0.044*
Week 16	25.6	14	0.130
Dry nose			
Baseline	0	0	
Week 4	33.3	12	0.010*
Week 8	24.1	10	0.003*
Week 12	14	2	0.020*
Week 16	11.1	0	0.001*
Dry skin			
Baseline	0	0	
Week 4	40.7	16	0.003*
Week 8	22.2	10	0.021*
Week 12	18.5	8	0.002*
Week 16	11.1	2	0.013*
Dry eyes			
Baseline	0	0	
Week 4	13	4	0.046*
Week 8	9.3	6	0.533
Week 12	3.7	0	0.169
Week 16	0	0	1.00

*P values less than 0.05 were considered significant.

There are few studies concerning administration of omega-3 PUFAs to reduce side effects of retinoids [30–32]. The only trial investigating the role of omega-3 on triglyceride levels in patients receiving isotretinoin found that supplementation with omega-3 may be a useful way to manage lipid levels in these patients [32].

In the present study, administration of omega-3 reduced isotretinoin-induced xerosis. This might be attributed to increased skin hydration. A recent study by Barcelos et al. demonstrated that fish oil supplementation reduces the transepidermal water loss, increases the skin hydration, and consequently decreases skin dryness and pruritus in rats [23].

We found that dryness of eyes was less frequent in patients receiving omega-3. There are several additional studies supporting our result. In a recent randomized, double-blind, multicentric trial, Bhargava and Kumar showed benefits of oral omega-3 in alleviating dry eye symptoms [22]. In another study by Kangari et al., oral administration of omega-3 fatty was associated with a decrease of tear evaporation, an increase in tear secretion, and eventually improvement of dry eye symptoms [21]. However, none of these studies were performed in patients receiving isotretinoin.

Furthermore, we demonstrated that cheilitis and dryness of nose mucosa improved by administration of omega-3 in

patients who were receiving isotretinoin. To our knowledge, the effects of omega-3 on these complications were not evaluated in any of the previous studies.

5. Conclusions

Since oral omega-3 reduces mucocutaneous side effects of isotretinoin, it is recommended in patients with acne vulgaris who are receiving this drug. Future prospective randomized placebo-controlled trials with different doses and formulations of isotretinoin and omega-3 are required to confirm this hypothesis.

References

[1] R. Vender and R. Vender, "Double-blinded, vehicle-controlled proof of concept study to investigate the recurrence of inflammatory and noninflammatory acne lesions using tretinoin gel (Microsphere) 0.04% in male patients after oral isotretinoin use," *Dermatology Research and Practice*, vol. 2012, Article ID 736532, 2012.

[2] D. Lynn, T. Umari, C. Dunnick, and R. Dellavalle, "The epidemiology of acne vulgaris in late adolescence," *Adolescent Health, Medicine and Therapeutics*, vol. 7, pp. 13–25, 2016.

[3] P. C. Durai and D. G. Nair, "Acne vulgaris and Quality of life among young aduils in south india," *Indian Journal of Dermatology*, vol. 60, pp. 33–40, 2015.

[4] J. Burris, W. Rietkerk, and K. Woolf, "Acne, the role of medical nutrition therapy," *Journal of the Academy of Nutrition and Dietetics*, vol. 113, pp. 416–430, 2013.

[5] E. Y. Gan, W.-P. Koh, A. Z. Jin, A. W. H. Tan, H. H. Tan, and M. B. Y. Tang, "Isotretinoin is safe and efficacious in Asians with acne vulgaris," *Journal of Dermatological Treatment*, vol. 24, no. 5, pp. 387–391, 2013.

[6] E. T. Landis, M. M. Levender, S. A. Davis, A. N. Feneran, K. R. Gerancher, and S. R. Feldman, "Isotretinoin and oral contraceptive use in female acne patients varies by physician specialty: Analysis of data from the National Ambulatory Medical Care Survey," *Journal of Dermatological Treatment*, vol. 23, no. 4, pp. 272–277, 2012.

[7] T. Mehra, C. Borelli, W. Burgdorf, M. Röcken, and M. Schaller, "Treatment of severe acne with low-dose isotretinoin," *Acta Dermato-Venereologica*, vol. 92, no. 3, pp. 247-248, 2012.

[8] M. Kotori, "Low-dose Vitamin "A" Tablets–treatment of Acne Vulgaris," *Medical Archives*, vol. 69, no. 1, pp. 28–30, 2015.

[9] C. Creuzot, M. Passemard, S. Viau et al., "Improvement of dry eye symptoms with polyunsaturated fatty acids," *Journal Français D'Ophtalmologie*, vol. 29, pp. 868–873, 2006.

[10] F. Goforoushan, H. Azimi, and M. Goldust, "Efficacy of vitamin E to prevent dermal complications of isotretinoin," *Pakistan Journal of Biological Sciences*, vol. 16, no. 11, pp. 548–550, 2013.

[11] B. Bergler-Czop and L. Brzezińska-Wcisło, "The new therapy schema of the various kinds of acne based on the mucosa-skin side effects of the retinoids," *Cutaneous and Ocular Toxicology*, vol. 31, no. 3, pp. 188–194, 2012.

[12] E. M. Balk and A. H. Lichtenstein, "Omega-3 fatty acids and cardiovascular disease: Summary of the 2016 agency of healthcare research and quality evidence review," *Nutrients*, vol. 9, no. 8, article no. 865, 2017.

[13] M. G. Duvall and B. D. Levy, "DHA- and EPA-derived resolvins, protectins, and maresins in airway inflammation," *European Journal of Pharmacology*, vol. 785, pp. 144–155, 2016.

[14] P. C. Calder, "N-3 Fatty acids, inflammation and immunity: new mechanisms to explain old actions," *Proceedings of the Nutrition Society*, vol. 72, no. 3, pp. 326–336, 2013.

[15] E. J. Baker, E. A. Miles, G. C. Burdge, P. Yaqoob, and P. C. Calder, "Metabolism and functional effects of plant-derived omega-3 fatty acids in humans," *Progress in Lipid Research*, vol. 64, pp. 30–56, 2016.

[16] J. K. Innes and P. C. Calder, "The Differential effects of eicosapentaenoic acid and docosahexaenoic acid on cardiometabolic risk factors: A systematic review," *International Journal of Molecular Sciences*, vol. 19, no. 2, p. 532, 2018.

[17] P. Bozzatello, E. Brignolo, E. De Grandi, and S. Bellino, "Supplementation with Omega-3 Fatty Acids in Psychiatric Disorders: A Review of Literature Data," *Journal of Clinical Medicine*, vol. 5, no. 8, p. 67, 2016.

[18] C. Weise, D. Ernst, E. A. F. van Tol, and M. Worm, "Dietary polyunsaturated fatty acids and non-digestible oligosaccharides reduce dermatitis in mice," *Pediatric Allergy and Immunology*, vol. 24, no. 4, pp. 361–367, 2013.

[19] Y. Miyake, K. Tanaka, S. Sasaki, and M. Arakawa, "Polyunsaturated fatty acid intake and prevalence of eczema and rhinoconjunctivitis in Japanese children: The Ryukyus Child Health Study," *BMC Public Health*, vol. 11, article no. 358, 2011.

[20] C. Anandan, U. Nurmatov, and A. Sheikh, "Omega 3 and 6 oils for primary prevention of allergic disease: systematic review and meta-analysis," *Allergy*, vol. 64, no. 6, pp. 840–848, 2009.

[21] H. Kangari, M. H. Eftekhari, S. Sardari et al., "Short-term consumption of oral omega-3 and dry eye syndrome," *Ophthalmology*, vol. 120, no. 11, pp. 2191–2196, 2013.

[22] R. Bhargava and P. Kumar, "Oral omega-3 fatty acid treatment for dry eye in contact lens wearers," *Cornea*, vol. 34, no. 4, pp. 413–420, 2015.

[23] R. C. S. Barcelos, C. de Mello-Sampayo, C. T. D. Antoniazzi et al., "Oral supplementation with fish oil reduces dryness and pruritus in the acetone-induced dry skin rat model," *Journal of Dermatological Science*, vol. 79, no. 3, pp. 298–304, 2015.

[24] X.-H. Tang and L. J. Gudas, "Retinoids, retinoic acid receptors, and cancer," *Annual Review of Pathology: Mechanisms of Disease*, vol. 6, pp. 345–364, 2011.

[25] N. K. Senftleber, S. M. Nielsen, J. R. Andersen et al., "Marine oil supplements for arthritis pain: A systematic review and meta-analysis of randomized trials," *Nutrients*, vol. 9, no. 1, article no. 42, 2017.

[26] L. Manzi, L. Costantini, R. Molinari, and N. Merendino, "Effect of Dietary ω-3 Polyunsaturated Fatty Acid DHA on Glycolytic Enzymes and Warburg Phenotypes in Cancer," *BioMed Research International*, vol. 2015, Article ID 137097, 2015.

[27] K. R. Zehr and M. K. Walker, "Omega-3 polyunsaturated fatty acids improve endothelial function in humans at risk for atherosclerosis: A review," *Prostaglandins & Other Lipid Mediators*, 2017.

[28] M. Newell, K. Baker, L. M. Postovit, and C. J. Field, "A critical review on the effect of docosahexaenoic acid (Dha) on cancer cell cycle progression," *International Journal of Molecular Sciences*, vol. 18, no. 8, article no. 1784, 2017.

[29] H.-W. Yum, H.-K. Na, and Y.-J. Surh, "Anti-inflammatory effects of docosahexaenoic acid: Implications for its cancer chemopreventive potential," *Seminars in Cancer Biology*, vol. 40, pp. 141–159, 2016.

[30] I. Cabello, O. Servitje, X. Corbella, I. Bardés, and X. Pintó, "Omega-3 fatty acids as adjunctive treatment for bexarotene-induced hypertriglyceridaemia in patients with cutaneous T-cell lymphoma," *Clinical and Experimental Dermatology*, vol. 42, no. 3, pp. 276–281, 2017.

[31] A. Musolino, M. Panebianco, E. Zendri, M. Santini, S. Di Nuzzo, and A. Ardizzoni, "Hypertriglyceridaemia with bexarotene in cutaneous T cell lymphoma: The role of omega-3 fatty acids," *British Journal of Haematology*, vol. 145, no. 1, pp. 84–86, 2009.

[32] S. Krishna, J.-P. Okhovat, J. Kim, and C. N. Kim, "Influence of ω-3 fatty acids on triglyceride levels in patients using isotretinoin," *JAMA Dermatology*, vol. 151, no. 1, pp. 101-102, 2015.

20

Cutaneous Tuberculosis: Clinicopathologic Arrays and Diagnostic Challenges

Priyatam Khadka ⓘ,[1,2] Soniya Koirala,[3,4] and Januka Thapaliya[2]

[1]*Department of Microbiology, Tribhuvan University Teaching Hospital, Kathmandu, Nepal*
[2]*M.Sc. Medical Microbiology, Tri-Chandra Multiple Campus, Tribhuvan University, Nepal*
[3]*Department of Dermatology and Venerology, Tribhuvan University Teaching Hospital, Kathmandu, Nepal*
[4]*M.D. Dermatology, Maharajgunj Medical Campus, Tribhuvan University, Nepal*

Correspondence should be addressed to Priyatam Khadka; khadka.priyatam@gmail.com

Academic Editor: Luigi Naldi

The clinicopathological manifestations of cutaneous tuberculosis are diverse. The precise diagnosis is often overlooked, due to clinical presentations as those of cutaneous diseases with different etiology and the relative paucity of the pathogens in the lesions. Meanwhile, almost all of the diagnostic methods confer lower sensitivity and specificities which augments further diagnostic challenges. This article revises the current scenario of the disease's physiopathology and underscores clinicopathological challenges, due to multifaceted presentations of cutaneous tuberculosis, in the diagnosis.

1. Background

Cutaneous tuberculosis is a relatively uncommon, comprising 1-1.5% of all extrapulmonary tuberculosis manifestations, which manifests only in 8.4-13.7% of all tuberculosis cases [1]. Although rare, given its global prevalence, it is imperative for the clinicians to distinguish the many clinical variants of cutaneous tuberculosis and the masquerading infections—granulomatous syphilis, discoid lupus erythematosus, psoriasis, tuberculoid leprosy, sarcoidosis, actinomycosis, mycetoma, bacterial abscesses, and other skin infections—to preclude missed or delayed diagnosis [2, 3]. Most of the diagnostic methods for cutaneous tuberculosis confer lower sensitivity and specificities. Therefore, the physicians must resort to every possible test along with broad clinical consideration; hence the summation of positive rudiments would be auxiliary in precise diagnosis.

2. Epidemiology

Tuberculosis represents a major public health problem in Southeast Asia, since a larger proportion (45%) of total estimated 10.4 million infective cases were listed in the region [4]. Compiling the toll death rate, Southeast Region and African Regions accounted for 85% of total death due to tuberculosis [4]. TB ranks the 6th leading cause of death in Nepal [5]. The prevalence study was not done in Nepal due to impassiveness of government participation in the health sector; however, annually, 34,122 cases of tuberculosis were reported to NTP [6].

Tuberculosis is endemic in Nepal; limited cases of cutaneous tuberculosis were reported, however. The incidence of cutaneous tuberculosis in Central Nepal was reported as 0.1%; nonetheless, the exact incidence is still anonymous over the country. The clinicoepidemiological study done in Nepal by Dwari et al. 2010 revealed tuberculosis verrucous (48%) as predominant clinical type [7]; however, on referencing to earlier studies, Lupus vulgaris was the most common (64%), followed by tuberculosis verrucosa cutis (19%) and papulonecrotic tuberculid (4%) [8]. Ironically, cases of cutaneous multidrug resistant tuberculosis (MDR-TB)—resistant with at least two of the most potent first-line anti-TB medications, isoniazid and rifampicin—and XDR-TB—MDR strains that are resistant to fluoroquinolones plus one of the injectables such as kanamycin, amikacin, and capreomycin—have also been reported from India and China abutting Nepal [9–11]. Nevertheless, the exact epidemiological entity of perchance MDR/XDR cutaneous tuberculosis cases is still unbeknownst or unreported from Nepal.

3. Etiological Agent

The main etiological agent of the Cutaneous tuberculosis is *Mycobacterium tuberculosis*—occasionally *M. bovis* or BCG vaccine (an attenuated strain of *M. bovis*) [12, 13].

Mycobacterium tuberculosis is a straight or slightly bent (rod-shaped), nonmotile, nonsporulated, bacillus, being 1 to 10 μm long and 0.2 to 0.6 μm wide; its most important feature is acid-fastness due to high lipid content in the cell wall. Approximately there are 4000 genes with most of them involved in the mechanism of immune system invasion and 200 of them for lipid metabolism; consequently, the pathogen is able to survive both inside and outside the phagocytic cells [14]. Meanwhile, as lipids are the main energy source of *Mycobacterium tuberculosis*, the pathogen is directly responsible for multiplying in host tissue and forming cellular walls [14, 15].

4. Route of Infection

Cutaneous tuberculosis can be acquired from hematogenous or lymphatic dissemination of a pulmonary focus or by direct inoculation. The pivotal factor for the clinical presentations prior to contact with bacilli is the host natural immune response, however.

Exogenous infection occurs with direct inoculation of bacilli into the skin of predisposed individuals (tuberculous chancre, tuberculosis verrucosa cutis) [1].

Endogenous infection is secondary to a preexisting primary focus and may result from contiguous (orificial tuberculosis, scrofuloderma), hematogenous (acute miliary tuberculosis, tuberculous gumma, and lupus vulgaris), or lymphatic dissemination (lupus vulgaris) [2, 16].

5. Classifications of Cutaneous Tuberculosis Based on a Load of Pathogens

Based on a load of the pathogens on skin, the tuberculosis variant can be classified into two broad categories.

Multibacillary forms (easily detected in cutaneous tissue) include tuberculous chancre, scrofuloderma, orificial tuberculosis, acute miliary tuberculosis, and tuberculous gumma [17, 18].

Paucibacillary forms (bacilli being sparse) include TB verrucosa cutis, tuberculoid, and lupus vulgaris [17, 18].

6. Clinical Manifestations of Cutaneous Tuberculosis

Cutaneous tuberculosis exhibits diverse clinical manifestations: inflammatory papules, verrucous plaques, suppurative nodules, chronic ulcers, and other atypical lesions [19].

7. Exogenous Cutaneous Tuberculosis

7.1. Tuberculosis Chancre. The direct inoculations of Mtb in the skin from the traumatic injuries or surgical procedures performed with unsterilized materials and even after tattoos or body piercing lead to acquired tuberculosis chancre. Progressing from a firm, painless, reddish-brown, slow-growing papule, or nodule, after 2 to 4 weeks it develops into the friable ulcers—tendency to bleed with a granular surface [20]. Furthermore, the bacilli disseminate to regional lymph nodes via lymph.

Presumptive identification can be done with histopathological examinations, where the acute neutrophilic inflammatory reaction prolific in AFB and necrotic areas are usually noticed [16]. Sequentially, the lesion acquires a granulomatous form with enlarged giant cells after 3 to 6 weeks with the reduced number of bacilli [20].

7.2. Tuberculosis Verrucosa Cutis. Tuberculosis verrucosa cutis, the usual exogenous form of tuberculosis, is more common in an anatomist, physicians, and bare-footed children of tropical zones, since the infection proceeds with an injured dermal layer [1]. The lesions—solitary, painless, and without adenopathy—are more seen commonly in the extremities prone to traumas [16]. The lesions jerk as erythematous papules to verrucous plaques with peripheral extension.

8. Endogenous Tuberculosis

8.1. Scrofuloderma. Scrofuloderma, also called colliquative cutis, is a common form of cutaneous tuberculosis; it results from direct extension from an underlying tuberculosis lesion in lymph node, bone, joints, or testicles [1, 2]. The neck, axillae, and groin are often involved, with the cervical lymph nodes as a common source of infection [1]. Early lesions appear as firm, painless, subcutaneous, and red-brown nodules which advanced to ulcers and discharging sinus [21]. Spontaneous healing may occur, leaving keloid scars, retractions, and the atrophic sequel [21].

8.2. Orificial Tuberculosis. Orificial tuberculosis—a very rare form of cutaneous tuberculosis— is clinically characterized by ulcerations at mucocutaneous orifices including mouth, nose, perianal region, and genitalia and adjacent skin, usually advanced form of lungs, intestinal, or genitourinary tuberculosis [22]. The lesions, about 1 to 3 cm in diameter, appear as friable, painful erythematous-to-yellowish papules and nodules, which may advance to painful ulcers [16]. Edema and inflammation are obvious in perilesional tissue.

8.3. Lupus Vulgaris. Lupus vulgaris is the most common form of cutaneous tuberculosis in Europe, India, and Nepal [8, 13, 16]. It is a chronic, progressive, paucibacillary form of cutaneous tuberculosis which occurs primarily in the previously sensitized individual [23, 24]. The infection occurs endogenously via lymphohematogenous route and occasionally via exogenous route—with drainage scar of scrofuloderma [25].

The most typical clinical feature of lupus vulgaris is a papulotubercular lesions commonly on the legs and buttocks, which eventually coalesce into a plaque (Figures 1, 2(a), and 2(b)) [12]. The plaques grow peripherally, with serpiginous or verrucous borders, accompanied by central discoloration and atrophy [25]. Besides, the classic appearance is described as "apple jelly nodules" observed on diascopy [24, 26].

8.4. Tuberculous Gumma. Tuberculous gumma, also known as metastatic tuberculosis abscess, is an outcome of hematogenous dissemination of mycobacteria from primary focus especially in an immunocompromised host, scarcely in an immunocompetent host too [17, 27]. Clinically it may bear a semblance to scrofuloderma; few lesions affecting trunks and extremities with inconsistent subcutaneous nodules having tendency to ulcerate and drain caseous secretion are seen in tuberculous gumma [23].

8.5. Acute Miliary Tuberculosis. It is a rare presentation of cutaneous tuberculosis predominantly in severely immunocompromised host, demonstrating anergy. The bulk of cases have been increasing primarily due to coinfection with HIV with declining CD4 count below 100 cells/μL [28]. Clinically, diverse cutaneous lesions—erythema and erythematous-whitish or erythematous-purplish papules—may be noticed which later on break to form umbilication and crust formation leaving hypochromic scars [17].

9. Tuberculids

Tuberculids are acute or chronic cutaneous forms of tuberculosis, appearing with diverse clinical forms, having a propensity of hyperergic expressions, active TB, or disseminated forms [20]. The discrete relationship between tuberculids and TB continues to be debated because the clinical forms usually have a symmetrical distribution, tuberculous involvement (usually inactive) of viscera or lymph nodes, and the absence of AFB (low positivity to culture and PCR) in the lesions [16, 26].

9.1. Papulonecrotic Tuberculids. Papulonecrotic tuberculids are the commonly observed form of cutaneous in children and young people [29]. They appear as painless, symmetrical erythematous, or violaceous papulonodular lesions noted particularly around the face, ears, extensor areas of the trunk, extremities, and buttocks, leaving a depressed scar [26].

9.2. Lichen Scrofulosorum. Lichen scrofulosorum is an eruption of multiple, small, grouped, asymptomatic, firm, perifollicular, lichenoid papules or plaques often affecting children and adults with underlying diseases of bone and lymph nodes [16, 26]. The dermatosis leaves no scar after months or years. The onset of this tuberculid was speculated, after BCG vaccinations and in the patient infected with *M. avium-intracellulare* [30].

9.3. Erythema Induratum of Bazin. Erythema induratum of Bazin is a granulomatous lobular panniculitis, which appears as erythematous-purplish subcutaneous nodules usually in legs and thighs [26]. The nodules advance few centimeters in diameter forming deep ulcers with caseous discharges and leave pigmented scar without or after successful treatment.

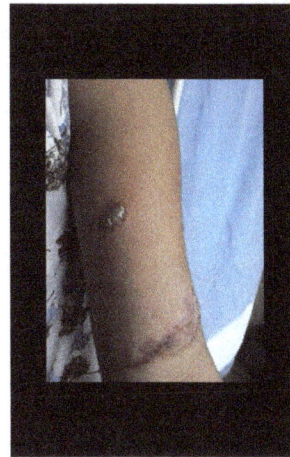

FIGURE 1: Erythematous plaque (2 ∗ 1 cm) of lupus vulgaris on right forearm of a 17-year-old female with a history of trauma forming a linear scar (4 ∗ 2 cm), visiting TUTH.

The relapse, however, may occur in flares every 3-4 months with similar clinical presentations [1]. Besides, the tendency of coinfectivity with systemic diseases like sarcoidosis is the differential clinical diagnosis of erythema nodosum [16, 21].

10. Diagnosis of Cutaneous Tuberculosis

10.1. Differential Diagnosis. The precise diagnosis is often significantly deferred and delayed, as cutaneous TB is not routinely considered in the differential diagnosis due to the relative paucity of pathogens in lesions and varied clinical manifestations (Table 1) [2, 16, 19, 31–33]. Hence, differential diagnosis is obligatory for the successful clinical management and treatment.

10.2. Laboratory Diagnosis

10.2.1. Tuberculin Skin Test. This technique involves an injection of 0.1 ml tuberculin, purified protein derivatives (PPD) derived from the attenuated strain of *M. tuberculosis*, intradermally, and read after 48 to 72 hours; on positive interpretation, the induration diameter exceeds the measuring of 10mm. The reaction is the classic example of delayed hypersensitivity reaction, where sensitized T-cells by prior infection are recruited thereby releasing the lymphokine [34]. These lymphokines induce indurations through local vasodilation, edema, fibrin deposition, and recruitment of other inflammatory cells to the area [34, 35]. TST has the sensitivity between 33% and 96% and specificity of 62.5% with cutoff 10mm for cutaneous tuberculosis; the sensitivity, however, exceeds 97% in an unvaccinated population [36, 37].

Furthermore, on analyzing clinical forms of cutaneous tuberculosis separately, positivity, intensity of the tuberculin skin test also diverges (Table 2). Conclusively, neither a positive TST necessarily indicates active infection nor a negative TST rules out the infection persistence.

10.2.2. Immunological Tests (Interferon Gamma-Release-Assay). The FDA approved immunological tests, QuantiFERON and

TABLE 1: Clinical manifestations of cutaneous tuberculosis and its differential diagnosis.

S. N	Classification of cutaneous tuberculosis		Diagnostic considerations
1	Exogenous cutaneous Tuberculosis	Tuberculosis chancre	sporotrichosis, leishmaniasis, atypical mycobacteriosis, syphilis, cat scratch disease and tularemia
		Tuberculosis verrucosa cutis	paracoccidioidomycosis, leishmaniasis, sporotrichosis, tuberculosis verrucosa and chromomycosis. Lobomycosis, atypical mycobacteriosis, hypertrophic lichen planus, verrucous carcinoma, iododerma, bromoderma, verruca vulgaris, keratoacanthoma centrifugum and pyoderma vegetans
2	Endogenous cutaneous tuberculosis	Scrofuloderma	tertiary syphilis, paracoccidioidomycosis, actinomycoses, lymphogranuloma venereum, bacterial abscesses, tumor metastasis, histiocytosis and hidradenitis
		Orificial tuberculosis	bullous diseases, trauma, fungal diseases, syphilis, sarcoidosis, or squamous cell carcinoma
		Lupus vulgaris	basal cell carcinoma, sarcoidosis, discoid lupus erythematosus, Leprosy, Deep Fungal infections
		Tuberculous gumma	leishmania, sporotrichosis, nocardiosis, atypical mycobacteria (*Mycobacterium marinum*), pyogenic infections (*Staphylococcus aureus, Streptococcus*), and deep fungal infections
		Acute miliary tuberculosis	metastatic carcinomas
3	Tuberculids	Papulonecrotic tuberculid	*pityriasis lichenoides et varioliformis acuta* (PLEVA), leukocytoclastic necrotizing vasculitis, pruritus and secondary syphilis
		Lichen scrofulosorum	lichen planus and lichen nitidus, syphilid lichenoides, eczematid, keratosis pilaris, pityriasis rubra pilaris (PRP) and micropapular sarcoidosis
		Erythema induratum of Bazin	erythema nodosum, cutaneous polyarteritis, pancreatic panniculitis, lupus profundus, subcutaneous sarcoidosis and cutaneous T-cell lymphoma

TABLE 2: TST result in different forms of cutaneous tuberculosis.

Clinical forms of cutaneous tuberculosis	Tuberculin skin test result
Tuberculosis chancre	initially negative, but becomes positive during course of disease (usually after 15 days)
Tuberculosis verrucosa	strongly positive
Lupus vulgaris	usually positive
Scrofuloderma	strongly positive
Orificial tuberculosis	negative
Acute cutaneous miliary tuberculosis	negative
Papulonecrotic tuberculoid	positive
Lichen scrofulosorum	positive
Erythema induratum of Bazin	positive

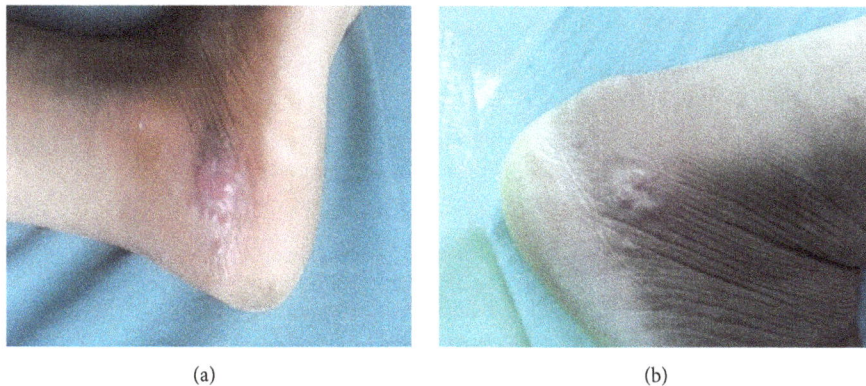

(a)   (b)

FIGURE 2: (a) Multiple erythematous papules of lupus vulgaris below lateral malleolus of right foot of 34-year-old female with a history of trauma on the right foot working in field 6 months earlier (before treatment). (b) The erythematous plaque reduced but did not resolve completely after antitubercular therapy; antitubercular therapy continued for three more months.

EliSpot, assess sensitizations to *M. tuberculosis* by measuring the amount of INF gamma released by lymphocytes confronted with *M. tuberculosis* specific antigens [16]. The sensitivity and specificity of QuantiFERON are 89% and 99%, respectively, while EliSpot has the sensitivity of 98.8% and a specificity of 100% [38]. Unlike tuberculin skin test (TST), it detects disease in patients who have been vaccinated against BCG (latent infection)—and active infection too.

These tests are still not in routine-practice in our midst, because of high cost and laborious cell extract procedure from culture to antigen preparation (particularly in EliSpot).

10.2.3. Histopathology. Histopathology of a skin biopsy shows granulomatous presentations as those of cutaneous diseases with different etiology—cutaneous leishmaniasis, tuberculid leprosy, superficial granulomatous pyoderma, cutaneous sarcoidosis, lupus miliaris disseminatus faciei, and chromomycosis [16, 19, 33]. Meanwhile, the exact elucidation in diagnosis of cutaneous tuberculosis could not be done; however, the characteristic feature (well-formed granulomas with absence of caseous necrosis, granulomas with caseous necrosis, and the presence of poorly formed granulomas with intense caseous necrosis) would be auxiliary to differentiate types of cutaneous tuberculosis (Table 3) [16, 19, 21, 26, 28, 33, 39].

The equivocal manifestation of cutaneous tuberculosis to correlate the histologic with clinical observations in an evidence-based diagnosis is imperfect and lacking pragmatics.

10.2.4. Diagnosis by Test: Staining and Culture. The mycobacterial cell wall is rich in complex lipids which resists the acid and alcohol; hence the pathogen is termed as acid-fast bacilli (AFB). Staining techniques include Ziehl-Neelsen (common in practice), Kinyoun, and fluorochrome-based techniques with auramine-rhodamine. Microscopic observation of AFB in staining of tissue or secretions enables the empiric therapy if there are sufficient clinical suspicions. However, this does not necessarily suggest the cutaneous tuberculosis, since the

other pathogens like *Nocardia*, *Corynebacterium*, nontuberculous mycobacteria, and even artifacts may reveal acid-fast characteristics [38, 40].

Furthermore, the lower sensitivities of staining results in extrapulmonary compared to pulmonary tuberculosis limit the applicability of the test [16, 37, 38]. The cultures of the pathogen, *Mycobacterium tuberculosis*, on specific solid media or by automatic detection of its metabolites in liquid media remain the gold standard method, for identifications and their drug sensitivities. However, the long generation time of the pathogens to grow and lower sensitivity of culture results for lesions and tissue samples attribute further challenges in prompt and accurate diagnosis of cutaneous tuberculosis [16, 38].

10.2.5. Amplifications of Nucleic Acids (PCR). The detection of Mycobacterium genus using bacterial 16S ribosomal DNA with PCR assays is now termed as a milestone in a diagnosis of pulmonary tuberculosis and several forms of cutaneous tuberculosis. DNA present in a sample of fresh tissues, blood, or a paraffin block even formalin fixed paraffin embedded sections, is amplified and it can then be identified, confirming the presence of mycobacteria [16, 33, 41].

PCR assay has augmented sensitivity and specificity in the diagnosis of cutaneous tuberculosis (Table 4) [42–55]; nevertheless, like other diagnostic approaches it is inconclusive in paucibacillary forms due to unevenly microbial distributions [25, 45].

10.2.6. Genotyping. Genotyping, the recent advance in the diagnosis of cutaneous tuberculosis, has a tendency to separate atypical mycobacteria from Mtb—and detect mutant if it persists inducing drug resistance in the pathogen. The major molecular typing methods—Spoligotyping, MIRU-VNTR (Mycobacterial Interspersed Repetitive Unit-Variable Number Tandem Repeats), and RFLP—detect *Mycobacterium tuberculosis*, DNA, or RNA in clinical specimens by in vitro nucleic acid amplifications, empowering investigations into epidemiology, transmission, and PTB outbreaks [56]. The

TABLE 3: Histopathological features of cutaneous tuberculosis.

Different forms of cutaneous tuberculosis	Histopathological features	Observation of AFB
Well-formed granulomas with absence of caseous necrosis		
Lupus vulgaris	epidermis may be atrophic or hypertrophic, featuring acanthosis, papillomatosis and even pseudo-epitheliomatous hyperplasia. Presence of well-formed tuberculous granulomas accompanied more often by Langhans giant cells, or foreign body-like granulomas in the reticular dermis.	infrequent
Lichen scrofulosorum	non-caseating, epithelioid cell granulomas in upper dermis and around dermal appendages	not seen
Intermediate forms: granulomas with caseous necrosis		
Tuberculosis verrucosa cutis	marked pseudoepitheliomatous hyperplasia of the epidermis with hyperkeratosis and dense inflammatory cell infiltrate consisting of neutrophils, lymphocytes, and giant cells. The presence of granulomatous infiltrates is a cardinal sign	can be seen
Primary cutaneous tuberculosis	it varies according to the time of inoculation; in recent lesions there is the presence of necrotizing neutrophilic infiltrate with numerous AFB. At a later stage there is organization of granulomas	decreased number
Acute miliary tuberculosis	skin consists of areas of an inflammatory infiltrate composed of lymphocytes, plasma cells, and neutrophils with focal superficial dermal areas of necrosis and abscess formation without true caseating granuloma. The presence of acid-fast bacilli with vascular thrombi is characteristic of these lesions	can be seen
Tuberculosis orificialis	there are tuberculoid granulomas, around a median, central, and superficial ulcer accompanied by caseous necrosis in the deep dermis	not usually found
Papulonecrotic tuberculid	lesions showed psoriasiform epidermal hyperplasia, and epithelioid granulomas with lymphocytes and Langhans giant cells with variable amounts of necrosis seen in the upper and mid dermis with a perifollicular distribution	not usually found
Poorly formed granulomas with intense caseous necrosis		
Scrofuloderma	Massive central necrosis with abscess formation and in many cases, suppuration, traces of granulomas can be observed at periphery of the lesions	may be found
Metastatic abscesses and gumma	Central ulceration with abundant caseous necrosis, surrounded by a rim of giant cells and macrophages can be observed	frequently detected

TABLE 4: Sensitivity and specificity of PCR in the diagnosis of cutaneous tuberculosis (literature review).

References and date	No. of samples	Sensitivity (%)	Specificity (%)
(Lee et al. 2016)	574	51.1	86.3
(Tan et al. 2001)	105	100	100 (multi-bacillary form)
		Overall 73 (positivity of 55% in cases of tuberculosis verrucosa and 60% in cases of lupus vulgaris; positivity of 54% for cases of erythema induratum)	not calculated (pauci-bacillary form)
(Chawla et al. 2009)	104	74.1	96.1
(Agarwal et al. 2017)	70	24.5	not calculated
(Salian et al. 1998)	60 (formalin fixed paraffin embedded)	73.6	100
(Ogusku et al. 2003)	37	43.7	90.4
(Negi et al. 2005)	37	95.2	100
(Abdalla et al. 2009)	34	88	83
(Hsiao et al. 2003)	34	56	not calculated
(Lall et al. 2017)	31	25.8	not calculated
(Khosravi et al. 2006)	30 (formaline fixed)	75	not calculated
(Ramam et al. 2013)	28	25	73.7
(Khine et al. 2017)	25	52	not calculated
(Quiros et al. 1996)	20	85	not calculated

clinical applicability testing of these genotyping techniques was also accessed in the patients with cutaneous tuberculosis in China by Ziang et al., 2017, with augmented sensitivity and specificity [57].

10.2.7. RFLP (Restriction Fragment Length Polymorphism). The gold standard in genotyping, IS6110-based restriction fragment length polymorphism (RFLP), has been for more than an epoch; however, it is laborious and costly and requires a large amount of chromosomal DNA [56].

10.2.8. Spoligotyping. Spoligotyping—commonly used to differentiate *Mycobacterium tuberculosis* complex strain—is based on polymorphisms of the chromosomal direct repeat (DR) locus, which contains a variable number of short DRs interspersed with nonrepetitive spacers [56, 57].

10.2.9. Mycobacterial Interspersed Repetitive Unit-Variable Number Tandem Repeat (MIRU-VNTR). Lately, the International consortium has proposed MIRU-VNTR as a standardized genotyping scheme, with 15- and 24-locus sets proven to have ample discriminatory power for tracing transmission and investigating the phylogenetics of tuberculosis [57].

11. Conclusions

In a limelight, almost all of the investigative methods confer lesser sensitivity and specificities for cutaneous tuberculosis, considering atypical erythema nodosum, nonspecific appearance, insufficiently elucidative radio-imaging approaches,

histopathology features, and even microbial culture techniques too. The genotyping techniques, nevertheless, could be an assistant to cope with this diagnostic challenge, paradoxically beyond reach to the third world like ours, due to expensive running cost and wanting equipped laboratory setup. In this perspective, the clinicians must resort to every possible test, so that supporting positive rudiments would be ancillary in the early and precise diagnosis of cutaneous tuberculosis.

Abbreviations

AFB: Acid-fast bacilli
MDR-TB: Multiple drug resistant tuberculosis
MIRU-VNTR: Mycobacterial Interspersed Repetitive Unit-Variable Number Tandem Repeat
Mtb: *Mycobacterium tuberculosis*
NTP: National Tuberculosis control Programme
PCR: Polymerase chain reaction
TST: Tuberculin skin test
XDR-TB: Extensively drug resistant tuberculosis.

Acknowledgments

The authors would like to thank Professor Dr. Jeevan Bahadur Sherchand (Department of Microbiology, Institute of Medicine) and Professor Dr. Dwarika Prasad Shrestha

(Department of Dermatology and Venerology, Institute of Medicine).

References

[1] L. van Zyl, J. du Plessis, and J. Viljoen, "Cutaneous tuberculosis overview and current treatment regimens," *Tuberculosis*, vol. 95, pp. 629–638, 2018.

[2] J. B. dos Santos, A. R. Figueiredo, C. E. Ferraz, M. H. de Oliveira, P. G. da Silva, and V. L. S. de Medeiros, "Cutaneous tuberculosis: Epidemiologic, etiopathogenic and clinical aspects - Part I," *Anais Brasileiros De Dermatologia Journal*, vol. 89, no. 2, pp. 219–228, 2014.

[3] N. Saxe, "Mycobacterial skin infections," *Journal of Cutaneous Pathology*, vol. 12(3–4), pp. 300–312, 1985.

[4] World Health Organization, *lobal Tuberculosis Report 2017: Leave no one behind - Unite to end TB*, 2017.

[5] Anonymous, "World TB day," *Nature Reviews Microbiology*, vol. 2, no. 5, Article ID 39490114, p. 360, 2004, http://ovidsp.ovid.com/ovidweb.cgi.

[6] Global Tuberculosis Report, *WHO Library Cataloguing-in-Publication*, 2016.

[7] B. Dwari, A. Ghosh, R. Paudel, and P. Kishore, "A clinicoepidemiological study of 50 cases of cutaneous tuberculosis in a tertiary care teaching hospital in Pokhara, Nepal," *Indian Journal of Dermatology*, vol. 55, no. 3, pp. 233–237, 2010.

[8] M. Mathur and S. N. Pandey, "Clinicohistological profile of cutaneous tuberculosis in Central Nepal," *Kathmandu University Medical Journal*, vol. 12, no. 48, pp. 238–241, 2014.

[9] Y. Pang, H. Dong, Y. Tan, Y. Deng, X. Cai, and H. Jing, "Rapid diagnosis of MDR and XDR tuberculosis with the MeltPro TB assay in China," *Nature Publishing Group*, pp. 1–8, 2016.

[10] X. Tao, Y. Guan, and Y. Mo, "Multidrug resistant Mycobacterium tuberculosis in cutaneous tuberculosis in China," *Annals of Nigerian Medicine*, vol. 7, no. 2, p. 71, 2013.

[11] V. Ramesh, M. K. Sen, and D. P. Sethuraman G, "Cutaneous tuberculosis due to multidrug-resistant tubercle bacilli and difficulties in clinical diagnosis," *Indian Journal of Dermatology*, vol. 8, no. 4, pp. 380–384, 2015.

[12] S. Ho, "Cutaneous Tuberculosis: Clinical Features, Diagnosis and Management," *Hongkong Dermatology Venereol Bull*, vol. 11, pp. 130–138, 2003.

[13] C. Aruna, A. L. Senthil, K. Sridevi, K. Swapna, and D. V. S. B. Ramamurthy, "A clinicoepidemiological study of cutaneous tuberculosis in a tertiary care teaching hospital in Andhra Pradesh, India," *International Journal of Research in Dermatology*, vol. 3, no. 1, pp. 88–93, 2017.

[14] I. Smith, "Mycobacterium tuberculosis pathogenesis and molecular determinants of virulence," *Clinical Microbiology Reviews*, vol. 16, no. 3, pp. 463–496, 2003.

[15] Z. Yang, D. Yang, Y. Kong et al., "Clinical relevance of Mycobacterium tuberculosis plcD gene mutations," *American Journal of Respiratory and Critical Care Medicine*, vol. 171, no. 12, pp. 1436–1442, 2005.

[16] M. F. R. G. Dias, F. Bernardes Filho, M. V. Quaresma, L. V. do Nascimento, J. A. D. C. Nery, and D. R. Azulay, "Update on cutaneous tuberculosis," *Anais Brasileiros de Dermatologia*, vol. 89, no. 6, pp. 925–938, 2014.

[17] F. Abebe and G. Bjune, "The protective role of antibody responses during *Mycobacterium tuberculosis* infection," *Clinical & Experimental Immunology*, vol. 157, no. 2, pp. 235–243, 2009.

[18] F. G. Bravo and E. Gotuzzo, "Cutaneous tuberculosis," *Clinics in Dermatology*, vol. 25, no. 2, pp. 173–180, 2007.

[19] S. Ramarao, J. N. Greene, B. C. Casanas, M. L. Carrington, J. Rice, and J. Kass, "Cutaneous Manifestation of Tuberculosis," *Infectious Diseases in Clinical Practice*, vol. 20, no. 6, pp. 376–383, 2012.

[20] M. Concha R, F. Fch S, R. Rabagliati B et al., "Tuberculosis cutánea: reporte de dos casos y revisión de la literatura," *Revista chilena de infectología*, vol. 28, no. 3, pp. 262–268, 2011.

[21] V. Ramesh, "Sporotrichoid cutaneous tuberculosis," *Clinical and Experimental Dermatology*, vol. 32, no. 6, pp. 680–682, 2007.

[22] N. N. Andrade and T. S. Mhatre, "Orofacial Tuberculosis—A 16-Year Experience With 46 Cases," *Journal of Oral and Maxillofacial Surgery*, vol. 70, no. 1, pp. e12–e22, 2012.

[23] R. R. Macgregor, "Cutaneous tuberculosis," *Clinics in Dermatology*, vol. 13, no. 3, pp. 245–255, 1995.

[24] A. H. Solis, N. E. González, F. Cazarez et al., "Skin biopsy: a pillar in the identification of cutaneous Mycobacterium tuberculosis infection," *The Journal of Infection in Developing Countries*, vol. 6, no. 08, 2012.

[25] A. Motta, C. Feliciani, A. De Benedetto, F. Morelli, and A. Tulli, "Lupus vulgaris developing at the site of misdiagnosed scrofuloderma," *Journal of the European Academy of Dermatology and Venereology*, vol. 17, no. 3, pp. 313–315, 2003.

[26] A. Frankel, C. Penrose, and J. Emer, "Cutaneous tuberculosis: a practical case report and review for the dermatologist," *The Journal of Clinical and Aesthetic Dermatology*, vol. 2, no. 10, Article ID 20725570, pp. 19–27, 2009.

[27] M. Almagro, J. Del Pozo, J. Rodríguez-Lozano, J. García Silva, M. T. Yebra-Pimentel, and E. Fonseca, "Metastatic tuberculous abscesses in an immunocompetent patient," *Clinical and Experimental Dermatology*, vol. 30, no. 3, pp. 247–249, 2005.

[28] P. del Giudice, E. Bernard, C. Perrin et al., "Unusual Cutaneous Manifestations of Miliary Tuberculosis," *Clinical Infectious Diseases*, vol. 30, no. 1, pp. 201–204, 2000.

[29] A. Singal and S. Sonthalia, "Cutaneous tuberculosis in children: The Indian perspective," *Indian Journal of Dermatology, Venereology and Leprology*, vol. 76, no. 5, pp. 494–503, 2010.

[30] G. Jacobsen, N. J. Samolitis, and R. M. Harris, "Lichenoid Eruption in a Patient With AIDS—Quiz Case," *JAMA Dermatology*, vol. 142, no. 3, 2006.

[31] I. Hadj, M. Meziane, O. Mikou, K. Inani, T. Harmouch, and F. Z. Mernissi, "Tuberculous gummas with sporotrichoid pattern in a 57-year-old female: A case report and review of the literature," *International Journal of Mycobacteriology*, vol. 3, no. 1, pp. 66–70, 2014.

[32] C. Chandrashekar, G. V. Anikethana, B. E. Kalinga, and I. S. Hasabi, "Cutaneous tuberculosis: a differential for chronic nonhealing ulcer," *Journal of Evolution of Medical and Dental Sciences*, vol. 3, no. 53, pp. 12366–12370, 2014.

[33] J. B. dos Santos, C. E. Ferraz, P. G. da Silva, A. R. Figueiredo, M. H. de Oliveira, and V. L. S. de Medeiros, "Cutaneous tuberculosis: Diagnosis, histopathology and treatment - Part II," *Anais Brasileiros de Dermatologia*, vol. 89, no. 4, pp. 545–555, 2014.

[34] "Targeted tuberculin testing and treatment of latent tuberculosis infection," *American Journal of Respiratory and Critical Care Medicine*, vol. 161, 3, pp. S221–S247, 2000.

[35] S. Nayak and B. Acharjya, "Mantoux test and its interpretation," *Indian Dermatology Online Journal (IDOJ)*, vol. 3, no. 1, p. 2, 2012.

[36] M. Ramam, A. Malhotra, T. Tejasvi et al., "How useful is the Mantoux test in the diagnosis of doubtful cases of cutaneous tuberculosis?" *International Journal of Dermatology*, vol. 50, no. 11, pp. 1379–1382, 2011.

[37] J. Barbagallo, P. Tager, R. Ingleton, R. J. Hirsch, and J. M. Weinberg, "Cutaneous tuberculosis: diagnosis and treatment," *American Journal of Clinical Dermatology*, vol. 3, no. 5, pp. 319–328, 2002.

[38] J. Almaguer-Chávez, J. Ocampo-Candiani, and A. Rendón, "Current panorama in the diagnosis of cutaneous tuberculosis," *Actas Dermo-Sifiliográficas*, vol. 100, no. 7, pp. 562–570, 2009.

[39] C. Aliağaoğlu, M. Atasoy, A. I. Güleç et al., "Tuberculosis verrucosa cutis," *European Journal of General Medicine*, vol. 6, no. 4, pp. 268–273, 2009.

[40] F. Peters, M. Batinica, G. Plum, S. A. Eming, and M. Fabri, "Bug or no bug: challenges in diagnosing cutaneous mycobacterial infections," *Journal of the German Society of Dermatology*, vol. 14, no. 12, pp. 1227–1236, 2016.

[41] T. Frevel, K. L. Schäfer, M. Tötsch, W. Böcker, and B. Dockhorn-Dworniczak, "PCR based detection of mycobacteria in paraffin wax embedded material routinely processed for morphological examination," *Journal of Clinical Pathology: Molecular Pathology*, vol. 52, no. 5, pp. 283–288, 1999.

[42] M. M. Ogusku, A. Sadahiro, M. H. Hirata, R. D. C. Hirata, C. Zaitz, and J. I. Salem, "PCR in the diagnosis of cutaneous tuberculosis," *Brazilian Journal of Microbiology*, vol. 34, no. 2, pp. 165–170, 2003.

[43] C. Suthar, T. Rana, U. B. Singh et al., "MRNA and DNA PCR tests in cutaneous tuberculosis," *Indian Journal of Dermatology, Venereology and Leprology*, vol. 79, no. 1, pp. 65–69, 2013.

[44] C. M. Z. Abdalla, Z. N. P. De Oliveira, M. N. Sotto, K. R. M. Leite, F. C. Canavez, and C. M. De Carvalho, "Polymerase chain reaction compared to other laboratory findings and to clinical evaluation in the diagnosis of cutaneous tuberculosis and atypical mycobacteria skin infection," *International Journal of Dermatology*, vol. 48, no. 1, pp. 27–35, 2009.

[45] S. H. Tan, H. H. Tan, and G. C. Sun YJ, "Clinical utility of polymerase chain reaction in the detection of Mycobacterium tuberculosis in different types of cutaneous tuberculosis and tuberculids," *ANNALS Academy of Medicine*, vol. 30, pp. 3–10, 2001.

[46] P.-F. Hsiao, C.-Y. Tzen, H.-C. Chen, and H.-Y. Su, "Polymerase chain reaction based detection of Mycobacterium tuberculosis in tissues showing granulomatous inflammation without demonstrable acid-fast bacilli," *International Journal of Dermatology*, vol. 42, no. 4, pp. 281–286, 2003.

[47] P. Agarwal, E. N. Singh, U. S. Agarwal, R. Meena, S. Purohit, and S. Kumar, "The role of DNA polymerase chain reaction, culture and histopathology in the diagnosis of cutaneous tuberculosis," *International Journal of Dermatology*, vol. 56, no. 11, pp. 1119–1124, 2017.

[48] E. Veringa, B. Van Harsselaar, and P. Hermans, "Polymerase chain reaction to detect Mycobacterium tuberculosis in a clinical microbiology laboratory," *Journal of Microbiological Methods*, vol. 16, no. 2, pp. 139–147, 1992.

[49] Y. J. Lee, S. Kim, Y. Kang et al., "Does polymerase chain reaction of tissue specimens aid in the diagnosis of tuberculosis?" *Journal of Pathology and Translational Medicine*, vol. 50, no. 6, pp. 451–458, 2016.

[50] E. Quiros, M. C. Maroto, A. Bettinardi, I. Gonzalez, and G. Piedrola, "Diagnosis of cutaneous tuberculosis in biopsy specimens by PCR and southern blotting," *Journal of Clinical Pathology*, vol. 49, no. 11, pp. 889–891, 1996.

[51] K. K. Zaw, A. G. WWA, and PWE, "Cutaneous TB: Different Clinical Types and Comparing the Values of its Diagnostic Tests," *Myanmar Health Sciences Research Journal*, vol. 29, no. 2, 2017.

[52] S. S. Negi, S. F. Basir, S. Gupta, S. T. Pasha, S. Khare, and S. Lal, "Comparative study of PCR, smear examination and culture for diagnosis of cutaneous tuberculosis," *Journal of Communicable Diseases*, vol. 37, no. 2, pp. 83–92, 2005.

[53] A. D. Khosravi and M. Omidian, "Application of polymerase chain reaction technique for laboratory diagnosis of cutaneous tuberculosis," *Pakistan Journal of Medical Sciences*, vol. 22, no. 3, pp. 291–294, 2006.

[54] H. Lall, N. Singh, M. Chaudhary, and I. Kaur, "Comparison of conventional and molecular methods in diagnosis of extrapulmonary (cutaneous) tuberculosis in a tertiary care hospital in Delhi," *International Journal of Medical Science and Public Health*, vol. 6, no. 1, p. 102, 2017.

[55] K. Chawla, S. Gupta, C. Mukhopadhyay, P. S. Rao, and S. S. Bhat, "PCR for M. tuberculosis in tissue samples," *The Journal of Infection in Developing Countries*, vol. 3, no. 02, 2009.

[56] Genotyping CA group on T. Guide to the Application of Genotyping to Tuberculosis Prevention and Control. 2004.

[57] H. Jiang, Y. Jin, V. Vissa et al., "Molecular characteristics of mycobacterium tuberculosis strains isolated from cutaneous tuberculosis patients in China," *Acta Dermato-Venereologica*, vol. 97, no. 4, pp. 472–477, 2017.

21

Dermatophytosis: Prevalence of Dermatophytes and Non-Dermatophyte Fungi from Patients Attending Arsho Advanced Medical Laboratory, Addis Ababa, Ethiopia

Adane Bitew (iD)

Department of Medical Laboratory Sciences, College of Health Sciences, Addis Ababa University, Addis Ababa, Ethiopia

Correspondence should be addressed to Adane Bitew; bitewadane@gmail.com

Academic Editor: Craig G. Burkhart

Background. Dermatophytosis is a disease of major public health problem around the globe causing a considerable morbidity. *Objective.* To study the prevalence of dermatophytosis and the spectrum of fungi implicated in causing the infection. *Methods.* Nail, skin, and scalp scrapings were collected from 318 patients and were used for microscopy and culture study. Fungal pathogens were identified by studying the macroscopic and microscopic characteristics of their colonies. *Result.* Tinea capitis was the predominant clinical manifestation consisting of 48.1% of the cases. Among 153 patients with tinea capitis, 73.2% were in the age group of 1-14 years. Of 318 study participants, 213 (67.98%) were found to be positive for dermatophytosis microbiologically. Out of 164 fungal isolates, 86 were dermatophytes and 78 were non-dermatophyte fungi. Among 86 dermatophytes, *T. violaceum* represented 38.4% of dermatophyte isolates and 89.7% of the isolates were recovered from tinea capitis. Of 76 non-dermatophyte molds, *Aspergillus* spp., *Scytalidium dimidiatum,* and *Cladosporium* spp. were the most common isolates, respectively. *Conclusions.* Failure to detect or isolate fungal pathogens in a large number of clinical samples revealed the limitation of clinical diagnosis in differentiating dermatophytosis from other skin infections demonstrating that clinical diagnosis should be coupled with laboratory methods. Recovery of large number of non-dermatophyte fungi along with dermatophytes in our study showed that non-dermatophyte fungi are emerging as important causes of dermatophytosis, warranting the implementation of intensive epidemiological studies of dermatophytosis across the country.

1. Introduction

Diseases caused by fungi can be divided into three broad groups: superficial mycosis, subcutaneous mycosis, and systemic mycosis. Among superficial mycosis, dermatophytosis is the most common contagious infection. It is a fungal infection of the outermost layer of skin and its appendages such as hair and nails with scalp ringworm being the most common in children of school age and adult males, respectively [1–4]. Dermatophytosis is currently a disease of worldwide importance and a public health problem in many parts of the world particularly in developing countries [5, 6]. Although the disease hardly causes death, it is a common refractory infection deleteriously affecting the quality of life via social stigma and upsetting day-to-day activities [1]. Large population size, low socioeconomic status, inadequate health facilities, and exchanging of foot-wears, clothes, and barber-shop materials among people in developing nation have been recognized as potential risk factors for the proliferation of the disease [1, 4].

Although species of *Epidermophyton, Microsporum,* and *Trichophyton* are the major cause of the mycosis [5, 7], an infection of skin and its appendage by non-dermatophyte molds and yeasts has been increasing [8–12]. Emergence of chronic diseases such as diabetes that resulted from an increase in the life expectancy of world population and suppression of host immune defense mechanisms by underlying diseases have made humans more susceptible not only to pathogenic fungi but also to all fungi that were once considered contaminants [13, 14].

Dermatophytes and non-dermatophyte fungi implicated as a cause of dermatophytosis have been recorded all over

TABLE 1: Frequency of clinical manifestation in relation to gender.

Clinical manifestation	Total number of samples	Sex	
	n (%)	Male n (%)	Female n (%)
Tinea capitis	153 (48.1)	63 (19.8)	90 (28.3)
Tinea corporis	57 (17.9)	19 (6.0)	38 (11.9)
Tinea unguium	60 (18.9)	21 (6.6)	39 (12.3)
Tinea pedis	14 (4.4)	4 (1.3)	10 (3.1)
Tinea faci	14 (4.4)	5 (1.6)	9 (2.8)
Tinea groin	8 (2.5)	6 (1.9)	2(0.6)
Tinea manum	12 (3.8)	3 (0.9)	9(2.8)
Total	318 (100)	122(38.4)	196(61.6)

the world, but with variation in distribution, incidence, epidemiology, clinical manifestations, and target hosts from one location to another. Differences in geographical location, health care, climatic factors, culture, and socioeconomic conditions are known to govern these discrepancies [15, 16].

In Ethiopia, studies conducted on dermatophytosis are few and these studies are concentrated on tinea capitis caused by dermatophytes primarily in children of school age [17–20]. There are only two studies of fungal infection of nails, skin, and scalp by dermatophytes and/or non-dermatophyte fungi [21, 22]. Furthermore, most of these studies were conducted before 2006. To this end, investigating human dermatophytosis regardless of age, site, and the distribution of fungi implicated in causing superficial mycosis appears to be one of the priorities in health related studies in Ethiopia.

2. Materials and Methods

2.1. Study Population. This prospective study was conducted from May 2017 to April 2018 at Arsho Advanced Medical Laboratory, Addis Ababa, Ethiopia. The study involved 318 patients that are clinically diagnosed for superficial mycosis and referred to Arsho from different health institutions for laboratory diagnosis.

2.2. Specimen Collection. Prior to sample collection, written informed consent was completed and signed by adult study subjects. Consent form was completed and signed by parents and/or guardians for those study subjects under 16 years of age. Patient information was collected using standard format. Nail, skin, and scalp scrapings were collected aseptically using sterile blades and transferred into sterile plastic petri-dishes.

2.3. Laboratory Diagnosis. Non-fungal elements were digested by placing clinical samples onto 20% potassium hydroxide (KOH) in a microscopic slide for about 5 to 10 minutes. The KOH preparation then was examined for the presence of fungal elements under low (×10) and high (×40) power magnification objective lenses. A portion of each clinical specimen was also streaked onto Mycosel agar and Sabouraud's dextrose agar containing chloramphenicol and gentamycin but without cycloheximide (BBL, Decton, Dickinsn and Company, USA). All plates were incubated at room temperature (25°C) for a minimum of 4 weeks

supervising them frequently for any fungal growth. Fungi were then identified by studying the macroscopic and microscopic characteristics of their culture. Texture, rate of growth, topography, and pigmentation of the front and the reverse side of the cultures were employed to characterize fungi macroscopically. Lactophenol cotton blue mount of each fungal isolate was used to characterize fungal isolates microscopically. Occasionally, urease test was used in the differentiation of *T. tonsurans*, *T. violaceum*, and *T. rubrum*. Many mycological laboratory texts and manuals [23–25] were used as reference materials in process of identification. Yeasts were identified by means of conventional routine diagnostic methods [25] and chromogenic medium, CHROMagar Candida (bioMérieux, France) as per the instruction of the manufacturer.

Ethical Clearance. All ethical considerations and obligations were duly addressed. The study was carried out after the approval of the research and ethical committee of Arsho Advanced Medical Laboratory private limited company (AAMLRERC). Data collection was started after obtaining written informed consent from study subjects and assent form was completed and signed by parents and/or guardians. All the information obtained from the study subjects was coded to maintain confidentially.

3. Results

In this study, a total of 318 clinical samples were collected from suspected cases of dermatophytosis of which 122(38.4%) were from male and 196 (61.6%) from female patients. Tinea capitis was the predominant clinical manifestation consisting of 48.1% (153/318) of the cases. This was followed by tinea unguium and tinea corporis representing 18.9% (60/318) and 17.9% (57/318) of the cases, respectively (Table 1).

As shown in Table 2, out of 318 study subjects enrolled, fungi were detected and/or isolated in 213 (67.98%). One hundred thirty-one (41.2%) clinical samples were KOH positive while 154 (48.4%) clinical samples were culture positive. Mixed infections were observed in 3.1% (n = 10) of the culture positive cases. Fungi were neither detected nor showed visible fungal growth in 105 (33.3%).

As depicted in Table 3, clinical manifestation in relation to age was the highest in study subjects with age group of 1-14

TABLE 2: Correlation of direct microscopy and culture (n= 318).

Test procedure	Number	Percentage
KOH positive	131	41.2
Culture positive	154	48.4
KOH negative culture positive	75	23.6
KOH positive culture negative	55	17.3
KOH and culture positive	62	19.5
KOH and culture negative	105	33.3

TABLE 3: Frequency of clinical manifestation in different age groups (n=318).

Clinical manifestation	Total sample	Age groups				
		1-14	15-24	25-44	45-64	>65
Tinea capitis	153	112	9	24	7	1
Tinea corporis	57	15	8	28	4	2
Tinea unguium	60	13	18	22	6	1
Tinea pedis	14	-	-	9	4	1
Tinea faciei	14	7	1	5	1	-
Tinea manum	12	3	1	7	1	-
Tinea groin	8	-	2	3	2	1
Total	318	150	39	98	25	6

(150) followed by age groups of 25-44 (98) and age groups of 15-24 (39), respectively. Out of 153 study subjects with tinea capitis, 73.2% (112/153) were ≤ 14 years of age. Study subjects in age group of 25-44 were the second most affected, tinea corporis being the highest. Tinea pedis was recorded in study subjects with an age of ≥ 25 years.

Among a total of 164 fungal isolates, dermatophytes were the most common isolates comprising 86 (52.4%) of the total isolates. *T. violaceum* was the dominant species involving 33 (38.4%) of the total dermatophyte isolates in which 29 (87.9%) of them were isolated from the scalp (Table 4). Seventy-eight isolates (47.6%) were non-dermatophyte fungi of which 69 (42.1%) were non-dermatophyte molds and the remaining 9 (5.5%) were yeasts. *Aspergillus* species (21), *Scytalidium dimidiatum (13)*, and *Cladosporium* spp. (13) were the 1st and the 2nd common isolates of non-dermatophyte fungi (Table 5). *Scytalidium dimidiatum* was isolated from patients only with tinea corporis and tinea unguium.

4. Discussion

In the current study, the prevalence of dermatophytosis was high (66.98%). This is understandable, given that Ethiopia is a tropical country with wet humid climate, large population size, low socioeconomic status, and inadequate health facilities that are conducive for the proliferation of dermatophytosis. Strong correlations between dermatological infections and low socioeconomic conditions, geographical locations, climate, overcrowding, health care, and hygiene have been demonstrated by many researchers [26–28].

Fungi were not detected and isolated in 33.3% study subjects suspected of having superficial mycosis indicating that differentiation of dermatophytosis from other related superficial infections by clinical means only is not reliable.

Coupling of clinical diagnosis with laboratory diagnosis appeared to be essential for better diagnosis as the cost and long duration of fungal therapy underline the significance of accurate diagnosis of the condition before starting therapy.

In our study, about seven different types of tinea were noted among which tinea capitis was the dominant clinical manifestation accounting for 48.1% of the total study subjects. According to Evans and Gentles [1], dermatophytosis affects both sexes, all ages, and all races, scalp ringworm being the predominant disease of children and tinea pedis being the predominant disease of adults, particularly adult males. Our result attested the work of Evans and his coworker [1] because, among study subjects with age ranging from 2 to 87 years, study subjects in the age range of 1-14 were the most affected with tinea capitis. Among 153 patients with tinea capits, 73.2% were in the age group of 1-14 years and tinea pedis was recorded in study subjects of ≥25 years of age. Differences in the amount of hormones before and after puberty [29] and insufficient production of fatty acids that have antifungal effect before puberty [30] are accountable for a difference in the prevalence of tinea capitis with age. Tinea capitis has been reported as the most frequent scalp infection affecting primary school children by previous studies conducted in Ethiopia [17–20]. These studies documented prevalence rates of tinea capitis in the range of 24.6-90%. In our study, tinea corporis, tinea unguium, and tinea pedis were less prevalent than tinea capitis. It has been reported that developing countries have high rates of tinea capitis, while developed ones have high rates of tinea pedis and onychomycosis [31]. High prevalence rates of tinea pedis and onychomycosis in developed countries have been related to increased urbanization of community showers, sports, and the use of occlusive footwear [16, 31, 32].

TABLE 4: Frequency and distribution of dermatophytes in relation to clinical manifestation.

Fungal isolates	Tinea capitis	Tinea corporis	Tinea unguium	Tinea pedis	Tinea faciei	Tinea groin	Tinea manuum	Total
				Clinical presentation				
T. violaceum	29	2	2	-	-	-	-	33
T. mentagrophytes	5	2	3	4	-	-	1	15
T. rubrum	2	3	-	2	1	1	1	10
T. tonsurans	-	3	1	1	-	-	-	5
T. soudanense	1	1	-	1	-	1	-	4
T. verrucosum	2	-	-	-	-	-	-	2
T. schoenleinii	5	-	-	-	-	-	-	5
M. audouinii	8	2	-	-	1	-	1	12
Total	47	10	5	7	2	2	3	86

TABLE 5: Frequency and distribution of non-dermatophyte fungi in relation to clinical manifestations.

Fungal isolates	Tinea capitis	Tinea corporis	Tinea unguium	Tinea pedis	Tinea faciei	Tinea groin	Tinea manum	Total
				Clinical presentation				
Scytalidium dimidiatum	-	2	10	-	1	-	-	13
Cladosporium spp	5	5	2	-	-	-	1	13
Alternaria spp	5	2	-	1	-	-	-	8
Fusarium spp	1	2	1	1	1	1	1	8
Scopulariopsis brevicaulis	-	1	4	-	-	-	1	6
Phialophora	-	3	-	-	-	-	-	3
Exophiala	1	2	-	-	-	-	-	3
Exophiala werneckii	-	-	-	-	-	-	2	2
Fonsecaea spp	-	1	-	-	-	-	-	1
Aspergillus niger	-	2	-	-	1	-	-	3
Aspergellus fumigatus	-	3	2	-	1	-	-	6
A.teresus	-	2	-	-	1	-	-	3
Candida albicans	1	1	7	-	-	-	-	9
Total	13	26	26	2	5	1	5	78

Out of 86 dermatophyte isolates in the present study, 69.8% were represented by *T. violaceum*, *T. mentagrophytes*, and *M. audouinii*, *T. violaceum* consisting of 38.4% of the total isolates and 89.7% isolated from patients with tinea capitis. Our finding was comparable with studies conducted in Ethiopia [17–20], many other African countries [33–35], and many Asian countries [36, 37]. According to Ameen [32], *T. violaceum* is an endemic dermatophyte in East Africa and Asia. Furthermore, 95.3% of the dermatophytes in our study were anthropophilic in contrast to developed countries where the major dermatophytes are zoophilic [38]. Differences in the mode of transmission of dermatophytes in developing and developed countries may explain the variation. In developing countries, transmission of dermatophytes from man to man is indirect via fomites (materials which are likely to carry infection, such as clothes, utensils, barbershop materials, and furniture). In addition to this, overcrowded human setting in developing countries has been noted as the main risk factor [37], whereas rearing and close proximity to domestic pets have been reported as significant risk factors for the transmission of dermatophytes in developed countries [39].

Non-dermatophytic molds were isolated from 44.8% culture positive study subjects, nails and skins being the most affected regions of the body. Our result was in line with the findings of Greer [40]. According to Greer [40], out of 691 nail infections, non-dermatophyte molds were recovered from 53% of the cases. The significance of non-dermatophyte mold species in skin-related infections has been highlighted in other many published studies [41–45]. However, the extent to which non-dermatophyte molds actually cause dermatophytosis particularly when a dermatophyte is present concurrently is still a subject of debate. Therefore, further investigations demonstrating how this group of fungi causes infection are needed.

Among non-dermatophyte molds isolated in the present study, *Aspergillus* species stood first. Our result supported the findings of Aikaterini et al. [46] and Nouripour-Sisakht et al. [47].

In the current study, *Scytalidium dimidiatum* represents a significant percentage of the non-dermatophyte mold isolates. They were isolated from skin and nail scrapings predominantly of toenails. *Scytalidium dimidiatum* and *Scytalidium hyalinum* are responsible for nearly 40% human superficial infections in tropical and subtropical regions [48]. *Cladosporium* spp., *Alternaria* spp., *Fusarium* spp., and *Scopulariopsis brevicaulis* were other most commonly isolated non-dermatophyte molds recorded in our study. The significance of such non-dermatophyte molds in causing skin-related infections has been demonstrated in many other studies [49–51]. Similarly, *Candida albicans* has been isolated in 9 subjects with nail infection. *Candida albicans* as a major cause of tinea unguium has been documented in many studies [8–10, 42, 44, 46, 47].

5. Conclusions

Failure to detect or isolate fungal pathogens in a large number of clinical samples revealed the limitation of clinical diagnosis in differentiating dermatophytosis from skin infection caused by other organisms noting that clinical diagnosis should be coupled with laboratory methods. Recovery of large number of non-dermatophyte fungi along with dermatophytes in our study showed that non-dermatophyte fungi are emerging as important causes of dermatophytosis, warranting the implementation of intensive epidemiological studies of dermatophytosis across the country.

Acknowledgments

The author would like to acknowledge Arsho Advanced Medical Laboratory for the provision of laboratory supplies and space. The author is also indebted to the patients.

References

[1] E. G. V. Evans and J. C. Gentles, *Essentials of Medical Mycology*, Churchill Livingstone, 1st edition, 1985.

[2] M. Ogutu, Z. Ng'ang'a, M. Namasaka, and M. Wambura, "Superficial mycoses among psychiatric patients in Mathari Hospital, Nairobi, Kenya," *East African Medical Journal*, vol. 87, no. 9, pp. 360–367, 2010.

[3] J. Del Boz-González, "Tinea capitis: Trends in Spain," *Actas Dermo-Sifiliográficas*, vol. 103, no. 4, pp. 288–293, 2012.

[4] J. N. Moto, J. M. Maingi, and A. K. Nyamache, "Prevalence of Tinea capitis in school going children from Mathare, informal settlement in Nairobi, Kenya," *BMC Research Notes*, vol. 8, article 274, 2015.

[5] E. I. Nweze, "Dermatophytosis in Western Africa: a review," *Pakistan Journal of Biological Sciences*, vol. 13, no. 13, pp. 649–656, 2010.

[6] E. I. Nweze and I. Eke, "Dermatophytosis in northern Africa," *Mycoses*, vol. 59, no. 3, pp. 137–144, 2016.

[7] S. A. Adefemi, L. O. Odeigah, and K. M. Alabi, "Prevalence of dermatophytosis among primary school children in Oke-oyi community of Kwara state," *Nigerian Journal of Clinical Practice*, vol. 14, no. 1, pp. 23–28, 2011.

[8] H. Al Shekh, "Epidemiology of dermatophtes in the eastern province of Saudi Arabia," *Research Journal of Microbiology*, vol. 4, pp. 229–234, 2009.

[9] Z. Erbagci, A. Tuncel, Y. Zer, and I. Balci, "A prospective epidemiologic survey on the prevalence of onychomycosis and dermatophytosis in male boarding school residents," *Mycopathologia*, vol. 159, no. 3, pp. 347–352, 2005.

[10] S. Beena, M. V. Sreeja, P. R. Bhavana, and S. Sreenivasa Babu, "Onychomycosis, prevalence and its etiology in a tertiary care hospital, south India," *International Journal of Health Sciences*, vol. 3, pp. 81–85, 2013.

[11] P. Satpathi, A. Achar, D. Banerjee, A. Maiti, M. Sengupta, and A. Mohata, "Onychomycosis in Eastern India - study in a peripheral tertiary care centre," *Journal of Pakistan Association of Dermatologists*, vol. 23, no. 1, pp. 14–19, 2013.

[12] M. Ali Asadi, R. Dehghani, and M. R. Sharif, "Epidemiologic study of onychomycosis and tinea pedis in kashan, Iran," *Jundishapur Journal of Microbiology*, vol. 2, no. 2, pp. 61–64, 2009.

[13] K. Bramono and U. Budimulja, "Epidemiology of Onychomycosis in Indonesia: Data Obtained from Three Individual Studies," *Nippon Ishinkin Gakkai Zasshi*, vol. 46, no. 3, pp. 171–176, 2005.

[14] M. M. Batawi, H. Arnaot, S. Shoeib, M. Bosseila, M. El Fangary, and A. S. Helmy, "Prevalence of non-dermatophyte molds in patients with abnormal nails," *Egyptian Journal of Dermatology and Venerology*, vol. 2, pp. 11–15, 2006.

[15] J. R. Hay, "Fungal infections," in *Oxford Textbook of Medicine*, D. A. Warrell, T. M. Cox, J. D. Firth, and E. J. Benz Jr., Eds., Oxford University Press, Oxford, UK, 2003.

[16] B. Havlickova, V. A. Czaika, and M. Friedrich, "Epidemiological trends in skin mycoses worldwide," *Mycoses*, vol. 51, supplement 4, pp. 2–15, 2008.

[17] Y. Woldeamanuel, Y. Mengitsu, E. Chryssanthou, and B. Petrini, "Dermatophytosis in Tulugudu Island, Ethiopia," *Medical Mycology*, vol. 43, no. 1, pp. 79–82, 2005.

[18] Y. Woldeamanuel, R. Leekassa, E. Chryssanthou, Y. Menghistu, and B. Petrini, "Prevalence of tinea capitis in Ethiopian schoolchildren," *Mycoses*, vol. 48, no. 2, pp. 137–141, 2005.

[19] Y. Woldeamanuel, R. Leekassa, E. Chryssanthou, Y. Mengistu, and B. Petrini, "Clinico-mycological profile of dermatophytosis in a reference centre for leprosy and dermatological diseases in Addis Ababa," *Mycopathologia*, vol. 161, no. 3, pp. 167–172, 2006.

[20] M. Leiva-Salinas, I. Marin-Cabanas, I. Betlloch et al., "Tinea capitis in schoolchildren in a rural area in southern Ethiopia," *International Journal of Dermatology*, vol. 54, no. 7, pp. 800–805, 2015.

[21] G. Teklebirhan and A. Bitew, "Prevalence of Dermatophytic Infection and the Spectrum of Dermatophytes in Patients Attending a Tertiary Hospital in Addis Ababa, Ethiopia," *International Journal of Microbiology*, vol. 2015, 2015.

[22] G. Teklebirhan, "Profile of Dermatophyte and Non Dermatophyte Fungi in Patients Suspected of Dermatophytosis," *American Journal of Life Sciences*, vol. 3, no. 5, p. 352, 2015.

[23] D. H. Larone, *Medically Important Fungi: A Guide to Identification*, American Society for Microbiology (ASM) Press, Washington, DC, USA, 5th edition, 1995.

[24] D. Frey, R. J. Oldfield, and R. C. Bridger, "A color Atlas of Pathogenic FungI," in *A color Atlas of Pathogenic Fungi*, Wolfe Medical Publications Ltd, London, 2nd edition, 1981.

[25] M. Kern, *Medical mycology, a self- instructional text*, F. D Davis Company, Philadelphia, Pennsylvania, 2nd edition, 1985.

[26] V. K. Bhatia and P. C. Sharma, "Epidemiological studies on dermatophytosis in human patients in Himachal Pradesh, India," *SpringerPlus*, vol. 3, no. 1, pp. 1–7, 2014.

[27] P. N. Chowdhry and S. L. Gupta, "Diversity of fungi as human pathogen," in *Recent Research in Science and Technology*, vol. 5, pp. 17–20, 2013.

[28] S. Accorsi, G. A. Barnabas, P. Farese et al., "Skin disorders and disease profile of poverty: analysis of medical records in Tigray, northern Ethiopia, 2005-2007," *Transactions of the Royal Society of Tropical Medicine and Hygiene*, vol. 103, no. 5, pp. 469–475, 2009.

[29] JAA. Oliveira, JA. Barros, ACA. Cortez, and JSRL. Oliveira, "Superficial mycoses in the city of Manaus," in *Superficial mycoses in the city of Manaus*, pp. 238–243, An. Bras. Dermatol, 2006.

[30] G. David, C. B. Richard, M. Barer, and W. Irving, *Medical Microbiology: a guide to microbial infections, pathogenesis, immunity, laboratory diagnosis and control*, Churchill Livingstone, 2003.

[31] C. Seebacher, J.-P. Bouchara, and B. Mignon, "Updates on the epidemiology of dermatophyte infections," *Mycopathologia*, vol. 166, no. 5-6, pp. 335–352, 2008.

[32] M. Ameen, "Epidemiology of superficial fungal infections," *Clinics in Dermatology*, vol. 28, no. 2, pp. 197–201, 2010.

[33] M. Lange, R. Nowicki, W. Barańska-Rybak, and B. Bykowska, "Dermatophytosis in children and adolescents in Gdańsk, Poland," *Mycoses*, vol. 47, no. 7, pp. 326–329, 2004.

[34] R. Caputo, K. De Boulle, J. Del Rosso, and R. Nowicki, "Prevalence of superficial fungal infections among sports-active individuals: Results from the Achilles survey, a review of the literature," *Journal of the European Academy of Dermatology and Venereology*, vol. 15, no. 4, pp. 312–316, 2001.

[35] A. M. Gargoom, M. B. Elyazachi, S. M. Al-Ani, and G. A. Duweb, "Tinea capitis in Benghazi, Libya," *International Journal of Dermatology*, vol. 39, no. 4, pp. 263–265, 2000.

[36] R. Kaur, B. Kashyap, and P. Bhalla, "Onychomycosis—epidemiology, diagnosis and management," *Indian Journal of Medical Microbiology*, vol. 26, no. 2, pp. 108–116, 2008.

[37] M. S. Ali-Shtayeh, A.-A. M. Salameh, S. I. Abu-Ghdeib, R. M. Jamous, and H. Khraim, "Prevalence of tinea capitis as well as of asymptomatic carriers in school children in Nablus area (Palestine)," *Mycoses*, vol. 45, no. 5-6, pp. 188–194, 2002.

[38] L. Triviño-Duran, J. M. Torres-Rodriguez, A. Martinez-Roig et al., "Prevalence of tinea capitis and tinea pedis in Barcelona Schoolchildren," *The Pediatric Infectious Disease Journal*, vol. 24, no. 2, pp. 137–141, 2005.

[39] J. G. Collee, A. G. Fraser, and J. G. Dugid, *Practical Medical Microbiology*, Churchill Livingstone Publishers, 14th edition, 1996.

[40] D. L. Greer, "Evolving role of non-dermatophytes in onchomycosis," *International Journal of Dermatology*, vol. 34, pp. 521–524, 1995.

[41] H.-H. Tan, "Superficial fungal infections seen at the National Skin Centre, Singapore," *Japanese Journal of Medical Mycology*, vol. 46, no. 2, pp. 77–80, 2005.

[42] R. C. Summerbell, J. Kane, and S. Krajden, "Onychomycosis, tinea pedis and tinea manuum casused by non-dermatophytic filamentous fungi," *Mycoses*, vol. 32, no. 12, pp. 609–619, 1989.

[43] R. J. Hay and M. K. Moore, "Clinical features of superficial fungal infections caused by Hendersonula toruloidea and Scytalidium hyalinum," *British Journal of Dermatology*, vol. 110, no. 6, pp. 677–683, 1984.

[44] F. Baudraz-Rosselet, C. Ruffieux, M. Lurati, O. Bontems, and M. Monod, "Onychomycosis insensitive to systemic terbinafine and azole treatments reveals non-dermatophyte moulds as infectious agents," *Dermatology*, vol. 220, no. 2, pp. 164–168, 2010.

[45] S. Bakheshwai, N. El Khizzi, A. Al Rasheed, A. Al Ajlan, and S. Parvez, "Isolation of Opportunistic Fungi from Dermatophytic Samples," *Asian Journal of Dermatology*, vol. 3, no. 1, pp. 13–19, 2011.

[46] A. Tsentemeidou, T.-A. Vyzantiadis, A. Kyriakou, D. Sotiriadis, and A. Patsatsi, "Prevalence of onychomycosis among patients with nail psoriasis who are not receiving immunosuppressive agents: Results of a pilot study," *Mycoses*, vol. 60, no. 12, pp. 830–835, 2017.

[47] S. Nouripour-Sisakht, H. Mirhendi, M. R. Shidfar et al., "Aspergillus species as emerging causative agents of onychomycosis," *Journal de Mycologie Médicale*, vol. 25, no. 2, pp. 101–107, 2015.

[48] M. Machouart, P. Menir, R. Helenon, D. Quist, and N. Desbois, "Scytalidium and scytalidiosis: What's new in 2012?" *Journal de Mycologie Médicale*, vol. 23, no. 1, pp. 40–46, 2013.

[49] E. Mercier, I. R. Peters, F. Billen et al., "Potential role of Alternaria and Cladosporium species in canine lymphoplasmacytic rhinitis," *Journal of Small Animal Practice*, vol. 54, no. 4, pp. 179–183, 2013.

[50] A. Tosti, B. M. Piraccini, C. Stinchi, and S. Lorenzi, "Onychomycosis due to Scopulariopsis brevicaulis: Clinical features and response to systemic antifungals," *British Journal of Dermatology*, vol. 135, no. 5, pp. 799–802, 1996.

[51] M. R. V. Straten, M. M. Balkis, and M. A. Ghannoun, "The role of non- dermatophyte Molds in onchomycosis: Diagnosis and treatment," in *Dermatologic Therapy*, vol. 15, pp. 89–95, 2002.

22

Confocal Microscopy Predicts the Risk of Recurrence and Malignant Transformation of Mucocutaneous Neurofibromas in NF-1: An Observational Study

Giuseppe Giudice,[1] **Giorgio Favia,**[1] **Angela Tempesta** (iD),[2]
Luisa Limongelli (iD),[2] **and Michelangelo Vestita** (iD)[1]

[1]*Section of Plastic and Reconstructive Surgery, Department of Emergency and Organ Transplantation, University of Bari, 11, Piazza Giulio Cesare, Bari, 70124, Italy*
[2]*Department of Interdisciplinary Medicine, Complex Operating Unit of Odontostomatology, "Aldo Moro" University, Piazza G. Cesare 11, 70124 Bari, Italy*

Correspondence should be addressed to Michelangelo Vestita; michelangelovestita@gmail.com

Academic Editor: E. Helen Kemp

From 2005 to 2010, 20 consecutive patients with fully manifested neurofibromatosis type 1 (NF1) underwent elective neurofibroma resection at our institution (Departments of Plastic Surgery and of Odontostomatology). Specimens were photographed under optical microscope and confocal laser scanning microscopy (CLSM) with ultra-high accuracy of detail, including depth of field. Patients were followed up for a minimum of 4 years and up to a maximum of 12 years, postsurgery. While all nonrecurring lesions showed intense fluorescence, six of the seven lesions with absence of fluorescence under CLSM recurred at a mean of 5.5 years after surgical excision. Among the re-excised lesions, 3 were diagnosed as malignant at the subsequent removal. Despite the limitation of a small cohort, CLSM appears to be a simple and low-cost technique to differentiate forms of neurofibromas with low and high risk of recurrence and malignant degeneration.

1. Introduction

We retrospectively describe our 5-year experience in using confocal laser scanning microscopy (CLSM) to differentiate the morphological features of Schwann cells at the time of first resection of neurofibromas arising in NF1 patients (study registration number: researchregistry3681). Based on our experience, we propose that CLSM could be a simple low-cost technique to differentiate neurofibromas with low or high risk of recurrence and malignant degeneration.

2. Report

From 2005 to 2010, 20 consecutive patients with fully manifested neurofibromatosis type 1 (NF1) underwent elective neurofibroma resection at our institution (Departments of Plastic Surgery and of Odontostomatology). The following demographic and clinical data were retrospectively included in our analysis: age, sex, location and type of neurofibroma excised, family history of NF1, recurrence after excision, time frame of recurrence, malignant degeneration, and other associated pathologies. All patients underwent wide (1.5 to 2 cm margins) surgical excision of burdening, symptomatic neurofibromas, with consequent direct surgical reconstruction of the defects, using local flaps or skin grafts. Excised specimens were fixed in 10% buffered formalin, paraffin-embedded, and cut in 8-12 μm thick sections and stained with hematoxylin and eosin, Masson's trichrome, and picrosirius red. Histological examination was carried out using Nikon Eclipse E-600 microscope, equipped with Argon-ion and Helium-neon lasers emitting 488 and 543 nm wavelengths, which allows both optical and confocal laser scanning analyses. Specimens were photographed and images were

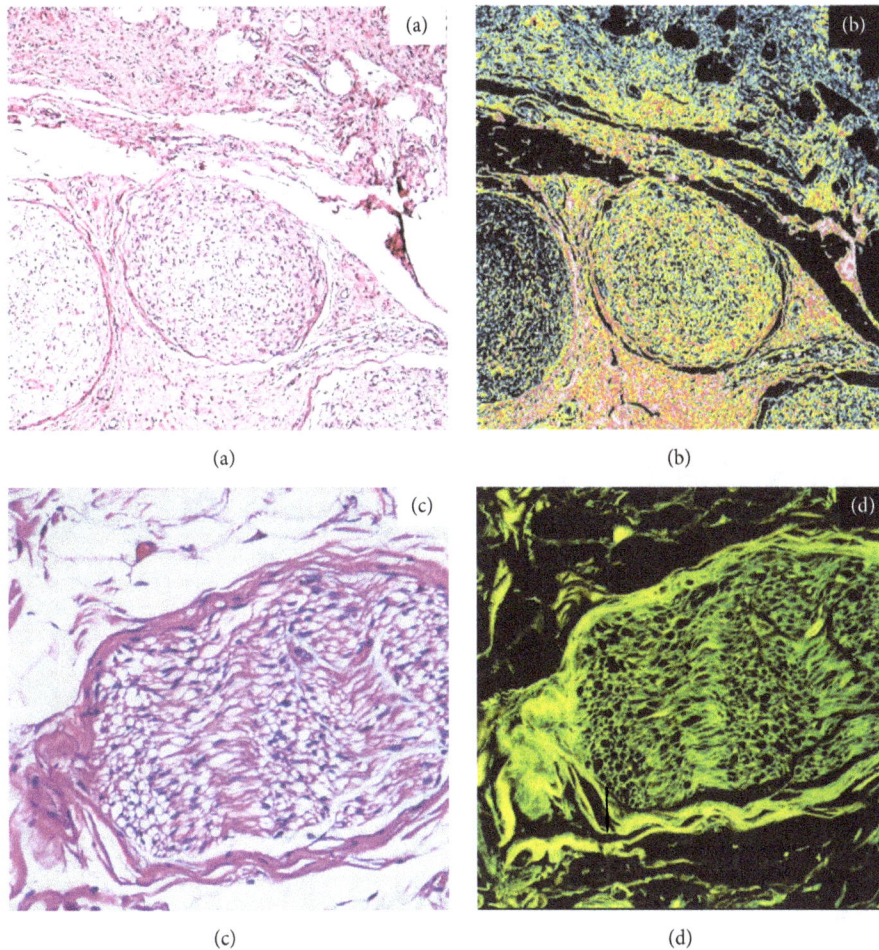

FIGURE 1: 45X. Traditional optical (a) and confocal laser scanning (b) analyses showing well differentiated Schwann cells in a multinodular plexiform neurofibroma and their intense fluorescence. Fields (c) and (d) show a normal nerve as comparison, respectively, in traditional optic and confocal laser scanning. A normal nerve also shows intense fluorescence. However, several features separate a neurofibroma from a normal nerve: an increase in cell density, an increase in the number of mitosis, and an increase in the number of spindle shaped cells, nuclear anomalies, and the presence of cells of a different nature (such as macrophages, mast cells, and histiocytes).

processed using the EC-1 software, with ultra-high accuracy of detail, including depth of field.

Patient characterics are summarized in Table 1.

Of the 20 lesions, 6 were subcutaneous/nodular, 9 were plexiform and 5 were diffuse. Schwann cells with similar morphological aspects under conventional microscopic investigation showed different patterns of endogenous autofluorescence during CLSM analyses at the time of first resection. These differences are due to their differentiation grade and to the percentage of residual neurofibromin in the cytoplasm: differentiated cells, rich in neurofibromin, showed an intense red and green fluorescence (Figures 1 and 2); less differentiated cells with minor neurofibromin content showed minimal fluorescence (Figure 3). Of the 20 lesions, 13 showed a high/medium grade of fluorescence, instead 7 showed a lack of fluorescence.

Patients were followed up for a minimum of 4 years and up to a maximum of 12 years, postsurgery. Six of the 7 lesions that showed a lack of fluorescence recurred at a mean of 5.5 years after surgical excision. The clinical-histological type of

recurrent lesions was as follows: 2 subcutaneous/nodular, 2 plexiform, and 2 diffuse lesions. All recurrent lesions were subsequently re-excised with larger margins, except in case 1 (Table 1) in which partial resolution of the neurofibroma was achieved with concomitant chemotherapy for the treatment of advanced melanoma [1]. Among the re-excised lesions, 3 were diagnosed as malignant at the subsequent removal (1 nodular, 1 diffuse, and 1 subcutaneous lesions). All recurring lesions showed absence of fluorescence under CLSM, with the exception of one case showing minimal fluorescence.

3. Discussion

CLSM appears to be a simple and low-cost technique to differentiate morphological features of apparently identical populations of Schwann cells and, thus, to differentiate forms of neurofibromas with low and high risk of recurrence and malignant degeneration. Specifically, we observed that neurofibromas that show negative laser fluorescence have a greater tendency to develop local recurrence and a greater

TABLE 1: Characteristics of the studied population and relative CLSM data.

Age	Sex	Excised neurofibroma site	Excised neurofibroma histo-type	Oral lesions	NF family history	Comorbidities	Recurrence	Time of recurrence (years)	Malignant degeneration	Schwann cells fluorescence
31	m	trunk	plexiform	x	x	advanced melanoma	x (regression with chemo)	6		none
47	f	lower limbs	subcutaneous/nodular							high
47	f	upper limb	diffuse	x			x	4	x	none
26	m	lower limbs	plexiform		x					high
42	f	upper limb	diffuse	x	x					high
73	f	trunk	plexiform	x		arterial hypertension, diabetes				high
44	m	trunk	Subcutaneous/nodular		x					high
16	m	oral	plexiform	x						high
59	f	upper limb	Subcutaneous/nodular	x			x	8		minimal
46	f	oral	plexiform	x						high
53	f	lower limbs	diffuse		x					high
53	f	face	plexiform			hypothyroidism				high
35	f	trunk	diffuse				x	7		none
41	m	oral	Subcutaneous/nodular	x	x					high
55	2	trunk	plexiform	x	x	arterial hypertension	x	3	x	none
50	2	face	diffuse	x						high
42	2	lower limbs	Subcutaneous/nodular		x					high
43	1	upper limb	plexiform	x						high
51	2	oral	Subcutaneous/nodular	x	x	arterial hypertension	x	5	x	none
47	2	lower limbs	plexiform		x					high

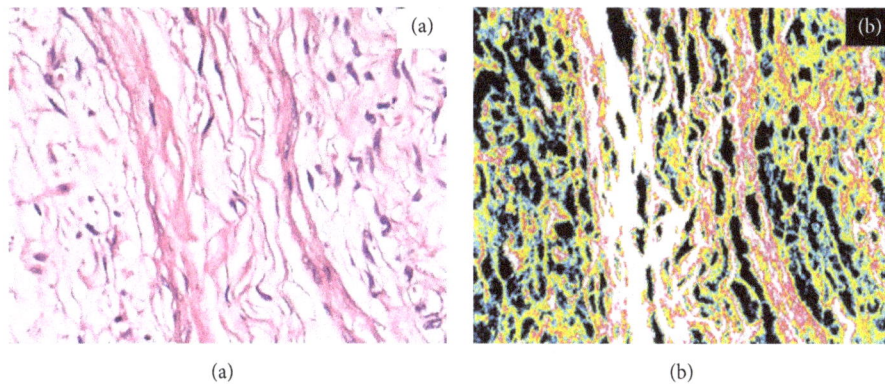

FIGURE 2: 150X. Traditional optical (a) and confocal laser scanning (b) analyses of a subcutaneous/nodular neurofibroma and its intense fluorescence due to the high content of neurofibromin in the well differentiated Shwann cells.

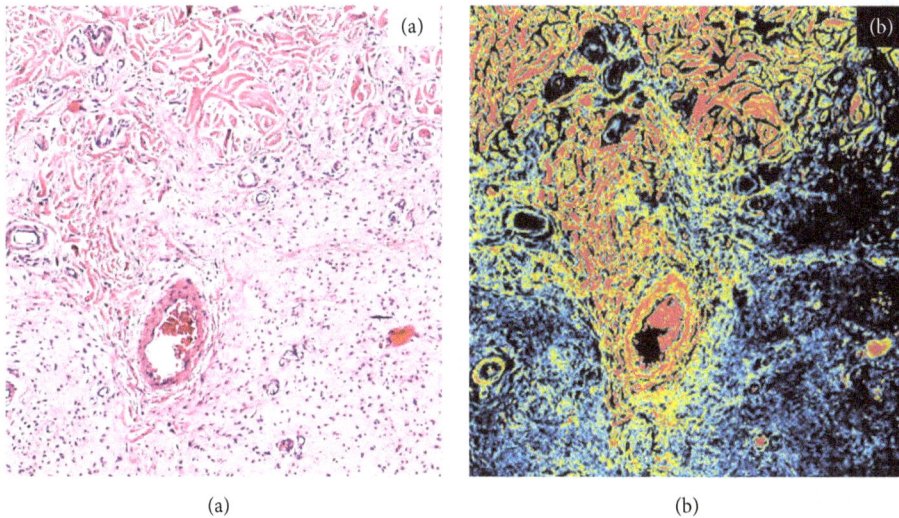

FIGURE 3: 50X. Traditional (a) and confocal laser scanning (b) analyses of an infiltrating plexiform neurofibroma with lack of fluorescence of proliferating Schwann cells in opposition with the high fluorescence of the fibroblasts of the deep dermis.

risk of malignant degeneration. Of note, there was no correlation between the incidence of recurrence\malignant degeneration and the clinical\histological type of neurofibroma in our cohort. These observations might tentatively be linked to peculiar aspects of the maturation and differentiation of Schwann cells in neurofibromas, which might translate into different concentrations of the cytoplasmatic content of neurofibromin, arising from differences in the morphological expression of genetic alterations of the NF1 gene (monoallelic or biallelic) [2–6] and the neural microenvironment [7]. Of course this is just speculation at present, and further immunohistochemical studies will need to demonstrate the possible link between neurofibromin content, fluorescence, and neurofibroma behavior. As a supplementary observation, the occurrence of a case of melanoma in our limited cohort seems to support the role NF1 and neurofibromin in neural crest-derived neoplasms, such as melanoma and other tumors [8–12]. More notable was the spontaneous partial regression of most neurofibromas (including a recurrent lesion after excision) when the patient underwent chemotherapy for his advanced melanoma [1].

In conclusion, despite the limitation of a small cohort, our preliminary data are encouraging and merit further assessment in a larger multicentre study. A correlation study to investigate the relationship between CLSM and molecular and genetic markers in Schwann cells would also be beneficial to further clarify the underlying structural and behavioral differences in these apparently indistinguishable cells.

Additional Points

(i) Confocal laser scanning microscopy might be able to differentiate the morphological features of Schwann cells in neurofibromas. Absence of fluorescence in Schwann cells was found in neurofibromas which later recur or undergo malignant degeneration. (ii) Confocal laser scanning microscopy could be used to identify neurofibromas that tend to recur or to degenerate and therefore need a more radical surgical management or closer follow-up.

References

[1] M. Guida, A. Cramarossa, E. Fistola et al., "High activity of sequential low dose chemo-modulating Temozolomide in combination with Fotemustine in metastatic melanoma. A feasibility study," *Journal of Translational Medicine*, vol. 8, article no. 115, 2010.

[2] N. Ratner and S. J. Miller, "A RASopathy gene commonly mutated in cancer: The neurofibromatosis type 1 tumour suppressor," *Nature Reviews Cancer*, vol. 15, no. 5, pp. 290–301, 2015.

[3] A. Cannon, M. Chen, P. Li et al., "Cutaneous neurofibromas in Neurofibromatosis type I: a quantitative natural history study," *Orphanet Journal of Rare Diseases*, vol. 13, no. 1, 2018.

[4] C. L. Monroe, S. Dahiya, and D. H. Gutmann, "Dissecting Clinical Heterogeneity in Neurofibromatosis Type 1," *Annual Review of Pathology: Mechanisms of Disease*, vol. 12, pp. 53–74, 2017.

[5] C. S. Higham, E. Dombi, A. Rogiers et al., "The characteristics of 76 atypical neurofibromas as precursors to neurofibromatosis 1 associated malignant peripheral nerve sheath tumors," *Neuro-Oncology*, vol. 20, no. 6, pp. 818–825, 2018.

[6] F. Calì, V. Chiavetta, G. Ruggeri et al., "Mutation spectrum of in Italian patients with neurofibromatosis type 1 using Ion Torrent PGM platform," *Eur J Med Genet*, vol. 60, no. 2, pp. 93–99, 2017.

[7] C.-P. Liao, S. Pradhan, Z. Chen, A. J. Patel, R. C. Booker, and L. Q. Le, "The role of nerve microenvironment for neurofibroma development," *Oncotarget* , vol. 7, no. 38, pp. 61500–61508, 2016.

[8] M. Mahalingam, "NF1 and Neurofibromin: Emerging Players in the Genetic Landscape of Desmoplastic Melanoma," *Advances in Anatomic Pathology*, vol. 24, no. 1, pp. 1–14, 2017.

[9] Á. Nagy, F. Garzuly, and B. Kßlmßn, "Pathogenic alterations within the neurofibromin gene in various cancers," *Magy Onkol*, vol. 61, no. 4, pp. 327–336, 2017.

[10] S. J. Howell, K. Hockenhull, Z. Salih, and D. G. Evans, "Increased risk of breast cancer in neurofibromatosis type 1: Current insights," *Breast Cancer : Targets and Therapy*, vol. 9, pp. 531–536, 2017.

[11] C. Philpott, H. Tovell, I. M. Frayling, D. N. Cooper, and M. Upadhyaya, "The NF1 somatic mutational landscape in sporadic human cancers," *Human Genomics*, vol. 11, no. 1, 2017.

[12] M. Kiuru and K. J. Busam, "The NF1 gene in tumor syndromes and melanoma," *Laboratory Investigation*, vol. 97, no. 2, pp. 146–157, 2017.

23

Evaluation of Therapeutic Efficacy and Safety of Tranexamic Acid Local Infiltration in Combination with Topical 4% Hydroquinone Cream Compared to Topical 4%Hydroquinone Cream Alone in Patients with Melasma: A Split-Face Study

Zohreh Tehranchinia, Bita Saghi ⓘ, and Hoda Rahimi ⓘ

Skin Research Center, Shahid Beheshti University of Medical Sciences, Tehran, Iran

Correspondence should be addressed to Bita Saghi; dr.saghi2020@yahoo.com

Academic Editor: Markus Stucker

Introduction. Melasma is an acquired pigmentary disorder characterized by hyperpigmented macules and/or patches affecting sun-exposed skin. Tranexamic acid (TA) can reduce melanin content of epidermis. Thus, we conducted this study to evaluate the efficacy and safety of tranexamic acid local infiltration in combination with topical 4% hydroquinone cream compared to topical 4% hydroquinone cream alone in patients with melasma. *Material and Methods.* This study was a prospective assessor- and analyst-blind, randomized split-face clinical trial which was performed on patients with bilateral malar epidermal melasma. A total of 55 patients were enrolled, and each side of their face was randomly allocated to either TA+HQ or HQ alone treatment. The MASI score was applied as an objective measurement to compare two treatment groups. The patient's satisfaction of melasma treatment was evaluated using a four-scale grading, as well. *Results.* The mean of MASI score in week 16 decreased in both groups significantly ($p < 0.01$). The therapeutic outcomes were significantly better in TA+HQ group than HQ group ($p=0.001$). Patients satisfaction with treatment was significantly higher in the TA + HQ group. The difference between the two groups regarding side effect occurrence was not statistically significant. *Conclusion.* Addition of tranexamic acid injections to conventional hydroquinone therapy can increase the efficacy of topical treatment. **This trial is registered with** IRCT2015110324865N1.

1. Introduction

Melasma, which may be symmetric or asymmetric, is an acquired pigmentary disorder characterized by hyperpigmented macules and/or patches affecting sun-exposed skin [1–4]. The precise etiology of melasma is unknown, but ultraviolet radiation, pregnancy, oral contraceptives (OCP), hormonal therapy, phototoxic and antiseizure drugs, and thyroid dysfunction are considered risk factors of melasma [1, 2, 4–6]. Melasma may impose major psychological and emotional burden on patients and affect their quality of life. Common therapeutic approaches for melasma include topical hydroquinone (HQ), azelaic acid, steroids, chemical peels, and lasers, most of which could not induce remarkable and constant satisfying outcomes [2, 3, 7].

Tranexamic acid (TA), an inhibitor of plasminogen activation, has been recently used in the treatment of melasma in different investigations [4–11]. The exact mechanism of action of tranexamic acid is still unknown, but the evidence shows that it can reduce the melanin content of epidermis, decrease the dermal vascularity, and mast cell numbers[7].

Although tranexamic acid is currently the only drug which can prevent hormonal, UV-induced, and keratinocyte-derived melanocyte activation and has shown promising results in treatment of melasma, blinded clinical trials that compare this drug with other conventional treatments are few. Thus, we conducted this study to evaluate the efficacy and safety of tranexamic acid local infiltration in combination with topical 4% hydroquinone cream compared to topical 4% hydroquinone cream alone in patients with melasma.

2. Patients and Methods

This study was a prospective assessor- and analyst-blind, randomized split-face clinical trial which was performed on patients with bilateral malar epidermal melasma. Exclusion criteria included pregnancy, lactation, any melasma treatment within 1 month prior to study, taking OCP or phototoxic drugs during 1 month prior to study, and history of vitiligo. The study was approved by our ethics committee and was registered on our national clinical trial registry (registration no. IRCT2015110324865N1). Informed consent was obtained from all patients before participation in the study.

A total of 55 patients were enrolled, and each side of their face was randomly allocated to either TA+HQ or HQ alone treatment. All patients applied topical HQ 4% cream (Merck Company, Germany) on his/her both malar sides every night, for 12 weeks. The TA+HQ side of the face received additional 1 mL TA (Caspian Tamin Company, 100 mg/ml) intradermal injection with 1 cm intervals by an insulin syringe with a 30-gauge needle at weeks 0, 4, 8, and 12. All patients were recommended to use a sunscreen cream with sun protection factor of 50.

The pretreatment assessment including comprehensive history, physical examination, melasma and severity index (MASI) scoring, and colour photographs were done by an expert dermatologist. The visit sessions were repeated at weeks 4, 8, 12, and 16, and at each session the new photographs were taken and patients were asked for any probable side effects.

The MASI score was applied as an objective measurement to compare two treatment groups more accurately. According to the MASI, the whole face is divided into four areas: 30% the forehead, 30% right malar (RM), 30% left malar (LM), and 10% chin (C). The grade of melasma severity was determined by 3 parameters: area (A), darkness (D), and homogeneity (H). A is scored from 0 (no involvement) to 6 (90-100% involvement) while D and H are scored from 0 (absent) to 4 (maximum). The MASI is then calculated by the following equation:

$$= 0.3\,(DF + HF)\,AF + 0.3\,(DMR + HMR)\,AMR$$
$$+ 0.3\,(DML + HML)\,AML \tag{1}$$
$$+ 0.1\,(DC + HC)\,AC \tag{9}$$

According to our study design, the MASI score was calculated for each malar area, separately. The MASI score for each side of the face was determined according to the photographs of baseline and week 16 (1 month after the completion of treatment) by a dermatologist who was blind to the treatment.

The patient's satisfaction of melasma treatment was evaluated using a four-scale grading: poor: response rate= 0-25%; fair: response rate= 25-50%; good: response rate=50-75%; excellent: response rate=75-100%.

TABLE 1: Baseline demographics and clinical characteristics of patients with melisma.

Gender, No. (%)	
Female	49 (89.1)
Male	6 (10.9)
Age, years	
Mean± SD	35.93±5.9
(Range)	(27-51)
Duration of disease , years	
Mean± SD	6.24±2.7
Fitzpatrick's skin type; N (%)	
2	9 (16.4)
3	35 (63.3)
4	11 (20)
Family history; N (%)	
Positive	28 (50.9)
Negative	27 (49.1)
History of oral contraceptive intake; N (%)	
Positive	30 (54.5)
Negative	25 (45.5)

All collected data were reported as number or frequency percentage for qualitative variables and mean ±standard deviation for quantitative variables. The data analyst was blind to treatment group allocation. Statistical analysis was performed by Statistical Package for the Social Sciences (SPSS 16.0.0, IBM, Chicago-IL, USA). Two sample t-test, paired samples t-test, and analysis of variance (ANOVA) were used to compare parameters. Variables were considered significant for a confidence interval of 95% (p<0.05).

3. Results

All 55 included patients completed the study. Baseline demographics and clinical characteristics of the patients are summarized in Table 1.

At baseline, the mean of MASI score was 5.165±1.875 in TA+HQ group 5.204±1.935 in HQ group with no significant difference between two groups (p=0.08). The mean of MASI score in week 16 decreased in both groups significantly (p < 0.01), which showed the efficacy of both therapeutic regimens. In week 16, the mean of MASI score was 1.769±0.981 in TA+HQ group (Figure 1) and 2.926±1.219 in HQ group (Figure 2). The therapeutic outcomes were significantly better in TA+HQ group than HQ group (p=0.001) (Table 2).

Patients satisfaction with treatment was significantly higher in the TA + HQ group with 55% of patients reporting good to excellent response compared to 16% in the HQ group (P < 0.001) (Figure 2).

The side effects in TA+ HQ group were minor and transient including erythema (47.3%) and pruritus at the site of injection (10.9%). The side effects in HQ group were erythema in 50.9% of cases and pruritus in 12.7% of cases.

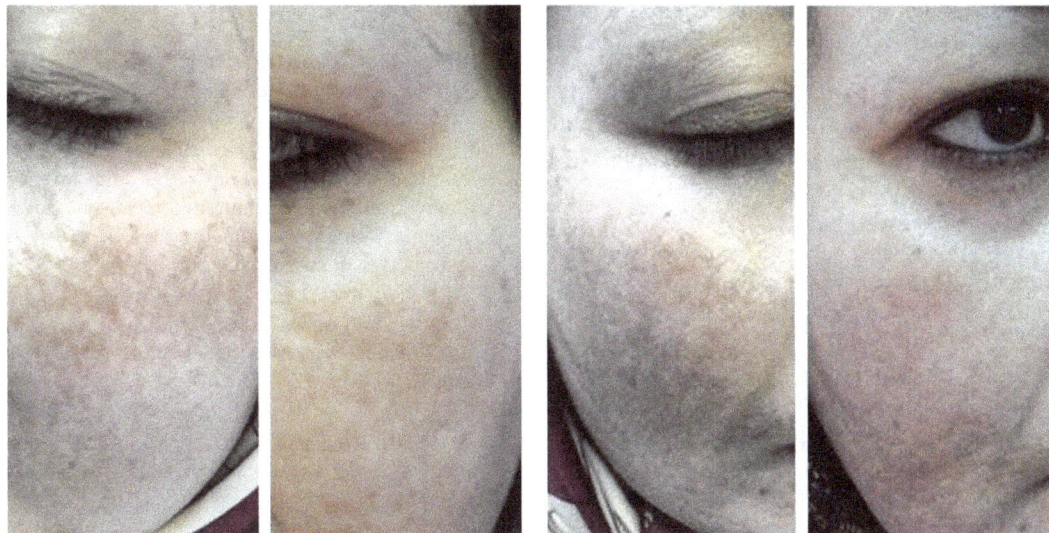

(a) Pretreatment (left picture) and posttreatment (right picture) photographs after 16-week administration of 4% hydroquinone cream

(b) Pretreatment (left picture) and posttreatment (right picture) photographs after 16-week combination therapy with intradermal tranexamic acid + 4% hydroquinone

FIGURE 1

TABLE 2: MASI score before and after treatment in two groups.

	Tranexamic acid + Hydroquinone	Hydroquinone	p-value
Baseline MASI Score (Mean±SD)	5.165±1.875	5.204±1.935	0.08
MASI Score in week 16 Mean±SD	1.769±0.981	2.926±1.219	0.001

The difference between the two groups regarding side effect occurrence was not statistically significant (P = 0.43).

4. Discussion

This study showed that combination therapy with intradermal tranexamic acid and topical hydroquinone was more effective than conventional therapy (hydroquinone) in the treatment of melasma with less side effects.

The mechanism of action of TA in treatment of melasma is not completely understood but it seems to suppress UV-induced plasmin activity in keratinocytes. Tranexamic acid inhibits the binding of plasminogen to keratinocytes, consequently reducing the synthesis of prostaglandins, which are well-known stimulators of tyrosinase activity [12]. Moreover, plasmin increases diffusible forms of vascular endothelial growth factor (VEGF), resulting in angiogenesis. Thus, inhibition of plasmin by TA leads to reduction of angiogenesis.

Several studies have demonstrated the efficacy of TA in treatment of melasma [4–11], but in a large number of these studies, TA have been used orally with numerous systemic side effects such as menstrual irregularities, gastrointestinal symptoms, and orthostatic imbalances [13–15].

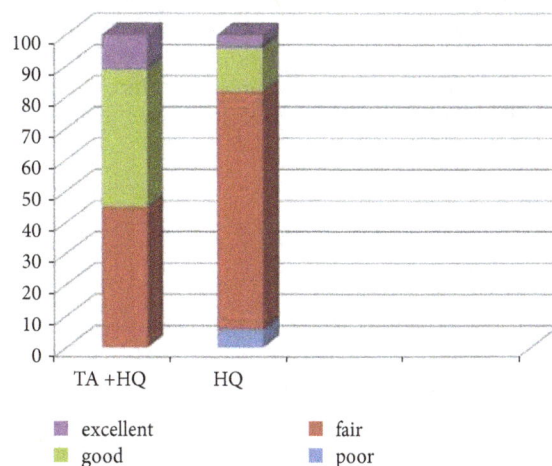

FIGURE 2: Comparison of patients satisfaction in two groups. HQ; hydroquinone, TA; tranexamic Acid. Poor: response rate = 0-25%; fair: response rate = 25-50%; good: response rate = 50-75%; excellent: response rate = 75-100%.

Topical administration of TA was assessed in a randomized double blind split-face trial study by Kanechorn Na

Ayuthaya et al. They reported that therapeutic effect of 5% TA gel on melasma was neither superior to nor different from its vehicle [16]. Na et al. reported that combination of oral and topical TA reduces epidermal pigmentation of melasma and reverses melasma related alterations in the dermis such as vessels and mast cells number [17]. In another split-face trial, Ebrahimi et al. used topical 3% TA suspension for one side of the face and a 3% hydroquinone, 2% vitamin C, and 0.01% dexamethasone suspension for the other side of the face. A significant decreasing in MASI score was observed in both groups, but with no significant difference between them [1].

There are only 4 trials which have investigated the effect of microneedling or microinjection in treatment of melasma. Lee et al. conducted a prospective open-label study to evaluate the effectiveness of weekly microinjection of TA in treatment of melasma. They observed statistically significant decline in MASI score from baseline to 8 and 12 weeks [18]. In another study, Steiner et al. evaluated the efficacy of intradermal injection of TA versus topical administration of 3% TA cream in treatment of melasma. They reported that both treatments improved melasma with no significant difference [19]. Budamakuntla et al. compared microinjection of TA with its microneedling and found no significant difference in MASI score and patient satisfaction between these two modalities [2].

In a recent study, Elfar et al. conducted a clinical trial to compare the therapeutic effect of intradermal injection of TA, glycolic acid peeling 50%, and topical silymarin cream in treatment of melasma. The participants were followed up for 3 months after the treatment. They reported that the microinjection of TA significantly decreased the MASI score; however, its response rate was less than glycolic acid peeling than silymarin cream [20].

Like most other studies, we found a better response rate with combination of TA and HQ. However, the limitation of our study was the short follow-up period of only 1 month. As recurrence of melasma is common in spite of appropriate treatment, studies with long-term follow-up are recommended.

5. Conclusion

In conclusion, addition of tranexamic acid injections to conventional hydroquinone therapy can increase the efficacy of topical treatment. In our study, major and statistically significant improvement in MASI scores was achieved by combining these two treatment regimens with fewer side effects. Therefore, it may be helpful in treatment of all cases of melasma, especially the refractory ones.

References

[1] B. Ebrahimi and F. F. Naeini, "Topical tranexamic acid as a promising treatment for melasma," *Journal of Research in Medical Sciences*, vol. 19, no. 8, pp. 753–757, 2014.

[2] L. Budamakuntla, E. Loganathan, D. Suresh et al., "A randomised, open-label, comparative study of tranexamic acid microinjections and tranexamic acid with microneedling in patients with melasma," *Journal of Cutaneous and Aesthetic Surgery*, vol. 6, no. 3, p. 139, 2013.

[3] H. J. Kim, S. H. Moon, S. H. Cho, J. D. Lee, and H. S. Kim, "Efficacy and safety of tranexamic acid in melasma: A meta-analysis and systematic review," *Acta Dermato-Venereologica*, vol. 97, no. 7, pp. 776–781, 2017.

[4] M. S. Kim, S. H. Ban, J.-H. Kim, H.-J. Shin, J.-H. Choi, and S. E. Chang, "Tranexamic acid diminishes laser-induced melanogenesis," *Annals of Dermatology*, vol. 27, no. 3, pp. 250–256, 2015.

[5] R. Sharma, V. K. Mahajan, K. S. Mehta, P. S. Chauhan, R. Rawat, and T. N. Shiny, "Therapeutic efficacy and safety of oral tranexamic acid and that of tranexamic acid local infiltration with microinjections in patients with melasma: a comparative study," *Clinical and Experimental Dermatology*, vol. 42, no. 7, pp. 728–734, 2017.

[6] H. Kato, J. Araki, H. Eto et al., "A prospective randomized controlled study of oral tranexamic acid for preventing postinflammatory hyperpigmentation after Q-switched ruby laser," *Dermatologic Surgery*, vol. 37, no. 5, pp. 605–610, 2011.

[7] T. Padhi and S. Pradhan, "Oral tranexamic acid with fluocinolone-based triple combination cream versus fluocinolone-based triple combination cream alone in melasma: An open labeled randomized comparative trial," *Indian Journal of Dermatology*, vol. 60, no. 5, p. 520, 2015.

[8] L. L. Zhou and A. Baibergenova, "Melasma: systematic review of the systemic treatments," *International Journal of Dermatology*, vol. 56, no. 9, pp. 902–908, 2017.

[9] D. Karn, S. KC, A. Amatya, E. A. Razouria, and M. Timalsina, "Oral tranexamic acid for the treatment of melasma," *Kathmandu University Medical Journal*, vol. 10, no. 40, pp. 40–43, 2014.

[10] M. Perper, A. E. Eber, R. Fayne et al., "Tranexamic Acid in the Treatment of Melasma: A Review of the Literature," *American Journal of Clinical Dermatology*, vol. 18, no. 3, pp. 373–381, 2017.

[11] M. Taraz, S. Niknam, and A. H. Ehsani, "Tranexamic acid in treatment of melasma: A comprehensive review of clinical studies," *Dermatologic Therapy*, vol. 30, no. 3, 2017.

[12] D. Li, Y. Shi, M. Li et al., "Tranexamic acid can treat ultraviolet radiation-induced pigmentation in guinea pigs," *The European Journal of Dermatology*, vol. 20, pp. 289–292, 2010.

[13] S. Wu, H. Shi, H. Wu et al., "Treatment of melasma with oral administration of tranexamic acid," *Aesthetic Plastic Surgery*, vol. 36, no. 4, pp. 964–970, 2012.

[14] H. C. Lee, T. G. Thng, and C. L. Goh, "Oral tranexamic acid in the treatment of melasma: A retrospective analysis," *Journal of the American Academy of Dermatology*, vol. 75, pp. 385–392, 2016.

[15] D. Karn, S. KC, A. Amatya, E. A. Razouria, and M. Timalsina, "Oral tranexamic acid for the treatment of melasma," *Kathmandu University Medical Journal*, vol. 10, no. 40, pp. 40–43, 2012.

[16] P. K. N. Ayuthaya, N. Niumphradit, A. Manosroi, and A. Nakakes, "Topical 5% tranexamic acid for the treatment of

melasma in Asians: A double-blind randomized controlled clinical trial," *Journal of Cosmetic and Laser Therapy*, vol. 14, no. 3, pp. 150–154, 2012.

[17] J. I. Na, S. Y. Choi, S. H. Yang, H. R. Choi, H. Y. Kang, and K.-C. Park, "Effect of tranexamic acid on melasma: A clinical trial with histological evaluation," *Journal of the European Academy of Dermatology and Venereology*, vol. 27, no. 8, pp. 1035–1039, 2013.

[18] J. H. Lee, J. G. Park, S. H. Lim et al., "Localized intradermal microinjection of tranexamic acid for treatment of melasma in Asian patients: A preliminary clinical trial," *Dermatologic Surgery*, vol. 32, no. 5, pp. 626–631, 2006.

[19] D. Steiner, C. Feola, N. Bialeski et al., "Study evaluating the efficacy of topical and injected tranexamic acid in treatment of melasma," *Surgical and Cosmetic Dermatology*, vol. 1, no. 4, pp. 174–177, 2009.

[20] N. N. Elfar and G. M. El-Maghraby, "Efficacy of Intradermal Injection of Tranexamic Acid, Topical Silymarin and Glycolic Acid Peeling in Treatment of Melasma: A Comparative Study," *Journal of Clinical & Experimental Dermatology Research*, vol. 06, no. 03, 2015.

24

Scabies Outbreak Investigation and Risk Factors in East Badewacho District, Southern Ethiopia: Unmatched Case Control Study

Jarso Sara,[1] Yusuf Haji ⓘ,[2] and Achamyelesh Gebretsadik ⓘ[2]

[1]Affiliate of School of Public and Environmental Health, College of Medicine and Health Sciences Hawassa University, Ethiopia
[2]School of Public and Environmental Health, College of Medicine and Health Sciences, Hawassa University, P.O. Box 1560, Hawassa, Ethiopia

Correspondence should be addressed to Yusuf Haji; yusufa2008@yahoo.com

Academic Editor: Luigi Naldi

Introduction. Scabies is one of the common public health problem but neglected parasitic diseases caused by *Sarcoptes scabiei* var. *hominis.* Global scabies prevalence in both sexes was 204 million. In Ethiopia, scabies is also a common public health issue but there is lack of studies regarding outbreak investigation and risk factors in the study area. This study was aimed to investigate the scabies suspected outbreak and risk factors in East Badewacho District, Southern Ethiopia, 2016. *Methods.* A community-based unmatched case control (1 : 2 ratios) study was conducted in East Badewacho District, using collected scabies line listed data and face-to-face interview to assess risk factors during October 23–30, 2016. The data were collected using structured questionnaire, and then the data were coded, entered, cleaned, and analyzed using SPSS statistical software, whereas, line listed data was entered into Microsoft excel for descriptive analyses. Odds ratios (OR) and 95% confidence interval (CI) were computed to determine associated factors. *Results.* A total of 4,532 scabies cases line listed with overall attack rate of 110/1,000 population. The mean age was 12 years, and most affected age group was 5–14 years. Independent risk factors found to be statistically associated with scabies infestation were age less than 15 years (AOR = 2.62, 95% CI: 1.31–5.22), family size greater than 5 members (AOR = 2.63, 95% CI: 1.10–6.27), bed sharing with scabies cases (AOR = 12.47, 95% CI: 3.05–50.94), and home being affected by flooding (AOR = 22.32, 95% CI: 8.46–58.90). *Conclusion.* Outbreak of scabies occurred in East Badewacho District. Age less than 15 years, family size greater than five members, sleeping with others, and home being affected by flooding are the risk factors. Providing risk factors related health education on prevention and controls especially, at community level and schools, is recommended.

1. Introduction

Scabies is one of the common but neglected parasitic diseases and is major public health problem globally and in resource-scarce countries in particular. Global scabies prevalence was about 204 million cases with 0.21% of total disability adjusted life years lost, and, in resource-poor tropical settings, the sheer burden of scabies infestation and their complications impose a major cost on healthcare systems [1, 2].

Scabies affects all age groups and both sexes but the most vulnerable age groups are young children and the elderly in resource-poor communities who are especially susceptible to scabies as well as to the secondary complications of infestation. The highest rates occur in countries with hot, tropical climates, where infestation is endemic, especially in communities where overcrowding and poverty coexist [1, 3].

The scabies mites usually spread by prolonged direct skin-to-skin contact with a person who has scabies. It can also spread easily to sexual partners and household members. Sometimes scabies can spread indirectly by sharing clothes, towels, or bedding used by infested individuals. A tiny scabies mite burrows into the epidermis of the skin where it lives and lays its eggs. The most common symptoms of scabies are severe itching especially at night and papular skin rash that may affect much of the body or be limited to common sites like interdigital space, flexor of the wrist, elbow, armpit, penis, nipple, and buttocks which usually begin 3–6 weeks after primary infestation [1, 4].

An outbreak of scabies could happen when cases are left untreated, and delayed diagnosis is linked with secondary bacterial infection which may lead to cellulitis, folliculitis, boils, impetigo, or lymphangitis and may also exacerbate other preexisting dermatoses such as eczema and psoriasis [5]. These secondary bacterial infections were mostly caused by group A streptococci and *Staphylococcus aureus*, which leads to nephritis, rheumatic fever, glomerulonephritis, chronic renal and rheumatic heart diseases, and sepsis especially in developing countries that causes for many deaths [6]. And evidence of renal damage is as high as 10% of children with infected scabies in resource-poor settings [1].

It is reported that overcrowded living conditions, sleeping together, sharing of clothes, sharing of towels, poor hygiene practices, malnutrition, and travel to scabies outbreak areas are common risk factors for scabies [1, 7, 8].

In Ethiopia, scabies is also common especially during natural or manmade disasters such as flooding, drought, civil war and conflict, poor water supply and sanitation, and overcrowding living condition. For example, according to public health emergency measures surveillance report scabies is becoming beyond sporadic clinical cases but is turn to be a public health concern and affecting wider geographic areas and population groups especially in drought affected nutrition hotspot woredas [9]. Previous study reported that the prevalence of scabies in tropical counties was high; for example, in Fiji the prevalence of scabies in school children was 18.5% [10]. A study in Northern Ethiopia, Gonder town, among "Yekolo Temari", revealed 22.5% scabies prevalence; however, another study conducted in southern Ethiopia revealed a prevalence of 5.5% among school children [11, 12]. Currently, Ethiopia is experiencing scabies outbreak in drought affected areas where there is shortage of safe water for drinking and poor personal hygiene as a result of direct impact of the drought caused by El Niño [13]. However, there is lack of studies regarding outbreak investigation and risk factors in the current study areas. Therefore, this study was aimed at investigating the scabies suspected outbreak and its risk factors in East Badewacho District, Southern Ethiopia.

2. Methods and Materials

2.1. Study Area and Population. The study was conducted in East Badewacho, one of the 11 districts of Hadiya Zone, Southern Nations Nationalities and Peoples (SNNPR) State of Ethiopia. Administratively, the district has 39 kebeles/subdistricts (1 urban versus 38 rural). As projected from 2007 Ethiopian Population Census, the 2016/17 population of the district is estimated to be 171,578 (85, 275 males, 86,303 women). Shone town, the district capital, is located at 90 km from Hosaina, the Zonal capital, and 115 km from Hawassa city, the Regional capital in the southwest, and 340 km from Addis Ababa, capital city of Ethiopia. The kebeles/subdistricts at which investigation conducted were 1st Chefa, 2nd Chefa, 1st Kerranso, 2nd Kerranso, and Gegara located nearly 15, 17, 23, 27, and 30 km, respectively, away from the Shone town and selected purposely (Figure 1). These kebeles/subdistricts were

affected by flooding disaster occurred in 2016 El Niño in the region [13].

Majority (80.6%) of district populations live in the rural while the remaining 19.4% were urban dwellers. The district has an area of 308.85 square kilometers with average population density of 555 people per square kilometers.

Currently, the district has 1 district hospital, 7 health centers, 41 health posts, and 21 private clinics which accounts for 98% of potential health services coverage. The overall water supply coverage of the district was 38%.

2.2. Study Design and Period. We conducted community-based unmatched case control (1 : 2 ratio) study from October 23–30/2016 to identify potential risk factors and ways of transmission. Line listed data analysis was performed.

2.3. Data Collection Methods and Tools. We used a structured questionnaire, which is adapted from different literatures, to collect information including sociodemographic characteristics, clinical features and management of the cases, and the possible risk factors. The data were collected through face-to-face interview with individual participants, or their families in case of children. Two unmatched controls were selected per each case. Line listing of cases was collected from health facilities and schools for further analysis. Data were collected by two trained diploma nurses.

2.4. Inclusion and Exclusion Criteria

2.4.1. Inclusion Criteria

Cases. Any resident of the kebeles, East Badewacho District, with sign and symptoms (specifically itching and rash) of scabies was selected for investigation and agreed to participate in the study during investigation period.

Diagnosis of a scabies infestation usually is clinical, made based upon presence of the typical rash and symptoms of unrelenting and worsening itch, particularly at night [9].

Controls. Any resident of community of kebeles without any signs and symptom of scabies was selected during the investigation period and agreed to participate in the study.

2.4.2. Exclusion Criteria

Cases. Those who refused to participate or none residents of the selected kebeles were excluded.

Controls. Those who refused to participate as well asfamily members from the same household were excluded from the study (if there are two or more persons in a single household, only one person randomly selected).

2.5. Data Analysis Procedures and Quality Control. Line listed data were entered and cleaned using Microsoft Office Excel 2007 for descriptive analysis, SPSS version 20 statistical software was used for risk factor identification and analysis. All line listed and interviewed data were checked for completeness before entry, cleaning, and analysis made.

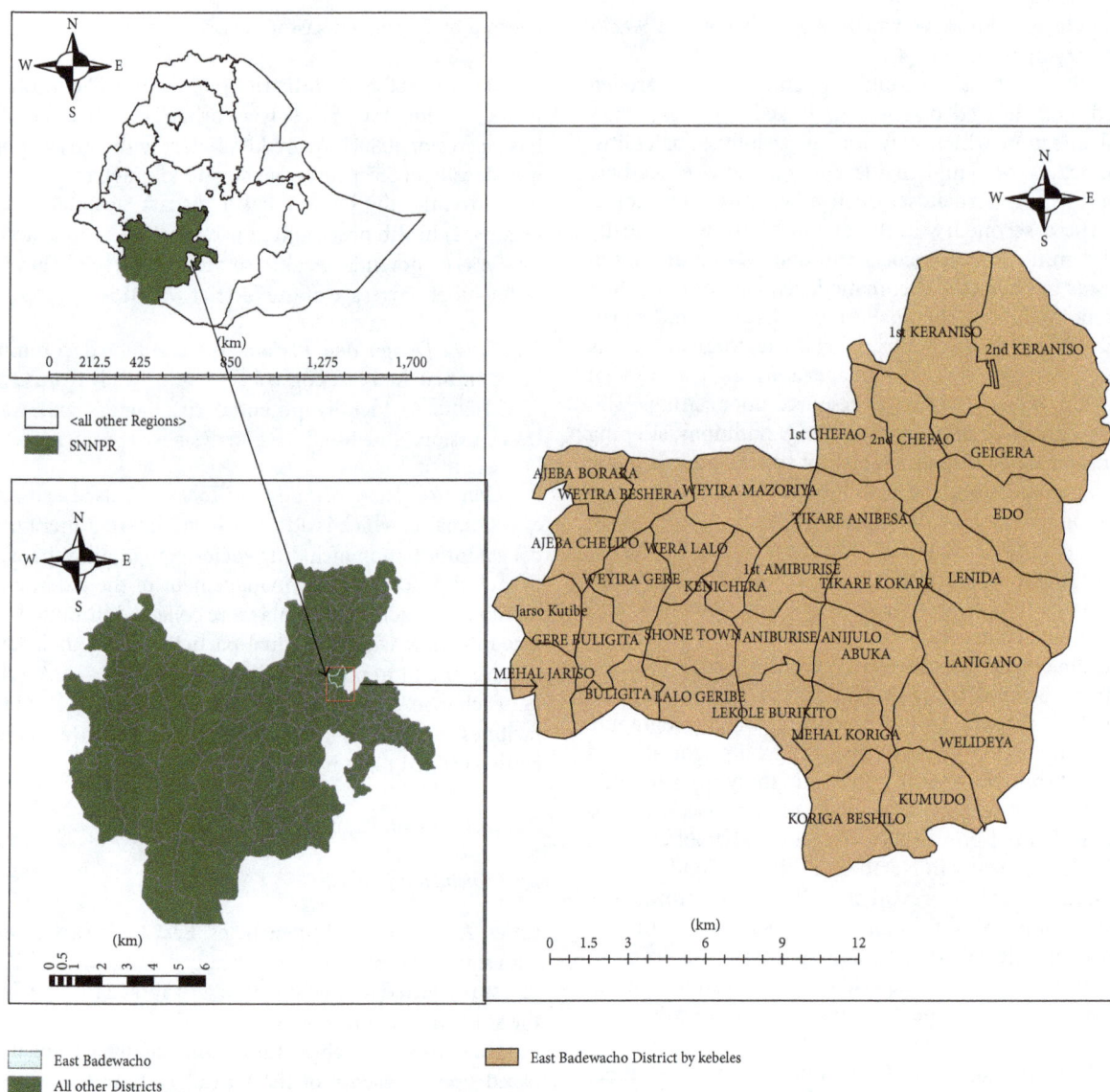

FIGURE 1: Administrative map of study kebeles, East Badewacho District, Southern Ethiopia, 2016.

Arc map was also used for mapping cases and the administrative area of the study. Results were presented using descriptive tables, charts, and choropleth map. Attack rate, *p*-value, and crude and adjusted ORs with 95% CI were used in deciding the strength and statistical significance of associations.

2.6. Study Variables

2.6.1. Dependent Variable.
Scabies infestation was a dependent variable.

2.6.2. Independent Variables.
Sociodemographic (age, sex, occupation, marital status, religion, and family size), travel history, contact history, adequacy of water for personal hygiene, and overcrowding condition were independent variables.

2.7. Ethical Consideration.
Letter of permission was obtained from SNNPR State Health Bureau, Public Health Emergency Management (PHEM) core process and other concerned organizations. Informed verbal consent was also obtained from all the study participants, or their parents in case of children. For the sake of confidentiality the names of participants were not recorded on the questionnaire. Regarding Figures 2, 3, and 7, informed consent was also obtained again from concerned participants orally and their names were not written on the figures.

2.8. Case Definition

2.8.1. Suspected Case.
A person with signs and symptoms consistent with scabies was suspected. The characteristic symptoms of a scabies infection include superficial burrows, intense pruritus (itching) especially at night, a generalized

TABLE 1: Scabies attack rate by age-group of affected kebeles, East Badewacho District, Hadiya Zone, SNNP region, Ethiopia, October 23–30, 2016.

Age group	Age group population	Number of cases	Attack rate per 1,000
0–4	6,445	137	21
5–14	13,319	3,509	263
15+	21,523	886	41
Total	*41,287*	*4,532*	*110*

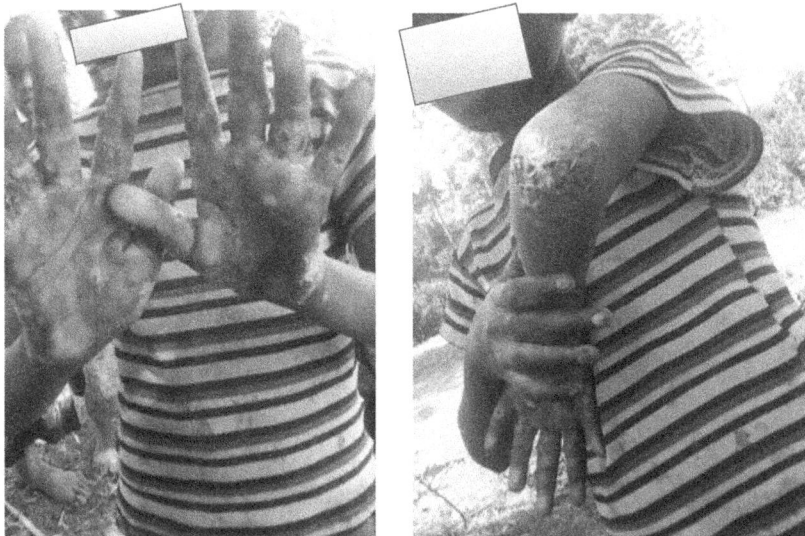

FIGURE 2: An 8-year-old girl of Gegara primary school student with secondary infection, Gegara kebele, East Badewacho District, Southern Ethiopia, 2016.

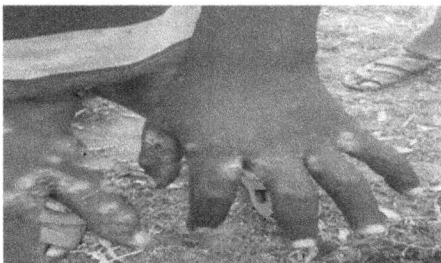

FIGURE 3: A 10-year-old boy's hands at 1st Kerenso primary school with secondary infection, 1st keranso kebele, East Badewacho District, Southern Ethiopia, 2016.

rash, and secondary infection on the head, face, neck, armpit, elbow, wrist, palms, buttocks, and soles [4, 9].

2.8.2. Confirmed Case. A person who has a skin scraping in which mites, mite eggs, or mite feces have been identified by a trained healthcare professional was considered a confirmed case [4, 9].

2.8.3. Contact. Contact is defined as a person without signs and symptoms consistent with scabies who has had direct contact (particularly prolonged, direct skin-to-skin contact) with a suspected or confirmed case in the two months preceding the onset of scabies signs and symptoms in the case [4, 9].

3. Result

3.1. Description of Line Lists. Rumors of scabies cases were reported from two primary schools (Gegara and 2nd keranso), East Badewacho District, on 17 October, 2016. From October 23 to 30, 2016, we identified a total of 4,532 suspected scabies cases line listed from 9 kebeles of the district with a prevalence of 11% (4532/41287). The overall attack rate of nine affected kebeles was 110 cases/1,000 populations, with no scabies related death (CFR = 0).

Out of 4,532 total suspected scabies cases, 2633 (58%) of them were males while 1,899 (42%) were females. The mean age was 12 years, ranging from 8 months to 70 years. Children of 5–14 years of age were the most affected age group with an attack rate of 263/1000 population followed by 15 years and above age groups which accounts for 41/1000 population (Table 1).

Most affected populations were children in the primary schools and most of them had shown sign of secondary infection attributable to scabies. For example, Figures 2 and 3 indicate cases with secondary infection captured during investigation.

During investigation period, 29% of the cases were reported from Gegara kebele followed by 1st Chefa (25%) and

TABLE 2: Distribution of scabies cases by affected kebeles, East Badewacho District, Southern Ethiopia 2016.

Kebeles	Total population	0–4		5–14		≥15	
		cases	ASAR/1000	cases	ASAR/1000	cases	ASAR/1000
1st Chefa	3,730	42	11	845	227	265	71
1st Keranso	6,167	0	0	325	53	17	3
2nd Chefa	4,944	32	6	527	107	101	20
2nd Keranso	6,502	8	1	872	134	51	8
Abuka	5,487	0	0	18	3	9	2
Gegara	3,833	70	18	842	220	409	107
kumudo	2,465	0	0	10	4	13	5
TikareAnbasa	4,225	0	0	52	12	6	1
Tikarekokare	3,934	0	0	11	3	7	2
Total	*41,287*	*152*	*4*	*3502*	*85*	*878*	*21*

TABLE 3: Sociodemographic characteristics of the cases and controls, East Badewacho District, Southern Ethiopia, 2016.

Variables	Case, n (%)	Control, n (%)	Total, n (%)	p. Value
Sex				0.65
Male	33 (60)	62 (56)	95 (58)	
Female	22 (40)	48 (44)	70 (42)	
Age in years				<0.01
0–4	11 (20)	8 (7)	19 (12)	
5–14	24 (44)	31 (28)	55 (33)	
15–44	19 (35)	64 (58)	83 (50)	
45+	1 (2)	7 (6)	8 (5)	
Religion				0.39
Protestant	12 (22)	18 (16)	30 (18)	
Muslim	43 (78)	92 (84)	135 (82)	
Occupation				0.78
Student	24 (44)	40 (36)	64 (39)	
Unemployed	1 (2)	2 (2)	3 (2)	
Merchant	1 (2)	4 (4)	5 (3)	
Farmer	29 (53)	64 (58)	93 (56)	
Educational Status				0.74
No formal education	21 (38)	45 (41)	66 (40)	
Formal education	34 (62)	65 (59)	99 (60)	
Marital status				0.82
Single	24 (44)	50 (45)	74 (45)	
Married	31 (56)	60 (55)	91 (55)	
Family members				0.01
>5 persons	47 (85)	72 (65)	119 (72)	
≤5 persons	8 (15)	38 (35)	46 (28)	

2nd Keranso (20.5%) kebeles, whereas small numbers of cases were reported from Tikare Kokare (0.4%) and Abuka (0.6%) kebeles. Figure 4 shows the spot map of cases by kebeles.

Age-specific attack rate (ASAR) was highest among the age group of 5–14 (85/1000 population) with 227/1000 population in 1st Chefa followed by Gegara (220/1000 population) kebele (Table 2).

On October 19, 2016, district heath office notified the situation to Hadiya Zone Health department. Then, Zonal Health Department notified the situation to Regional Health Bureau (RHB) on October 20, 2016, and investigation team was deployed to assess the situation (Figure 5).

3.2. *Case Control Analysis.* A total of 165 (55 cases and 110 controls) participants were randomly selected from the community to identify the risk factors for scabies outbreak in affected 9 kebeles with case to control ratio of 1 : 2. Almost all cases had a history of rash and itching, and 33 (60%) of them had sign of secondary infection. Among the total 55 interviewed cases, 33 (60%) of them were males and 22 (40%) were females; and of 110 controls, 62 (56%) were males and 48 (44%) of them females. The mean age of study subjects was 12.62 (6 months–65 years) years of age among cases, while the mean age for controls was 20.8 years (3 months to 50 years), p. value < 0.01 (Table 3).

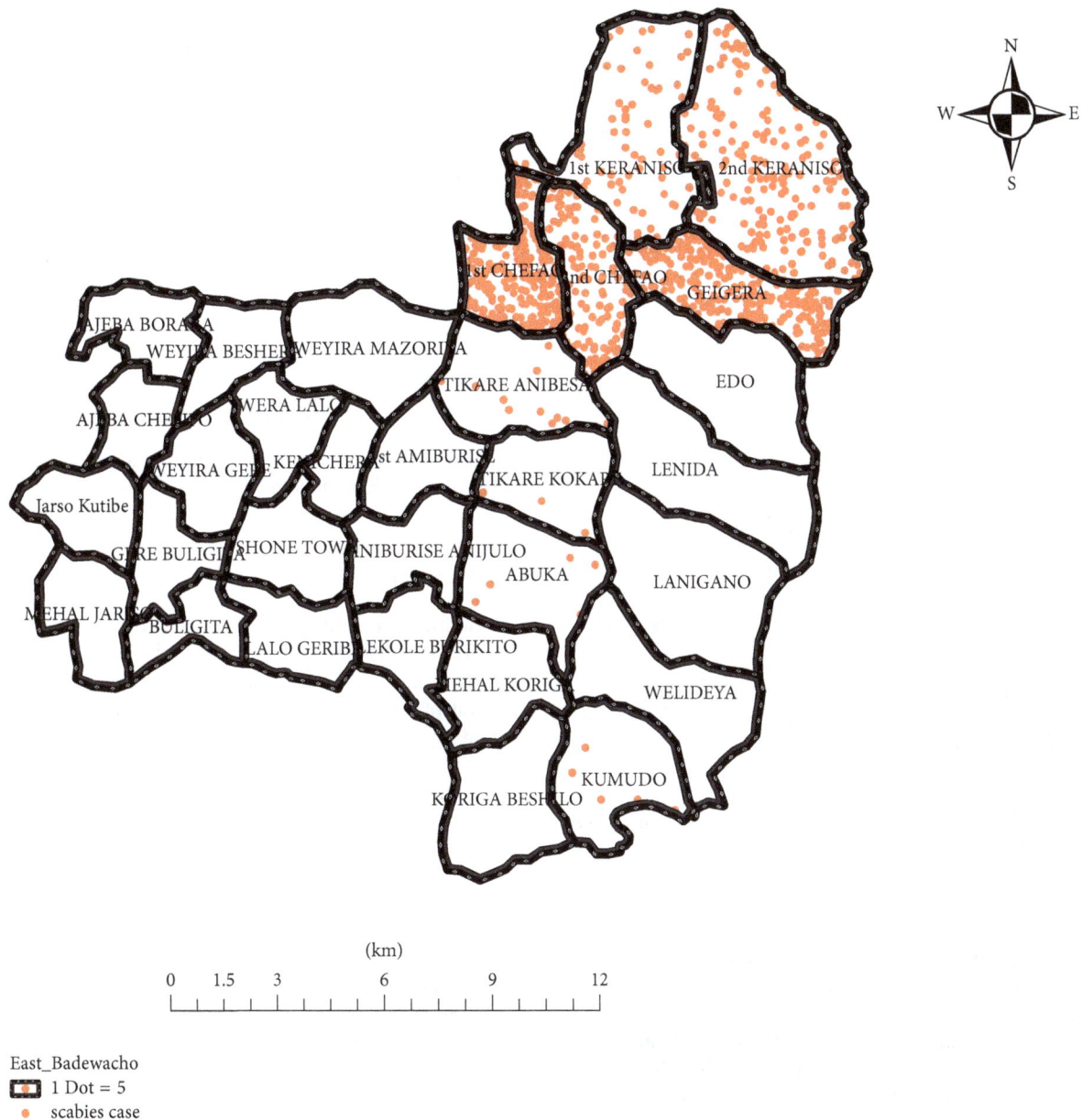

FIGURE 4: Spot map of scabies cases by kebeles, East Badewacho District, Southern Ethiopia, 2016.

3.2.1. Presence of Clinical Features of Scabies. Figure 6 shows clinical features of scabies diagnosed subjects (cases). Accordingly, of 55 cases, 54 (98%) of them had both itching and scabies related skin rash, followed by crusts on the skin that was not yet ascertained as that of scabies crusts 44 (80%) and secondary bacterial infection 33 (60%).

Of the total cases, 35 (64%) of them did not visit health facility to get treatment for infestation. Thirteen percent of cases and 14% of controls had travel history within past 2 months prior to the onset of symptoms. Fifty-two (94%) of cases responded that they had contact history with active case of scabies. However, 84 (76%) of controls reported that they had no history of contact with scabies cases. Among the cases those who had a contact history, 32 (58%) of them had history

of sleeping together, 30 (54%) playing together, and 18 (33%) sharing clothes as types of contacts.

Regarding site of the rash on the body, 41 (75%) of cases had it on buttocks, 39 (71%) had it on interdigital space, 35 (64%) of cases had rash on the flexor wrist surface, and the rest are stated in table (Table 4).

3.2.2. Factors Associated with Scabies Outbreak. Concerning risk factors, variables such as sex, age, educational status, religious, marital status, family size, travelling history to scabies epidemic area within the last 2 months, sleeping with scabies cases, water source for daily bases, and home being affected by flooding in last disaster were entered into binary logistic regression model.

TABLE 4: Site of the rash on the body of investigated cases, East Badewacho District, Southern Ethiopia, 2016.

Site of Rash	Number of cases ($n = 55$)	Percentage (%)
Flexor wrist surface	35	64
Inter digital spaces	39	71
Abdomen	30	55
Inter gluteal	33	60
Buttocks	41	75
Elbow	25	45

Note. Multiple responses possible.

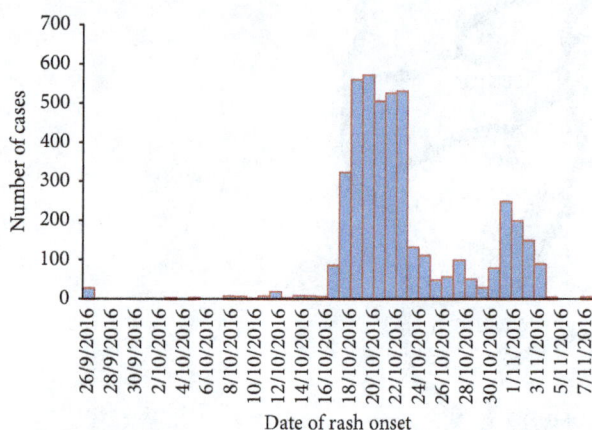

FIGURE 5: Epidemic curve of scabies outbreak by date of onset, East Badewacho District, Southern Ethiopia, 2016.

In bivariate analysis, age group, family size > 5 members, sleeping with person infested with scabies cases, water source for daily bases, and home being affected by flooding were significantly associated with scabies infestation (Table 5).

Age in years, family size, sharing beds with scabies cases, source of water for daily bases, and home being affected by flood were entered into multivariate logistic regression model to control for confounding factor.

After adjusting for possible confounding factors the result of multiple logistic regression analysis showed that age group less than fifteen years, family size > greater 5 members, sleeping with scabies cases, and home being affected with flood were found to be the final independent variables significantly associated with scabies infestation. Accordingly, those persons aged less than 15 years were 2.6 times more likely to develop scabies with [AOR (95% CI) = 2.62 (1.31–5.22)] compared with age >= 15 years of age. The odd of developing scabies infestation was 2.6 among family members with size >= 5 persons compared to those whose family size <= 5 members with [AOR (95%) = 2.63 (1.10–6.27)]. There is also strong association between the home being affected by flooding and scabies infestation. Thus, the odd of acquiring scabies was about 22 times among households affected by flooding than their counterparts [AOR (95% CI) = 22.32 (8.46–58.90)].

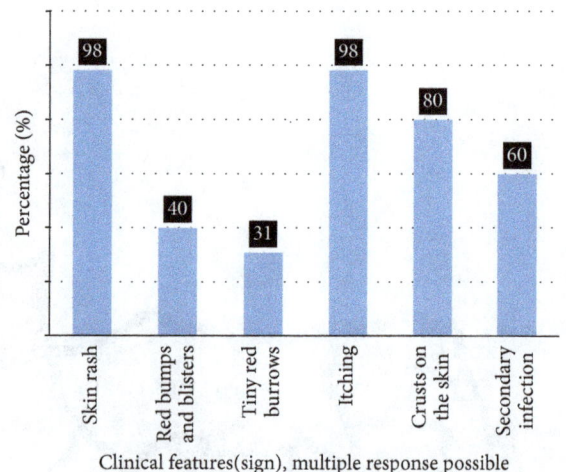

FIGURE 6: Percentage of cases with clinical features of scabies, East Badewacho District, Southern Ethiopia, 2016.

4. Discussion

We identified a total of 4,532 suspected scabies cases line lists from 9 kebeles, and 165 individuals were randomly selected from the community as case-controls (55 cases and 110 controls) from 5 purposely selected kebeles/subdistricts during investigation period. The overall prevalence rate was 11% with school-aged children being affected more (26%). This result is lower to the findings of studies conducted in Northern Ethiopia among "Yekolo temeri" which is reported to be 22.5% and study among school children in Fiji where the overall prevalence of scabies infection was 23.6% [10, 11]. The relative lower prevalence observed in our study could be due to the fact the study population mostly institutionalized, for example, "yekolo temeri", in Ethiopia was mostly living in single institution (church), while this study conducted among the general rural community, and, as to Fiji study, the climatic variation might have existed as Fiji is tropical climate and ours is subtropical area.

However, the finding of this study is higher than other study conducted in southern Ethiopia reporting 5.5% scabies prevalence among school children [12]. This is because, our study conducted in drought hit areas, El Nino was the case in the study area [13].

In this study 75% of cases were found in the age group of 5 to 14 years, and age groups less than 15 years are at risk of acquiring scabies compared to age greater than 15 years. Our findings are similar to studies conducted in Fiji and Cameroon where the school-aged children commonly affected [10, 14]. Children in primary school were most affected populations, and most of them had sign of secondary infection attributable to scabies. This might be due to the fact that younger children, particularly, those at school are at high risk of scabies infestations as the school environments may increase the susceptibility of cross-infestation and increase contacts which can be passed to family members and other.

Regarding the sites of rash, interdigital spaces (71%), flexor wrists (64%), and buttocks (75%) were the main sites in the current study. This is nearly similar to the study conducted

TABLE 5: Bivariate and multivariate analysis of Scabies outbreak, East Badewacho District, Southern Ethiopia, 2016.

Variables/Risk factors	Case, n (%)	Control, n (%)	COR (95% CI)	AOR (95% CI)	Adjusted p-values
Sex					
Male	33 (60)	62 (56)	1		
Female	22 (40)	48 (44)	1.16 (0.601–2.24)		
Age in years					
<15	19 (35)	67 (61)	2.95 (1.503–5.798)	2.624 (1.31–5.22)	0.006
≥15	36 (65)	43 (39)	1	1	
Educational status					
Formal education	21 (38)	45 (41)	1		
No formal education	34 (62)	65 (59)	0.892 (0.459–1.732)		
Religious					
Muslim	43 (78)	92 (84)	1		
Protestant	12 (22)	18 (16)	1.426 (0.63–3.22)		
Marital status					
Single	24 (44)	50 (45)	1		
Married	31 (56)	60 (55)	1.098 (0.525–2.296)		
Family Size					
≤5	8 (15)	38 (35)	**1**		0.028
>5	47 (85)	72 (65)	4.10 (1.33–7.22)	2.63 (1.10–6.27)	
Travel history to scabies epidemic area within the last 2 months					
No	48 (87)	94 (85)	1		
Yes	7 (13)	16 (15)	0.857 (0.330–224)		
Sleeping with scabies cases					
Yes	32 (62)	4 (17)	7.6 (2.25–25.59)	12.4 (3.05–50.9)	<0.0001
No	20 (38)	19 (83)	1	1	
Source of water for daily bases					
Pipe Water	28 (51)	84 (76)	1	1	
Spring	4 (7)	2 (2)	3 (1.13–7.95)	5.57 (0.57–53.75)	0.137
Pond	10 (18)	10 (9)	6 (1.04–34.54)	2.36 (0.68–8.11)	0.171
River	13 (24)	14 (13)	2.786 (1.170–6.63)	1.63 (0.57–4.69)	0.358
Home affected by flooding					
Yes	49 (89)	82 (75)	23.9 (9.24–61.84)	22.32 (8.46–58.90)	<0.0001
No	6 (11)	28 (25)	1	1	

at boarding schools in Cameroon with the interdigital spaces and flexor wrists were the common sites affected by scabies [14]. This might be true as these parts of the body might be softer than the other body parties which is favorable for mites [1].

Concerning the risk factors for scabies, there is statistically significant associations between family sizes and scabies infestation that the odds of acquiring scabies are higher in those having more than five family members. This finding is consistent with study done in Solomon Islands indicating households with six to ten persons per household were 1.4 times more likely to acquire scabies compared to those households having less than 5 family members [15]. In addition, this result is also supported by other similar study conducted in west of Iran which revealed that scabies had been directly associated with family size [16]. This might be due to overcrowding among larger families compared to the smaller ones, which increases sharing of cloths, beds, etc. It

is well known that scabies can spread easily under crowded conditions where close body and skin contact is common [7].

Another factor showing strong association is sleeping with cases of scabies. Hence, those who had reported to have slept with scabies infested individuals were twice more likely to have developing scabies infestations than their counterparts. This result is in line with systematic reviews done on scabies in developing countries showing that having skin contact in the past 2 months with a person infested with scabies and sleeping with others were risk factors for scabies [17]. Moreover, study conducted among solders in Pakistan shows sharing of beds among male soldiers was one of the risk factors for scabies [8]. This is supported by a body of science that mites of scabies can be frequently transmitted by skin-to-skin contacts, as well as through infected closes and bedding [1, 4, 5].

Moreover, strong association was seen between homes being affected by flooding and scabies infestations in the

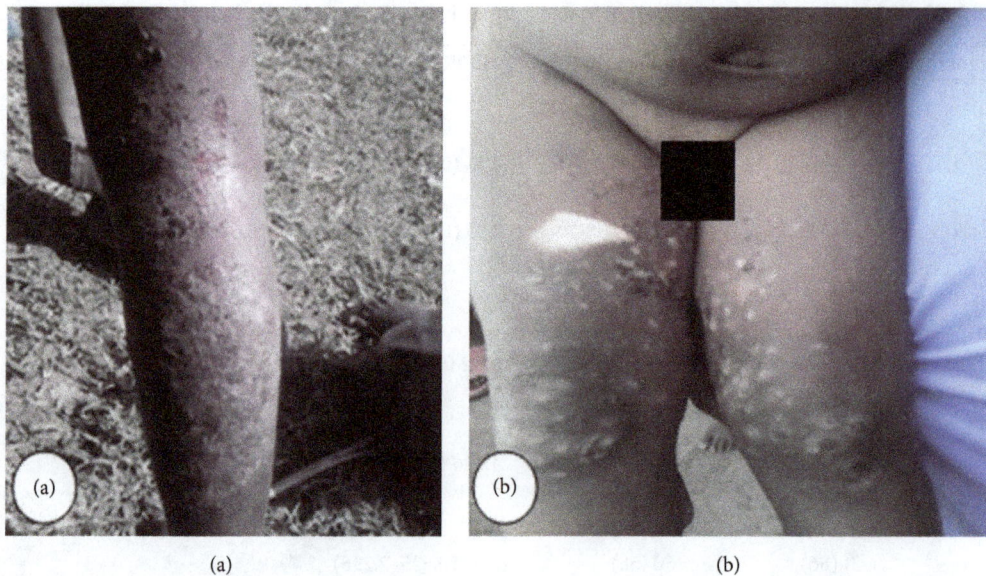

FIGURE 7: Posterior leg (a) and intergluteal (b) scabies rash on the body, East Badewacho District, Southern Ethiopia, 2016.

current study. Compared to controls, the odds of households being affected by flooding were 22 times among that of cases. This might be a result of the displacements, overcrowding, and impairment in personal hygiene and may increase susceptibility to different skin problems like scabies infestation.

Finally, we recommend the following:

(i) Strong and continuous active case search should be strengthened at all levels.

(ii) Providing risk factors related health education on prevention and control especially is recommended, at schools and community level.

(iii) Scabies mass drug treatment should be initiated as soon as possible in kebeles with prevalence ≥ 15%.

(iv) As long as each scabies outbreak is unique and requires an individualized approach, we recommend maintaining social mobilizing at health facilities, schools, and any public gathering areas to alleviate the spread of scabies.

Our study is not free from limitations. First of all, as the study conducted is based on only a clinical signs and symptoms while lacking laboratory confirmation, ascertainment of cases could be a problem. Second, due to small sample size some confidence intervals are wider, for assessing risk factors for scabies. Another limitation of our study is ascertainment of clinical presentations of cases of scabies; for example, secondary bacterial infections, crusts, and presence of burrows are difficult as we did not employ any laboratory or microscopic test. Furthermore, as we employed case control study, the role of recall bias could not be ruled out.

5. Conclusions

In conclusion, it is confirmed that scabies outbreak occurred in East Badewacho District, Southern Ethiopia. Age less than 15 years, family size > 5 members, contact history with scabies cases, sleeping with others, and home being affected by flooding are the independent risk factors associated with scabies in the district.

Authors' Contributions

Jarso Sara initiated the study, collected the data, and analyzed and prepared manuscript. Yusuf Haji and Achamyelesh Gebretsadik conceived the study analyzed and revised and finalized the manuscript. All authors read and approved the final version of the manuscript.

Acknowledgments

We would like to acknowledge East Badewacho District and investigation catchment area Heath centers staffs for their support to conduct the investigation. Our gratitude is also goes to Federal ministry of health and Hawassa University School of Public and Environmental Health for their financial and logistic support. Finally, our thank goes to data collectors and respondents without whom our work could not be accomplished.

References

[1] World Health Organization, "Scabies epidemiology," WHO, 2017, http://www.who.int/lymphatic_filariasis/epidemiology/scabies/en/.

[2] C. Karimkhani, D. V. Colombara, A. M. Drucker et al., "The global burden of scabies: a cross-sectional analysis from the global burden of disease study 2015," *The Lancet Infectious Diseases*, vol. 17, no. 12, pp. 1247–1254, 2017.

[3] O. Chosidow, "Clinical practice. Scabies," *The New England Journal of Medicine*, vol. 354, no. 16, pp. 1718–1727, 2006.

[4] "Scabies: Centers for Disease Control and Prevention guide line: 2010," https://www.cdc.gov/parasites/scabies/gen_info/index .html.

[5] *Scabies Infestations/Outbreaks and Management: A Guide for General Practitioners*, 2015.

[6] D. Engelman, K. Kiang, O. Chosidow et al., "Toward the global control of human scabies: introducing the international alliance for the control of scabies," *PLOS Neglected Tropical Diseases*, vol. 7, no. 8, Article ID e2167, 2013.

[7] FDRE MOH, *Scabies Outbreak Preparedness and Response Plan*, 2015.

[8] N. Raza, S. N. R. Qadir, and H. Agha, "Risk factors for scabies among male soldiers in Pakistan: Case-control study," *Eastern Mediterranean Health Journal*, vol. 15, no. 5, pp. 1105–1110, 2009.

[9] Federal Democratic Republic of Ethiopia, *Federal Democratic Republic of Ethiopia. Interim-guideline for multi-sectorial scabies outbreak emergency response*, 2015.

[10] A. C. Steer, A. W. J. Jenney, J. Kado et al., "High burden of impetigo and scabies in a tropical country," *PLOS Neglected Tropical Diseases*, vol. 3, no. 6, article no. e467, 2009.

[11] Z. J. Yassin, A. F. Dadi, H. Y. Nega et al., "Scabies Outbreak Investigation among "Yekolo Temaris" in Gondar Town, North Western Ethiopia," *Electronic Journal of Biology*, vol. 13, no. 3, 2015.

[12] S. L. Walker, E. Lebas, V. De Sario et al., "The prevalence and association with health-related quality of life of tungiasis and scabies in schoolchildren in southern Ethiopia," *PLOS Neglected Tropical Diseases*, vol. 11, no. 8, Article ID e0005808, 2017.

[13] WHO, *El Niño and health ETHIOPIA overview*, WHO, NFORM index 13, 2016.

[14] A. K. Emmanuel, R. N. Jobert, M. K. Kouawa et al., "Prevalence and drivers of human scabies among children and adolescents living and studying in Cameroonian boarding schools," *Parasites & Vectors*, 2016.

[15] D. S. Mason, M. Marks, O. Sokana et al., "The prevalence of scabies and impetigo in the solomon islands: a population-based survey," *PLOS Neglected Tropical Diseases*, vol. 10, no. 6, Article ID e0004803, 2016.

[16] M. Nazari and A. Azizi, "Epidemiological pattern of scabies and its social determinant factors in West of Iran," *Health*, vol. 06, no. 15, pp. 1972–1977, 2014.

[17] R. J. Hay, A. C. Steer, D. Engelman, and S. Walton, "Scabies in the developing world—its prevalence, complications, and management," *Clinical Microbiology and Infection*, vol. 8, 2012.

25

Magnetic Resonance Imaging Evaluation in Patients with Linear Morphea Treated with Methotrexate and High-Dose Corticosteroid

Mohammad Shahidi-Dadras,[1] **Fahimeh Abdollahimajd**[ID],[1] **Razieh Jahangard**[ID],[1]
Ali Javinani,[2] **Amir Ashraf-Ganjouei,**[2] **and Parviz Toossi**[1]

[1]*Skin Research Center, Shahid Beheshti University of Medical Sciences, Tehran, Iran*
[2]*Rheumatology Research Center, Tehran University of Medical Sciences, Tehran, Iran*

Correspondence should be addressed to Fahimeh Abdollahimajd; fabdollahimajd@sbmu.ac.ir
and Razieh Jahangard; razi_jahan@yahoo.com

Academic Editor: E. Helen Kemp

Background. Morphea is an inflammatory disease of the connective tissue that may lead to thickening and hardening of the skin due to fibrosis. The aim of this study was to document magnetic resonance imaging (MRI) changes in patients with linear morphea who were treated with methotrexate (MTX) and high-dose corticosteroid. *Methods.* This study was conducted on 33 patients from the outpatient's dermatology clinic of our institute, who fulfilled the inclusion criteria. Patients received 15 mg/week of MTX and monthly pulses of methylprednisolone for three days in six months. The effectiveness of the treatment was evaluated by MRI, modified LS skin severity index (mLoSSI), and localized scleroderma damage index (LoSDI). *Results.* All parameters of mLoSSI and LoSDI including erythema, skin thickness, new lesion/lesion extension, dermal atrophy, subcutaneous atrophy, and dyspigmentation were also noticeably improved after treatment. Subcutaneous fat enhancement was the most common finding in MRI. MRI scores were significantly associated with clinical markers both before and after the treatment with the exception of skin thickness and new lesion/lesion extension which were not associated with MRI scores before and after the treatment, respectively. *Limitations.* The lack of correlative laboratory disease activity markers, control group, and clearly defined criteria to judge the MRI changes. *Conclusion.* MRI could be a promising tool for the assessment of musculoskeletal and dermal involvement and also monitoring treatment response in patients with morphea.

1. Introduction

Morphea, localized scleroderma (LS), is an inflammatory connective tissue disease that may lead to skin thickening and hardening due to fibrosis. The course of LS includes an early inflammatory stage. It starts with hyperaemia of the skin and is followed by fibrosis, sclerosis, and, finally, atrophy [1]. LS has a diverse clinical presentation [2] and has been classified into circumscribed (superficial and deep), linear (including scleroderma en coup de sabre), generalized (four or more and larger than 3 cm individual plaques), pansclerotic, and mixed forms [3].

Morphea affects the underlying structures [3], in which case it may be associated with flexion contractures, pain, and considerable impairment [4, 5]. At the more severe end of the spectrum, the disease can progress over the years and cause significant atrophy, joint contractures, irreversible structural deformities, growth retardation, and severe functional, cosmetic, and psychological disabilities [6].

Although numerous therapeutic modalities including methotrexate (MTX) in combination with systemic corticosteroid have been discussed for these debilitating forms of morphea, optimal treatment is unknown maybe due to a lack of consensus as to the methods of evaluation and monitoring of treatment response [7–13].

Although several clinical and paraclinical diagnostic and assessment tools including the modified LS skin severity index (mLoSSI), the localized scleroderma cutaneous assessment tool (LoSCAT), ultrasonography (US), elastography, and skin biopsy have been documented, all of them have some limitations; for example, only a limited subset of the clinical parameters is evaluated by each mLoSSI and LoSCAT, or elastography is so hard to perform, US is usually not so helpful on the scalp/face due to a thin tissue, and finally no one really wants to biopsy the face. Magnetic Resonance Imaging (MRI) has recently been shown to be a useful diagnostic tool for identifying the musculoskeletal involvement in patients with morphea [14–16].

The aim of this study was to document the MRI changes in patients with morphea who were treated with MTX and high-dose corticosteroid.

2. Materials and Methods

2.1. Study Population. The study was approved by the ethics committee of Shahid Beheshti University of Medical Sciences. Informed consent was sought from the patients in accordance with legal requirements.

This study was conducted on 33 patients from the outpatient's dermatology clinic, who fulfilled the inclusion criteria. The inclusion criteria were immunocompetent patients 10 years old or older with confirmed morphea (generalized or linear forms), normal bone mineral density, and being negative for latent infections, endocrinopathies, and cardiovascular, renal, and pulmonary disorders. The patients were excluded if they had systemic sclerosis, major concomitant medical conditions, leukopenia $<3.0 \times 10^9$/l, thrombocytopenia $<100 \times 10^9$/l, liver transaminase levels more than twice the upper limit of normal, or renal impairment defined as creatinine clearance <90 ml/min/1.73 m^2, osteopenia, and osteoporosis, or if the patient was unwilling or unable to adhere to the protocol.

Morphea diagnosis was confirmed by histological examination. Owing to the activation of latent infections during immunosuppressive treatment regimens, the patients were also examined for tuberculosis, viral hepatitis, and HIV infections.

2.2. Treatment Protocol. Treatment protocol and duration encompassed six months and, in this period, the patients received MTX, methylprednisolone, and folic acid. MTX was started with a weekly oral dosage of 15 mg, and 1 mg of daily folic acid was prescribed to diminish its toxicity. At the beginning of each month, patients were hospitalized for three days to administer 20–30 mg/kg (500–1000 mg/m^2) per pulse, up to a maximum dose of 1 g intravenous methylprednisolone (or 2 mg/kg/day of prednisolone with a maximum dose of 60 mg and 1 mg/kg/week of MTX with a maximum dose of 15 mg/week in pediatrics). On the other hand, all patients were followed up to 18 months and methotrexate (15 mg/wk) was continued in this period.

2.3. Clinical Assessment. The localized scleroderma assessment tool (LoSCAT) assesses 18 cutaneous anatomic sites, capturing both disease activity and damage parameters. Scores for each site are based on the most severe score for each parameter. To minimize intersubject variability, all skin changes are compared with the contralateral or ipsilateral skin area.

The modified LS skin severity index (mLoSSI) includes the total of three separate activity scores as follows: (A) erythema (ER), (B) skin thickness (ST), and (C) new lesion/lesion extension (N/E). Three cutaneous damage domains are summated to obtain the localized scleroderma damage index (LoSDI) as follows: (A) dermal atrophy (DAT), (B) subcutaneous atrophy (SAT), and (C) dyspigmentation (DP) [17].

Patients were visited monthly with complete laboratory data to check for probable adverse side-effects. Efficacy of the treatment was assessed clinically by mLoSSI and LoSDI before starting the medication. MRI was also performed before and after 6 months of the treatment by 1.5T closed-bore MRI body scanner which elucidates the depth and thickness of the soft-tissue structures and the degree of inflammation and edema. MRI scans were performed for all patients using high-performance gradients (maximum amplitude, 45 mT/m; minimum rise time, 200 μs; maximum slew rate, 200 T/m/s) with integrated parallel acquisition techniques in three spatial directions. The imaging protocol consisted of gradient-echo localizers on each table position, followed by coronal whole-body STIR images for assessment of pathological signal changes occurring in the musculoskeletal system. MRI images were graded from 0 to 10 by an experienced and blinded radiologist. Also MRI scores (before and after treatment) were compared and scored from 0 (no improvement) to 10 (total healing) by investigators.

2.4. Statistical Methods. The variables were checked for having normal distribution by using Shapiro-Wilk test. According to nonparametric clinical variables (LoSDI, mLoSSI, and MRI), the Wilcoxon signed-rank test was used instead of paired-samples t-test. The correlation of these clinical markers with MRI scores before and after treatment was also assessed separately using Spearman's correlation test. Variations in clinical indices were analyzed by two-tailed Student's t-test with odds ratio (OR) and 95% confidence interval (CI). P-values which were adjusted with Benjamini–Hochberg method to control the false discovery rate lower than 0.05 were considered statistically significant. SPSS software for Windows (version 19.0, IBM SPSS Inc., USA) was used to perform all statistical analyses.

3. Results

3.1. Demographic Features. In present study, the female to male ratio was 5.6:1 (28 women and five men). The median age was 29.00 with IQR$_{25-75}$ of 19.00 to 37.50, with an age range of 10–61 years. Eight patients (24.2%) were <18 years. The mean duration of skin stiffness or atrophy was 5.81 ± 3.31 months, and the minimum and maximum durations were two and 13 months, respectively. Linear morphea was diagnosed in 28 cases that all of them had the en coup de sabre subtype; none of these patients had neurological involvement. The remaining five individuals were diagnosed with generalized type.

TABLE 1: Efficacy of the treatment regimen.

Clinical or Paraclinical Indices		Shapiro-Wilk Test	Before treatment Median (IQR$_{25-75}$)	After treatment Median (IQR$_{25-75}$)	P-value[*]
mLoSSI	Erythema	<0.001	2.00 (2.00-2.00)	1.00 (1.00-1.50)	<0.001
	Skin thickness	<0.001	1.00 (1.00-2.00)	1.00 (1.00-1.50)	0.002
	New lesion/lesion extension	<0.001	1.00 (1.00-1.50)	0.00 (0.00-0.00)	<0.001
LoSDI	Dermal atrophy	<0.001	2.00 (2.00-2.00)	1.00 (1.00-1.00)	<0.001
	Subcutaneous atrophy	<0.001	1.00 (0.00-2.00)	1.00 (0.00-2.00)	0.014
	Dyspigmentation	<0.001	2.00 (2.00-3.00)	1.00 (1.00-2.00)	<0.001
Magnetic Resonance Imaging		0.004	4.00 (3.00-6.00)	2.00 (1.00-3.00)	<0.001

LoSDI: localized scleroderma damage index; mLoSSI: modified localized skin severity index; * the Wilcoxon signed-rank test was used and adjusted P-value is reported according to Benjamini and Hochberg test.

TABLE 2: The association between MRI and mLoSSI and LoSDI.

Variables	Before treatment[*]	P-value[+]	After treatment[*]	P-value[+]
Erythema	0.479	0.008	0.467	0.008
Skin thickness	0.345	0.053	0.466	0.008
New lesion/lesion extension	0.451	0.009	0.322	0.068
Dermal atrophy	0.528	0.004	0.558	0.002
Subcutaneous atrophy	0.642	<0.001	0.585	<0.001
Dyspigmentation	0.536	0.002	0.596	<0.001

* correlation coefficient with MRI scores is shown in these columns. ‡ P-values are adjusted by Benjamini and Hochberg method.

3.2. Efficacy of Treatment. As mentioned previously, the efficacy of the treatment was evaluated by mLoSSI, LoSDI, and MRI, which is shown in Table 1. Based on statistically acceptable number of linear morpheae, the efficacy of the treatment has been evaluated separately in this group of patients and shown in Table 1. The number of cases with generalized morphea was negligible to analyze them distinctly.

According to mLoSSI, erythema, skin thickness, and new lesion/lesion extension were significantly improved after the treatment. Furthermore, all parameters of LoSDI including dermal atrophy, subcutaneous atrophy, and dyspigmentation were also noticeably improved after treatment. The treatment regimen was evaluated to be an effective method according to MRI by a P-value <0.001 (Figure 1). The results identified subcutaneous fat enhancement as the most common finding. The association of MRI scores with clinical markers (erythema, skin thickness, new lesion/lesion extension, dermal atrophy, subcutaneous atrophy, and dyspigmentation) before and after treatment is shown separately in Table 2. As it is evident, all of these clinical markers have an accepted and significant correlation with MRI modality, either before and after the treatment. The two exceptions were skin thickness and new lesion/lesion extension which were not associated with MRI scores before and after the treatment, respectively.

3.3. Safety and Tolerability. Among the 33 patients who received treatment, all of them experienced some adverse side-effects. According to the precise inclusion criteria, which excluded patients with latent infection, none of them experienced any severe adverse effect of immunosuppression.

Weight gain and acne vulgaris were the most prevalent side-effects, detected in 26 and 23 patients, respectively. These were primarily due to high dosages of glucocorticoid. Constitutional side-effects such as fatigue (n=13), nausea (n=11), and headache (n=5) were also reported in less than half of the patients, which could probably be due to MTX. Striae rubrae and alopecia were two cosmetically important adverse effects, respectively, observed in seven and six patients. Secondary Cushing syndrome was observed in approximately 10% of the patients (three individuals) as the most important adverse effect in this study. Finally, hypokalemia (n=8), leukopenia (n=2), and anorexia (n=1) were other reported side-effects.

4. Discussion

It is worth noting that this study demonstrated the effectiveness and sensitivity of MRI to treatment and its association with LoSCAT that would definitely be more novel and unique in the treatment of these patients.

Over the years, a variety of therapeutic options has been reported for morphea, topical and systemic corticosteroids, topical and systemic calcipotriol, topical tacrolimus, phototherapy, and MTX [12, 18–23]. One of the most challenging problems in the treatment of patients with morphea is the assessment of treatment efficacy and duration of the treatment. A valuable follow-up instrument should be able to differentiate between therapy responders, patients with stable disease, and those who are unresponsive to treatment. Mertens et al. showed that recurrences in morphea can occur even after many years of quiescence [24].

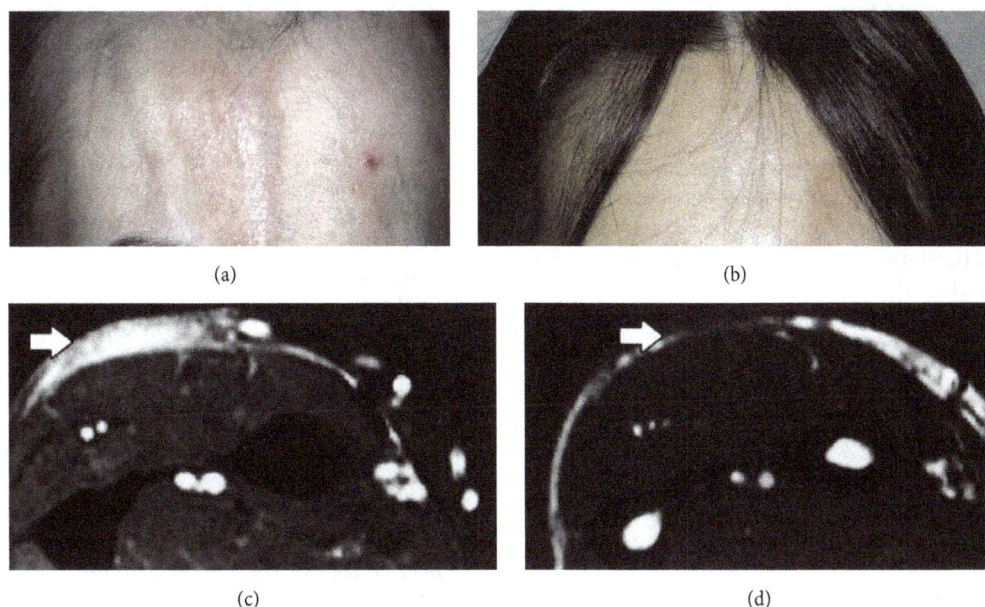

FIGURE 1: A patient with linear morphea before (a) and after (b) treatment. MRI results before (c) and after (d) treatment.

In the study conducted by Kreuter et al., fourteen LS patients were treated with 15 mg/week of MTX and monthly methylprednisolone pulse (1000 mg for three days) for six months. The effectiveness of the treatment was evaluated by ultrasound (US) and histological findings. Almost all of the patients had achieved clinical improvement, which was confirmed by paraclinical criteria [11]. In another study, Torok et al. examined the effectiveness of 1 mg/kg/week of MTX (a maximum dose of 25 mg/week) and 2 mg/kg/day of prednisone (a maximum dose of 60 mg). This treatment regimen was prescribed for 36 pediatrics patients who were followed up for an average of 36 months. The effectiveness was measured by physician general assessment (PGA) and mLoSSI, which showed clinical improvement in all patients [25]. Another study performed by Seyger et al. analyzed the effectiveness of 15 mg/week of MTX using visual analogue scale (VAS), durometer score, and modified skin score (MSS). After 36 weeks of follow-up, improvement in all patients was observed [26]. A multicenter study was published in 2006, in which methylprednisolone pulse (a maximum dosage of 500 mg) and 10 mg /m^2/week of MTX were given to 34 patients. The effectiveness of the treatment was measured by thermography and clinical criteria, and, ultimately, 71% of patients had entered the remission phase [6].

Several clinical and laboratory methods have been reported to measure morphea disease activity. One of these criteria is LoSCAT. Arkachaisri et al. [27] in 2008 examined the reliability of these criteria. In this study, two rheumatologists registered these symptoms for 22 patients and reported a significant association of LoSSI with medical interventions. Also they showed a significant association of mLoSSI with PGA, patients' quality of life, and medical interventions over time [28].

In 2010, a new standard was designed for the measurement of damage that was composed of DT, SAT, and DP. The reliability of this score with mLoSSL and PGA was acceptable. In our study, mLoSSI and LoSDI were significantly improved after treatment. Similar to earlier studies [25], we also used LoSCAT which was significantly improved. But as mentioned earlier, each evaluates only a limited subset of the clinical parameters especially that they are not so sensitive in the en coup de sabre subtype.

An important issue is the lack of a universal agreement on the optimal tools to be used for assessment of disease activity and damage severity or monitoring of the treatment response. Skin scores and recently more sensitive tools including laser Doppler flowmetry, Doppler US, and MRI have been used for evaluation and monitoring of the lesions [29].

Ultrasonography has been utilized for assessment of the superficial linear and circumscribed lesions because of its availability and excellent soft-tissue resolution, but evaluation of deep tissues may be impossible by US [14] and also US is usually not helpful as much as MRI on the scalp/face due to a thin tissue.

The data clearly show that MRI plays a key role and is able to document both dermal and musculoskeletal involvement at the initial presentation, as well as the changes occurring during these therapies. A valuable follow-up instrument should be able to differentiate between therapy responders, patients with stable disease, and those who are unresponsive to treatment. In our series, we found treatment success, which is in line with previous studies. Schanz et al. [15] showed that, in patients with morphea, MRI is a useful tool for the detection of clinical manifestations. Consistent with findings of Schanz et al. [16], our results showed that MRI is a suitable tool for patients with morphea and also the musculoskeletal and dermal manifestations in MRI improved in parallel with clinical improvement after systemic treatment.

Schanz et al. [16] mentioned that MRI provided complementary information about the depth of involvement of underlying morphological structures, contrary to clinical examination, which generally reveals information about the superficial involvement in this disorder. Thus, MRI may confirm the findings from the physical examination, and its findings are generally easier to interpret. It is better to evaluate the depth of involvement in generalized or deep morphea (also its subtypes) by imaging techniques (particularly MRI). The signal intensity is based on the grade and level of involvement, but there are no clearly defined criteria to judge the MRI changes [15, 16].

This study is subject to a number of important limitations: the lack of correlative laboratory disease activity markers and clearly defined criteria to judge the MRI changes; lack of a control group can be mentioned as another limitation, but it should be noted that it is inconsistent with ethical principles for patients not treated for several months.

5. Conclusions

We demonstrate the ability of MRI to capture disease improvement in patients with linear morphea responding to a methotrexate and corticosteroid regimen as defined by a significant change in the mLoSSI and LoSDI scores. Larger and comparative studies are needed to elucidate the diagnostic and monitoring applications of MRI in different types of morphea.

Abbreviations

LS: Localized scleroderma
MTX: Methotrexate
MRI: Magnetic resonance imaging
mLoSSI: Modified LS skin severity index
LoSDI: Localized scleroderma damage index.

Acknowledgments

The study was supported by the Skin Research Center of Shahid Beheshti University of Medical Sciences, and the authors wish to add that this article is the result of a dermatology specialty thesis of Dr. Razieh Jahangard in Shahid Beheshti University of Medical Sciences, Tehran, Iran.

References

[1] L. Weibel and J. Harper, *Harper's Textbook of Pediatric Dermatology*, A. Irvine, P. Hoeger, and A. Yan, Eds., Blackwell Publishing, Oxford, UK, 3rd edition, 2011.

[2] L. S. Peterson, A. M. Nelson, and W. P. D. Su, "Classification of morphea (localized scleroderma)," *Mayo Clinic Proceedings*, vol. 70, no. 11, pp. 1068–1076, 1995.

[3] R. M. Laxer and F. Zulian, "Localized scleroderma," *Current Opinion in Rheumatology*, vol. 18, no. 6, pp. 606–613, 2006.

[4] E. B. M. Kroft, E. M. G. J. De Jong, and A. W. M. Evers, "Physical burden of symptoms in patients with localized scleroderma and eosinophilic fasciitis," *JAMA Dermatology*, vol. 144, no. 10, pp. 1394-1395, 2008.

[5] G. Martini, A. V. Ramanan, F. Falcini, H. Girschick, D. P. Goldsmith, and F. Zulian, "Successful treatment of severe or methotrexate-resistant juvenile localized scleroderma with mycophenolate mofetil," *Rheumatology*, vol. 48, no. 11, pp. 1410–1413, 2009.

[6] L. Weibel, M. C. Sampaio, M. T. Visentin, K. J. Howell, P. Woo, and J. I. Harper, "Evaluation of methotrexate and corticosteroids for the treatment of localized scleroderma (morphoea) in children," *British Journal of Dermatology*, vol. 155, no. 5, pp. 1013–1020, 2006.

[7] Y. Uziel, B. M. Feldman, B. R. Krafchik, R. S. M. Yeung, and R. M. Laxer, "Methotrexate and corticosteroid therapy for pediatric localized scleroderma," *Journal of Pediatrics*, vol. 136, no. 1, pp. 91–95, 2000.

[8] V. Falanga and T. A. Medsger, "D-Penicillamine in the Treatment of Localized Scleroderma," *JAMA Dermatology*, vol. 126, no. 5, pp. 609–612, 1990.

[9] S. C. Li, K. S. Torok, E. Pope et al., "Development of consensus treatment plans for juvenile localized scleroderma: a roadmap toward comparative effectiveness studies in juvenile localized scleroderma," *Arthritis Care & Research*, vol. 64, no. 8, pp. 1175–1185, 2012.

[10] A. Kreuter, T. Krieg, M. Worm et al., "German guidelines for the diagnosis and therapy of localized scleroderma," *JDDG: Journal der Deutschen Dermatologischen Gesellschaft*, vol. 14, no. 2, pp. 199–216, 2016.

[11] A. Kreuter, T. Gambichler, F. Breuckmann et al., "Pulsed high-dose corticosteroids combined with low-dose methotrexate in severe localized scleroderma," *JAMA Dermatology*, vol. 141, no. 7, pp. 847–852, 2005.

[12] E. B. M. Kroft, M. C. W. Creemers, F. H. J. Van Den Hoogen, J. B. M. Boezeman, and E. M. G. J. De Jong, "Effectiveness, side-effects and period of remission after treatment with methotrexate in localized scleroderma and related sclerotic skin diseases: An inception cohort study," *British Journal of Dermatology*, vol. 160, no. 5, pp. 1075–1082, 2009.

[13] F. Zulian, G. Martini, C. Vallongo et al., "Methotrexate treatment in juvenile localized scleroderma: A randomized, double-blind, placebo-controlled trial," *Arthritis & Rheumatology*, vol. 63, no. 7, pp. 1998–2006, 2011.

[14] E. P. Eutsler, D. B. Horton, M. Epelman, T. Finkel, and L. W. Averill, "Musculoskeletal MRI findings of juvenile localized scleroderma," *Pediatric Radiology*, vol. 47, no. 4, pp. 442–449, 2017.

[15] S. Schanz, G. Fierlbeck, A. Ulmer et al., "Localized scleroderma: MR findings and clinical features," *Radiology*, vol. 260, no. 3, pp. 817–824, 2011.

[16] S. Schanz, J. Henes, A. Ulmer et al., "Response evaluation of musculoskeletal involvement in patients with deep morphea treated with methotrexate and prednisolone: A combined MRI and clinical approach," *American Journal of Roentgenology*, vol. 200, no. 4, pp. W376–W382, 2013.

[17] C. E. Kelsey and K. S. Torok, "The Localized Scleroderma Cutaneous Assessment Tool: Responsiveness to change in a pediatric clinical population," *Journal of the American Academy of Dermatology*, vol. 69, no. 2, pp. 214–220, 2013.

[18] A. Kreuter, "Localized scleroderma," *Dermatologic Therapy*, vol. 25, no. 2, pp. 135–147, 2012.

[19] M. T. Dytoc, I. Kossintseva, and P. T. Ting, "First case series on the use of calcipotriol-betamethasone dipropionate for morphoea [5]," *British Journal of Dermatology*, vol. 157, no. 3, pp. 615–618, 2007.

[20] M. M. Hulshof, J. N. B. Bavinck, W. Bergman et al., "Double-blind, placebo-controlled study of oral calcitriol for the treatment of localized and systemic scleroderma," *Journal of the American Academy of Dermatology*, vol. 43, no. 6, pp. 1017–1023, 2000.

[21] N. Hunzelmann, S. Anders, G. Fierlbeck et al., "Double-blind, placebo-controlled study of intralesional interferon gamma for the treatment of localized scleroderma," *Journal of the American Academy of Dermatology*, vol. 36, no. 3, pp. 433–435, 1997.

[22] E. B. M. Kroft, T. J. Groeneveld, M. M. B. Seyger, and E. M. G. J. De Jong, "Efficacy of topical tacrolimus 0.1 in active plaque morphea: Randomized, double-blind, emollient-controlled pilot study," *American Journal of Clinical Dermatology*, vol. 10, no. 3, pp. 181–187, 2009.

[23] M. Kerscher, M. Volkenandt, C. Gruss et al., "Low-dose UVA1 phototherapy for treatment of localized scleroderma," *Journal of the American Academy of Dermatology*, vol. 38, no. 1, pp. 21–26, 1998.

[24] J. Mertens, M. Seyger, W. Kievit et al., "Disease recurrence in localized scleroderma: a retrospective analysis of 344 patients with paediatric- or adult-onset disease," *British Journal of Dermatology*, vol. 172, no. 3, pp. 722–728, 2015.

[25] K. S. Torok and T. Arkachaisri, "Methotrexate and corticosteroids in the treatment of localized scleroderma: A standardized prospective longitudinal single-center study," *The Journal of Rheumatology*, vol. 39, no. 2, pp. 286–294, 2012.

[26] M. M. B. Seyger, F. H. J. Van Den Hoogen, I. M. J. J. Van Vlijmen-Willems, P. C. M. Van De Kerkhof, and E. M. G. J. De Jong, "Localized and systemic scleroderma show different histological responses to methotrexate therapy," *The Journal of Pathology*, vol. 193, no. 4, pp. 511–516, 2001.

[27] T. Arkachaisri and S. Pino, "Localized scleroderma severity index and global assessments: A pilot study of outcome instruments," *The Journal of Rheumatology*, vol. 35, no. 4, pp. 650–657, 2008.

[28] T. Arkachaisri, S. Vilaiyuk, S. Li et al., "The localized scleroderma skin severity index and physician global assessment of disease activity: A work in progress toward development of localized scleroderma outcome measures," *The Journal of Rheumatology*, vol. 36, no. 12, pp. 2819–2829, 2009.

[29] D. P. Hawley, C. E. Pain, E. M. Baildam, R. Murphy, A. E. M. Taylor, and H. E. Foster, "United Kingdom survey of current management of juvenile localized scleroderma," *Rheumatology*, vol. 53, no. 10, pp. 1849–1854, 2014.

26

The Antibacterial Effect *In Vitro* of Honey Derived from Various Danish Flora

Reem Dina Matzen ⓘ,[1] Julie Zinck Leth-Espensen,[2] Therese Jansson,[2] Dennis Sandris Nielsen ⓘ,[2] Marianne N. Lund,[2,3] and Steen Matzen ⓘ[1]

[1]*Department of Plastic Surgery and Breast Surgery, Zealand University Hospital, Roskilde, Denmark*
[2]*Department of Food Science, Faculty of Science, University of Copenhagen, Denmark*
[3]*Department of Biomedical Sciences, Faculty of Health and Medical Sciences, University of Copenhagen, Denmark*

Correspondence should be addressed to Steen Matzen; shm@regionsjaelland.dk

Academic Editor: Bruno A. Bernard

The mechanism behind the biologic actions of honey as a wound remedy has been intensively studied; however, there is no published data regarding any antibacterial effect of honey derived from Danish flora. We surveyed 11 honeys of various Danish floral sources for their antibacterial activity and compared them to a culinary processed commercial honey (Jakobsens) and a raw and a medical grade Manuka (*Leptospermum scoparium*) honey using the agar-well diffusion method. We tested the effect on three gram-positive bacteria (two strains of *Staphylococcus aureus* and one strain of *Staphylococcus epidermidis*) and two gram-negative bacteria (*Pseudomonas aeruginosa* and *Escherichia coli*). All samples, except the commercial honey, exhibited antibacterial activity, and samples derived from Water Mint (*Mentha aquatica*), Organic 2 (mixed organic flora), and Linden (*Tilia cordata*) honey had consistent effects on all bacteria tested and showed greater effect than medical grade and raw Manuka (*L. scoparium*) honey. The content of methylglyoxal was low in the Danish honey (< 2 μg/mL) and significantly (p<0.05) higher in both the raw and the medical grade Manuka (*L. scoparium*) honey, where the concentrations were, respectively, 6.29 μg/mL and 54.33 μg/mL. The antibacterial effect of Danish honeys was mostly due to hydrogen peroxide. We conclude that honeys derived from Danish flora possess antibacterial effect, probably by a hurdle effect of viscosity, osmolality, acidity, bioactive peptides, and most importantly the content of hydrogen peroxide. These findings indicate that honeys of various Danish floral sources may have clinical potential, although further studies are necessary to elucidate this in order to determine whether the results of our *in vitro* experiments also apply to a clinical setting.

1. Introduction

Honey has drawn increasing attention as a remedy for wound treatment of different kinds, mainly due to a verified antibacterial activity [1]. Antibiotic resistance and chronic wound infections have increased the interest in antimicrobial treatments, including honey-based wound care products, and these have been registered with medical regulatory authorities as wound care agents in many countries, among others, the European Union, USA, and New Zealand. These products are mainly based on Manuka (*Leptospermum scoparium*) honey from New Zealand.

Honey is a collection of nectar and consists of sugar (75–79%), water (20%), proteins, vitamins, minerals, and antioxidants [2]. The mechanisms of action of honey have been studied intensively, and it is acknowledged that it exerts a wound healing effect through a series of physical and bioactive properties [1]. The antibacterial activity of honey can be attributed to the natural occurrence of the enzymatic production of hydrogen peroxide (H_2O_2) and a varied presence of phytochemical components such as methylglyoxal (MGO) [3, 4]. The concentration of H_2O_2 in honey is low while still having a disinfectant and tissue debridement effect without being cytotoxic and causing tissue damage [5]. Furthermore, honey has a low pH, high osmolality, and viscous properties, which inhibits the growth of microorganisms [6].

Honey of different geographical and floral origins may possess differences in antibacterial properties, which may be related to different chemical compositions of honeys [5, 6]. Honey derived from the *Leptospermum* species in New Zealand (Manuka) and Australia is characterized by a high antibacterial activity even in the presence of catalase, which is an enzyme destroying H_2O_2. This nonperoxide activity is attributed to the high concentration of MGO, which is derived from dihydroxyacetone, present in large amount in the nectar from *Leptospermum* species [5, 7]. But other factors, such as phytochemical substances and polypeptides like bee-defensin-1, may contribute to the overall biological effects of honey as well [8, 9].

The raw Danish honeys which are sold via farmer's markets or local shops are characterized by not being heated in the process of production. This is mainly due to the fact that the raw Danish honey submerges from local beekeepers that process the honey immediately in glasses ready for sale, unlike commercial honeys, which are heated in order to liquefy after being stored. This immediate processing without heating preserves the natural enzymatic properties of the honey, but there is also a small risk of bacterial contamination. In order to not jeopardize the antibacterial effect of honey and to eradicate microorganisms, such as *Clostridium botulinum* spores which are sometimes found in honey, medical grade honey should be sterilized by gamma-irradiation, and not by heating which destroys the enzyme glucose oxidase [10, 11].

Interestingly, there is no published data regarding any antibacterial effect of honey derived from Danish flora, despite a large tradition for production and sale of raw honey in Denmark and the obvious interest in developing a local, biological, and therapeutically useful remedy for wound care.

The aim of this study was to examine the biological activities of Danish honey of different floral sources, determine the antibacterial activity of the various types *in vitro*, and correlate this with the presence of H_2O_2 and MGO. Furthermore, we analyzed a commercial (heated) honey and a medical grade Manuka (*L. scoparium*) honey as well as a raw Manuka (*L. scoparium*) honey from New Zealand for comparison.

2. Material and Methods

2.1. Honey Samples. Honey samples of different floral sources (**Table 1**) were collected from local beekeepers between July and August 2016. In addition, one sample was a commercial culinary processed honey from a Danish manufacturer Jakobsens and consisted of a blend of acacia honeys originating from different areas in Eastern Europe. Also, a raw Manuka (*L. scoparium*) honey was obtained from a local producer from New Zealand and a commercial medical grade Manuka (*L. scoparium*) honey (*"Activon"*, *Advancis Medical*) was included. All samples were stored in sterilized containers in the dark at room temperature (20-22°C). All tests were performed blinded, and labels were given after the experimental work and statistical analysis were completed. The source of floral identity was provided by the beekeepers

TABLE 1: Honey samples included in the study. The Danish samples were obtained by two local beekeepers from the Zealand Region. The Activon Manuka is a medical grade honey and was obtained from Advancis Medical. The raw Manuka was obtained from a local beekeeper in New Zealand.

Sample no.	Floral source Common name (Scientific name)
1	Heather (*Calluna vulgaris*)
2	Organic 1-mixed organic flora
3	Raspberry (*Rubus odoratus*)
4	Rapeseed (*Brassica napus*)
5	Organic 2-mixed organic flora
6	Water mint (*Mentha aquatica*)
7	Linden (*Tilia cordata*)
8	Hawthorn (*Crataegus monogyna*)
9	Raw Manuka (*Leptospermum scoparium*)
10	Bell Heather (*Erica tetralix*)
11	White clover (*Trifolium repens*)
12	Sand heather (*Hudsonia tomentosa*)
13	Activon Manuka (*Leptospermum scoparium*)
14	Jakobsens

based on availability of different sources for the nectar at the time of collection, the location of the apiary, and the organoleptic properties of the honey. The samples were diluted for handling by adding sterile Milli-Q water at 37°C to reach the desired dilutions. Throughout the antibacterial experiments, a solution of 75% honey was used, unless otherwise stated.

2.2. Pathogens. The pathogens (Culture collection of Food Microbiology and Fermentation, Department of Food Science at University of Copenhagen, Denmark) used for this study included

    (i) *Staphylococcus aureus* CCUG 1800;

    (ii) *Staphylococcus aureus* 1094-7;

    (iii) *Staphylococcus epidermidis* CCUG 39508;

    (iv) *Pseudomonas aeruginosa* SKN 1317;

    (v) *Escherichia coli* K 12.

2.3. Procedure and Measurement. For testing the antibacterial effects of the honey samples the agar-well diffusion method was applied using Brain Heart Infusion (BHI) broth (CM0113) and BHI Agar (CM1136) as medium, prepared according to the instructions of the manufacturer (OXOID Ltd. Basingstoke, Hampshire, England).

The BHI agar was heated in microwave, then cooled to 50°C, and transferred into sterile tubes of 30 mL agar and 100 μL of the tested pathogen (propagated in BHI broth overnight). The agar was stirred before pouring into sterile Petri-dishes and kept to solidify at room temperature for 30 min.

Wells (5 mm) were cut into the agar-dishes and 50 μL of the honey samples was pipetted into each well. Milli-Q water served as reference. The dishes were incubated at 37°C for 48 h and the diameters of the growth inhibition zones were measured in centimeters to the nearest 0.05 cm.

To identify the primary antibacterial substance of the honey, following tests were performed: osmotic stress, dilution of the samples, thermal sensitivity, the effect of MGO, and enzyme sensitivity. All experiments were performed with duplicate samples of the honey, unless otherwise stated.

2.4. Osmotic Effect. A sample of 75% sucrose (w/w), corresponding to the amount of sugar in honey, was made by diluting 7.5 g sucrose in 2.5 g sterile Milli-Q water. A sample of 15% sucrose (w/w), corresponding to the amount of sugar in 20% honey samples, was made by diluting 1.5 g sucrose into 8.5 g sterile Milli-Q water. 50 μl of the pure sugar samples was placed in the agar wells and procedure followed as described above.

2.5. Testing Thermal Sensitivity. 500 μL of each sample was added to Eppendorf tubes and heated in either a 60°C water bath or in a pot with boiling water (100°C) for 30 min. before testing.

2.6. Testing the Effect of Methylglyoxal. Two dilutions of 40% methylglyoxal in water solution (CAS 78-98-8, SIGMA-ALDRICH) were prepared. For a 0.02% concentration (200 μg/mL), 10 μl methylglyoxal was added to 19.99 mL sterilized water. For a 0.04% concentration (400 μg/mL), 20 μl methylglyoxal was added to 19.98 mL sterilized water.

2.7. Testing Enzyme Sensitivity. The honey samples were treated with two different enzymes, proteinase-K and catalase, to investigate the significance of a possible bioactive polypeptide and H_2O_2. 500 μl of each honey sample (75% honey) was pipetted into two Eppendorf tubes. One sample was added 50 μl of a 10 mg/ml proteinase-K solution K (CAS No. 39450-01-6, SIGMA-ALDRICH) for a 1 mg/mL solution. The other 500 μl of each honey sample was added 10 μl of a 50 mg/ml catalase solution (CAS No. 9001-05-2, SIGMA-ALDRICH) for a 1 mg/mL solution.

All samples were incubated at 37°C for 2 hours before being filled in the wells and tested as described previously. The experiments were only carried out on four out of the five pathogens mentioned in Section 2.2, thereby excluding *Pseudomonas aeruginosa* SKN 1317, due to no remarkably inhibiting activity in the previous experiments.

2.8. pH Measurement. pH measurements were carried out using a calibrated PHM250 Ion Analyzer-Radiometer Analytical.

2.9. Determination of MGO Concentration in Honeys. The determination of dicarbonyls in honey was performed according to Adams [12]. Briefly, 2 mL of Milli-Q water was mixed with 0.6 g of honey. Subsequently, 1.5 mL of the diluted honey was mixed with 0.75 mL 2% o-phenyl

diamine (OPD) (98%; Sigma, Steinheim, Germany) in phosphate buffer (0.5 M, pH 6.5; Merck, Darmstadt, Germany), in triplicate, and left over night to derivatize (19 hours). After the derivatization, the samples were filtered through 0.2 μm filters and analyzed by a method based on ultrahigh performance liquid chromatography (UHPLC) described by Hellwig et al. [13]. In short, the samples were separated on a Prontosil 60 phenyl material (250 mm*4.6 mm, 5 μm), with a guard column (Knauer, Berlin Germany, 5*4 mm) filled with the same material and an online filter (3 μm). The injection volume was 50 μL, flow rate was 0.7 mL/min, and the UV detection was 312 nm. Eluent A consisted of 0.075% acetic acid (Sigma, Steinheim, Germany), and eluent B was 80% methanol (Sigma, Steinheim, Germany) and 20% of eluent A. The gradient was as follows: 10% B to 50% B from 0 to 27 min. by a linear gradient, 50% B kept constant from 27 to 30 min., increase from 50% to 70% B from 30 to 34 min. by a linear gradient followed by an increase to 100% B to 44 min., which was kept constant from 44 to 48 min., and finally back to 10% B from 48 to 50 min. by a linear gradient. A standard curve was prepared with the quinoxaline of MGO (Sigma, Steinheim, Germany) in the range between 0.4 μg/mL and 20 μg/mL.

2.10. Statistical Analyses. As the distribution of data was assumed normal, the statistical analysis was carried out using Excel v15.26 and StatPlus 2016 v6.1.60 for t-tests and one-way ANOVA tests. In addition, measurements of least squares means (lsmeans) were applied on the data for pairwise comparison of the MGO data (alfa=0.05) by the software RStudio (RStudio Team (2015), version 0.99.446, RStudio: Integrated development for R. RStudio, Inc., Boston, MA).

3. Results

All the Danish honeys had antibacterial effect (p<0.05), and the honey samples Organic 2 (mixed organic flora), Water Mint (*Mentha aquatica*), and Linden (*Tilia cordata*) even possessed specific activity against *E. coli* and *P. aeruginosa*, while the medical grade Manuka (*L. Scoparium*) honey showed no activity at all towards these species. There were no significant differences (p>0.05) between the duplicate testing of all samples and all controls did not show any significant value throughout the various experiments. An example of the test results after agar diffusion method is presented in **Figure 1**.

The bar charts in **Figures 2 and 3** disclose the antibacterial effect of the honey samples. The Water Mint (*M. aquatica*), Linden (*T. cordata*), and Organic 2 (mixed organic flora) were able to inhibit all of the tested pathogens, showed the greatest inhibition zones and had a significant (p<0.05) effect on the gram-negative pathogens. The antibacterial effect of the honeys was greatest on the three gram-positive pathogens as compared to the gram-negative pathogens. The two honeys Hawthorn (*Crataegus monogyna*) and Activon Manuka (*L. scoparium*) showed the least inhibitory effect on the three gram-positive *Staphylococci* and were not able to inhibit the two gram-negative bacteria *P. aeruginosa* and *E. coli*. The

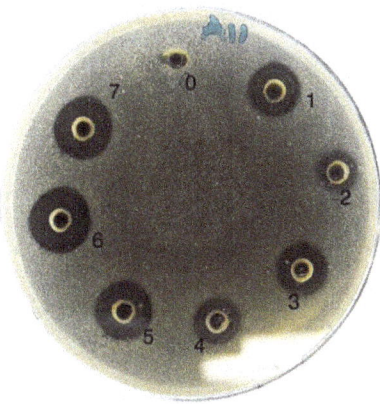

FIGURE 1: Photo of an agar-dish after agar-well diffusion assay. The dish is inoculated with *Staphylococcus aureus* (CCUG 1800) and honeys 1-7 are added in the wells. Milli-Q water serves as reference [0].

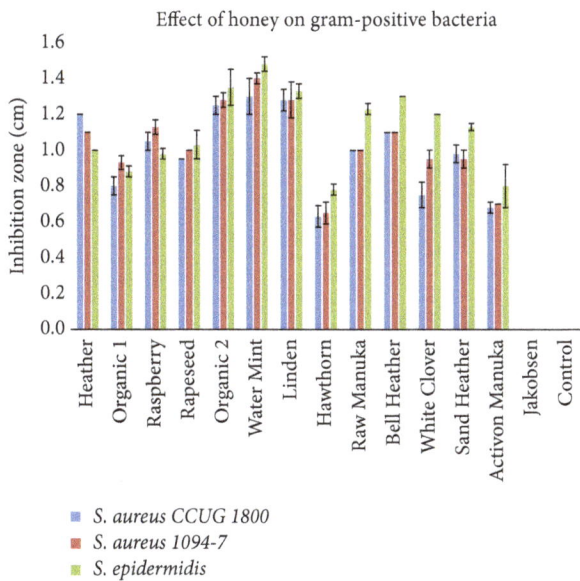

FIGURE 2: Effect of different floral sources of honey on growth of gram-positive bacteria (mean ± SD; n = 2).

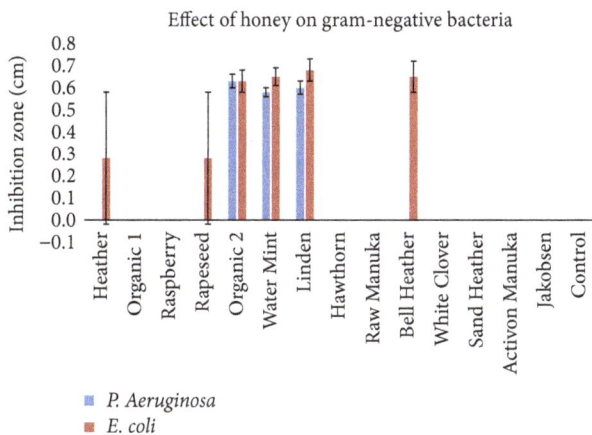

FIGURE 3: Effect of different floral sources of honey on growth of gram-negative bacteria (mean ± SD; n = 2).

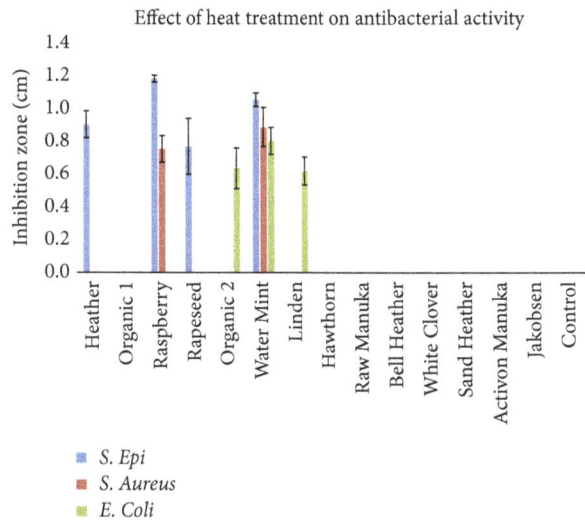

FIGURE 4: Antimicrobial effect of honey samples after heat treatment at 60°C/30 min. Some samples still showed antibacterial activity. These samples include Heather, Raspberry, Rapeseed, Organic 2, Water Mint, and Linden (mean ± SD; n = 2).

commercial honey, Jakobsens, had no antibacterial effect in any of the tests.

3.1. Osmotic Effect. The pure sugar samples (75% and 15% sucrose) did not show any inhibition on the five selected pathogens.

3.2. Thermal Sensitivity. The heat treatment of the honey samples revealed a reduction in the inhibitory effect on the tested pathogens. The heat treatment of the honey samples at 100°C in 30 min. inhibited all antimicrobial effect in all honey samples; however, honey samples Heather (*Calluna vulgaris*), Raspberry (*Rubus odoratus*), Rapeseed (*Brassica napus*), Organic 2 (mixed organic flora), Water Mint (*M. aquatica)*, and Linden (*T. cordata*) were able to inhibit microbial growth of some of the pathogens after heat treatment at 60°C (**Figure 4**).

3.3. Effect of MGO. Pure MGO solutions containing 200 μg/mL or 400 μg/mL showed an inhibitory effect on four out of the five tested pathogens, as *P. aeruginosa* samples were excluded from the study due to contamination. At a concentration of 400 μg/mL MGO, an inhibitory effect was seen on all four tested pathogens and significantly ($p<0.05$) higher compared to the 200 μg/mL MGO in three of the tested pathogens (*S. aureus* (1094-7), *S. epidermidis*, and *E. coli*).

3.4. Effect of Proteinase-K. All samples showed varying inhibitory effects on the different bacteria. For *S. aureus* (1094-7), honey samples Organic 1 (mixed organic flora), Rapeseed (*B. napus*), Water Mint (*M. aquatica*), Hawthorn (*C. monogyna*), and Bell Heather (*Erica tetralix*) had significantly ($p<0.05$) reduced activity after proteinase-K treatment.

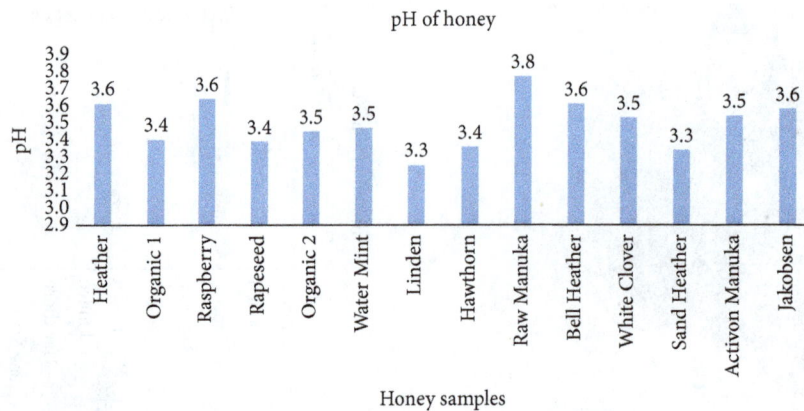

FIGURE 5: pH values of the 14 tested honey samples. The measurements are performed on a solution of 20% honey ($n = 1$).

For *S. epidermidis,* comparable results were observed with Raspberry (*R. odoratus*), Hawthorn (*C. monogyna*), and Bell Heater (*E. tetralix*) ($p<0.05$). For *E. coli,* proteinase-K treatment resulted in a significant ($p<0.05$) decrease in nine of the 13 honey samples, and in six of the samples the inhibitory effect was lost completely (**Table 2**).

3.5. Effect of Catalase. Treatment with catalase abolished the antimicrobial effect of all the Danish honey samples, while the Activon Manuka (*L. scoparium*) maintained a significant antibacterial effect on S. aureus (1094-7) and *epidermidis* ($p<0.05$) (**Table 3**).

3.6. pH in Honey. The 14 honey samples had a pH varying between 3.25 and 3.77 (mean: 3.49 and standard variation: 0.14) (**Figure 5**).

3.7. Methylglyoxal in Honey Samples. The concentrations of MGO in Activon Manuka (*L. scoparium*) and in raw Manuka honey (*L. scoparium*) were, respectively, 54.33 μg/mL and 6.29 μg/mL, and these concentrations were significantly higher than the other honey samples (**Figure 6**).

4. Discussion

This is the first study demonstrating that honey derived from Danish flora exhibit antimicrobial effects. This biological effect was for some honeys similar to or higher than the antibacterial effect of Manuka (*L. scoparium*) honey, especially regarding the inhibition of gram-negative microorganisms. The mechanism of action is mainly due to the content of H_2O_2 present in the Danish honey. The content of MGO is low in the Danish honeys compared to the medical grade Manuka (*L. scoparium*) honey, and the influence of this phytochemical substance on the antimicrobial effect of Danish honeys is probably of minor significance.

Clear differences could be observed in the antibacterial effect of the floral sources of honey with the Water Mint (*M. aquatica*), Linden (*T. cordata*), and Organic 2 (mixed organic flora) having the most consistent antibacterial effects on all tested pathogens. Also, the commercial culinary processed

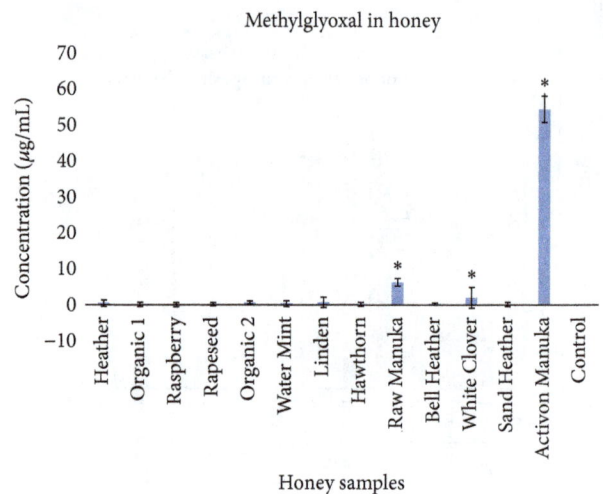

FIGURE 6: Concentration of methylglyoxal in 13 of the tested honey samples (mean ± SD, n=3). Symbol (∗) denotes statistical difference ($p<0.05$).

honey does not show any inhibition of the pathogens. This result, in conjunction to the results from the pure sugar samples, indicates that the antimicrobial effect is not simply conditional to the sugar content in the honey.

The gram-positive target strains were the most susceptible to honey whereas the gram-negative microbes were less sensitive to all honey samples including Manuka (*L. scoparium*), which is in accordance with previous observations [9, 14]. The difference in susceptibility to honey and other antibacterial agents between gram-positive and gram-negative microbes may be due to the composition of the cell wall. Gram-positive bacteria do not have an outer membrane protecting the peptidoglycan layer in contrast to gram-negative bacteria making it easier for antimicrobial agents to penetrate and cause damage [15].

The production of H_2O_2 by the presence of the enzyme glucose oxidase in honey is considered to be an important factor for the overall antibacterial effect of honeys [16]. But the concentration does not reach levels that are considered

TABLE 2: Mean zones of inhibition (mm) before (-) and after (+) treatment with the proteolytic enzyme proteinase-K on the 14 different honey samples.

Bacteria	1	2	3	4	5	6	7	8	9	10	11	12	13	14
Staph. aureus CCUG 1800														
-	10.5 ± 0.7	3.5 ± 0.4	9.5 ± 0.7	9.0 ± 1.4	13.8 ± 1.1	15.0 ± 2.1	12.5 ± 0.4	6.3 ± 0.4	8.8 ± 0.4	11.2 ± 1.1	9.3 ± 0.4	10.8 ± 1.8	0.0 ± 0.0	0.0 ± 0.0
+	7.5 ± 0.7	0.0 ± 0.0	8.0 ± 0.7	7.3 ± 0.4	11.0 ± 1.4	12.3 ± 1.1	10.0 ± 0.7	0.0 ± 0.0*	7.7 ± 0.4	8.5 ± 0.7	8.0 ± 1.4	9.0 ± 0.7	0.0 ± 0.0	0.0 ± 0.0
Staph. aureus (1094-7)														
-	9.5 ± 0.7	7.7 ± 0.4	10.0 ± 0.4	7.7 ± 0.4	-	-	12.0 ± 0.0	6.8 ± 0.4	10.8 ± 1.1	11.3 ± 0.4	-	-	-	-
+	8.5 ± 0.7	0.0 ± 0.0*	8.5 ± 0.4	0.0 ± 0.0*	-	-	11.0 ± 0.1	0.0 ± 0.0*	8.3 ± 0.4	8.3 ± 0.4*	-	-	-	-
Staph. epi (CCUG 39508)														
-	10.5 ± 0.7	3.8 ± 5.3	10.3 ± 0.4	9.0 ± 1.4	14.3 ± 1.1	15.0 ± 1.4	11.5 ± 0.7	6.0 ± 0.0	9.9 ± 0.7	10.0 ± 0.0	10.0 ± 1.4	9.7 ± 1.1	7.3 ± 0.4	0.0 ± 0.0
+	8.0 ± 0.7	0.0 ± 0.0	7.8 ± 0.4*	3.8 ± 5.3	11.3 ± 1.1	11.0 ± 1.1	9.5 ± 0.0	0.0 ± 0.0*	7.8 ± 0.4	7.5 ± 0.7*	7.0 ± 0.0	7.7 ± 0.7	6.5 ± 0.0	0.0 ± 0.0
E. coli (K 12)														
-	8.3 ± 0.4	3.3 ± 4.6	7.3 ± 0.4	7.3 ± 0.0	10.5 ± 8.0	11.3 ± 0.4	9.5 ± 0.7	6.0 ± 0.3	7.8 ± 0.4	8.0 ± 0.2	7.5 ± 0.2	8.0 ± 0.5	6.3 ± 0.4	-
+	7.0 ± 0.0*	0.0 ± 0.0	0.0 ± 0.0*	0.0 ± 0.0*	8.0 ± 0.0*	8.5 ± 0.0*	7.8 ± 0.4	0.0 ± 0.0*	7.0 ± 0.0*	7.0 ± 0.0*	0.0 ± 0.0*	7.0 ± .4*	3.0 ± 4.2	-

The antibacterial effect of different honey types on four different bacteria was assessed by the agar well diffusion method on duplicate samples and the mean ± SD are presented.
Symbol (-) indicates insufficient samples (n=1 or 0).
Symbol (∗) denotes statistically significance (p< 0.05; enzyme treatment versus no treatment).

TABLE 3: Mean zones of inhibition (mm) before (−) and after (+) treatment with the enzyme catalase on the 14 different honey samples.

Bacteria	1	2	3	4	5	6	7	8	9	10	11	12	13	14
Staph. aureus CCUG 1800														
−	8.0 ± 0.7	6.3 ± 0.4	7.5 ± 0.0	7.5 ± 0.0	7.0 ± 0.0	11.0 ± 2.1	8.8 ± 0.4	6.0 ± 0.4	7.8 ± 0.4	8.8 ± 0.4	-	-	-	0.0 ± 0.0
+	0.0 ± 0.0*	0.0 ± 0.0*	0.0 ± 0.0*	0.0 ± 0.0*	0.0 ± 0.0*	0.0 ± 0.0*	0.0 ± 0.0*	0.0 ± 0.0*	0.0 ± 0.0*	0.0 ± 0.0*	00 ± 0.0	0.0 ± 0.0	-	0.0 ± 0.0
Staph. aureus (1094-7)														
−	9.8 ± 2.5	7.8 ± 0.4	10.5 ± 0.7	787 ± 1.8	13.3 ± 1.1	13.5 ± 0.7	12.0 ± 0.0	6.0 ± 0.0	10.0 ± 0.0	10.0 ± 0.0	9.3 ± 0.4	10.5 ± 0.7	7.5 ± 0.1	0.0 ± 0.0
+	0.0 ± 0.0*	0.0 ± 0.0*	0.0 ± 0.0*	0.0 ± 0.0*	0.0 ± 0.0*	0.0 ± 0.0*	0.0 ± 0.0*	0.0 ± 0.0*	0.0 ± 0.0*	0.0 ± 0.0*	0.0 ± 0.0*	0.0 ± 0.0*	6.5 ± 0.1*	0.0 ± 0.0
Staph. epi (CCUG 39508)														
−	7.5 ± 0.0	0.0 ± 0.0	7.0 ± 0.0	7.0 ± 0.0	8.0 ± 0.0	9.0 ± 0.7	7.3 ± 0.4	6.0 ± 0.0	7.8 ± 0.4	7.8 ± 0.4	7.5 ± 0.4	7.8 ± 0.4	6.5 ± 0.1	0.0 ± 0.0
+	0.0 ± 0.0*	0.0 ± 0.0*	0.0 ± 0.0*	0.0 ± 0.0*	0.0 ± 0.0*	0.0 ± 0.0*	0.0 ± 0.0*	0.0 ± 0.0*	0.0 ± 0.0*	0.0 ± 0.0*	0.0 ± 0.0*	0.0 ± 0.0*	6.0 ± 0.1	0.0 ± 0.0
E. coli (K12)														
−	0.0 ± 0.0	0.0 ± 0.0	0.0 ± 0.0	0.0 ± 0.0	6.0 ± 0.0	6.8 ± 0.4	6.3 ± 0.4	0.0 ± 0.0	0.0 ± 0.0	6.0 ± 0.0	0.0 ± 0.0	0.0 ± 0.0	0.0 ± 0.0	0.0 ± 0.0
+	0.0 ± 0.0	0.0 ± 0.0	0.0 ± 0.0	0.0 ± 0.0	0.0 ± 0.0*	0.0 ± 0.0*	0.0 ± 0.0*	0.0 ± 0.0	0.0 ± 0.0	0.0 ± 0.0*	0.0 ± 0.0	0.0 ± 0.0	0.0 ± 0.0	0.0 ± 0.0

The antibacterial effect of different honey types on four different bacteria was assessed by the agar well diffusion method on duplicate samples and the mean ± SD are presented.
Symbol (−) indicates insufficient samples (n=1 or 0).
Symbol (∗) denotes statistically significance (p< 0.05; enzyme treatment versus no treatment).

cytotoxic [17], which could be of relevance in case of applying honey as a remedy for wound care [18]. In the present study it was observed that treating the honey samples with catalase, an enzyme inhibiting glucose oxidase and thereby the production of H_2O_2, significantly reduced the antibacterial effect of all the Danish honeys. However, the antibacterial effect of the Manuka (*L. scoparium*) honey on some of the gram-positive strains was unaffected. This finding is in accordance with previous observations that more important factors than the level of H_2O_2 accounts for the antibacterial effect of this sort of honey [1, 19]. It was confirmed that MGO, at least in the higher concentration (400 $\mu g/mL$), had an antibacterial effect, and together with the finding of a high level of MGO in the Manuka (*L. scoparium*) honey samples, this substance can be accountable for most of the antibacterial effect of this honey as reported previously [19]. In contrast, the Danish honeys had very low MGO levels, which is why this substance has little or no significance to the antibacterial effects of these particular honey types. On the other hand, studies have indicated that honeys with H_2O_2-dependent activity may be more broad spectrum and therapeutically useful as antifungal agents than Manuka honey, because they were found to be more effective than Manuka honey at inhibiting dermatophyte fungi [20] and species of the yeast *Candida* [21].

Besides the production and content of H_2O_2 or MGO, other properties of honey may contribute to the overall effects on bacteria. The low water content of honey and high osmolality and viscosity, acidic pH, and presence of leptosin and polypeptides like bee-defensin-1 have all been found to contribute to the reduced bacterial growth [22]. The low pH of honey did not seem to be an important factor in the present study. High osmolality is presumed to add to the antimicrobial effect of honey. However, from our experiments, high concentrations of glucose alone did not show any inhibition of bacterial growth. Furthermore, the heated preprocessed commercial honey had no antibacterial effect at all, despite a presumed high level of sugar. Other studies also indicate that solutions of glucose has less antimicrobial effect than honey [23], and the sugar-induced osmolality in honey is merely regarded as contributing to an unfavorable environment for pathogens, rather than being a primary inhibiting factor on bacterial growth by itself.

For further characterization of the mechanisms behind the antibacterial effect observed in the Danish honeys, the involvement of bioactive peptides was investigated by adding proteinase-K to the different honey samples. Proteinase-K was expected to cleave the proteins and thereby inactivate bioactive peptides such as defensin-1 [5]. Defensins are antibacterial peptides created to protect the host cells from invasion and infection by pathogens [24]. We found overall smaller inhibition zones on the agar plates with some differences between pathogens tested and the honey types after application of proteinase-K. It has previously been reported that there are differences in the presence of bee-defensin-1 in different sorts of honeys [9]. Our study shows a reduced effect on bacterial growth after adding a proteolytic enzyme and this is indicative of involvement of a biologic active peptide. However, further studies and other methods are necessary to elucidate if Danish honeys contain bioactive bee-defensin-1.

Throughout the experiments, the agar-well diffusion method was applied and used with a 75% solution of honey, for practical reasons, to determine the antibacterial effects of the honey samples. The 75% solution of honey had significant effect on the bacterial growth, while no effect was seen for the 20% solution of honey. This finding was also applied for the Manuka (*L. scoparium*) honey. It is well established that the agar-well diffusion method is suited for testing antibacterial effect, but if minimum inhibitory concentrations (MIC) are to be calculated, a more sensitive method like agar or broth dilution, where the honey is incorporated directly into the agar growth media must be used [25]. By this method the microbes are brought into direct contact with the testing inhibiting substance, and thereby not relying on the agent's ability to diffuse through the agar media [26].

Due to the physical characteristics of honey, it may contribute to a moist environment, which is beneficial for wound healing [27]. Furthermore, honey has been shown to stimulate the immune response and reduce inflammation, which in turn leads to an accelerated wound healing [1, 28, 29]. In addition, honey may also reduce the need for surgical wound debridement in selected cases [18, 30]. However, if honey is to be applied as a medical remedy for wound care it is necessary to process the honey for sterilization in order to eliminate a possible presence of pathogens or *C. botulinum* spores [11], why sterilization by gamma-irradiation should be performed [10]. No significant change in the antibacterial activity of honey was found caused by this method of sterilization of honey, neither in the honeys with H_2O_2-dependent activity or in the Manuka honeys [10]. Additionally, no significant changes were found in the physiochemical and mineral contents of honey resulting from sterilization by gamma-irradiation [31]. The process of heating honey will eliminate pathogens but also reduce the activity of H_2O_2 and other antibacterial substances. This is verified in the present study where the antibacterial activity was inhibited in most of the samples by heating the honey to 60°C.

5. Conclusion

This is the first study providing a substantial *in vitro* investigation of the antibacterial effect of honey derived from various Danish flora. We verified great variation in different floral sources with the Water Mint (*M. aquatica*), Linden (*T. cordata*), and Organic 2 (mixed organic flora) possessing the highest antibacterial activity on all the tested pathogens. These Danish honeys were comparable and even superior to commercial medical grade honey. The antibacterial effect was probably due to the activity of H_2O_2, though no direct measurements of the concentration of this substance was performed. Other studies have also been able to verify variation in antibacterial activity of honey depending on geographical location and floral source [26, 32].

Since the foraging of bees is not completely controllable and depends on the dominant floral source at the time of collection, it will be almost impossible to standardize a natural monofloral honey. Therefore, it is reasonable to assume that a specific floral source of honey also builds on a certain percentage of nonspecific nectar. However, while the antibacterial activity of honey might be a result of a hurdle effect of the honey's phytochemical characteristics, pH, viscosity, and content of H_2O_2, the mixture of different honey types might prove superior to a monofloral honey. Further studies are necessary to elucidate this hypothesis and to determine whether the results of our *in vitro* experiments also apply to a clinical setting.

Authors' Contributions

All authors have contributed equally to the above.

References

[1] P. Molan and T. Rhodes, "Honey: a biologic wound dressing," *Wounds*, vol. 27, no. 6, pp. 141–151, 2015.

[2] V. Bansal, B. Medhi, and P. Pandhi, "Honey—a remedy rediscovered and its therapeutic utility," *Kathmandu University Medical Journal*, vol. 3, no. 3, pp. 305–309, 2005.

[3] F. Alam, M. A. Islam, S. H. Gan, and M. I. Khalil, "Honey: a potential therapeutic agent for managing diabetic wounds," *Evidence-Based Complementary and Alternative Medicine*, vol. 2014, Article ID 169130, 16 pages, 2014.

[4] R. Jenkins, N. Burton, and R. Cooper, "Proteomic and genomic analysis of methicillin-resistant staphylococcus aureus (MRSA) exposed to manuka honey in vitro demonstrated down-regulation of virulence markers," *Journal of Antimicrobial Chemotherapy*, vol. 69, no. 3, pp. 603–615, 2014.

[5] J. Irish, S. Blair, and D. A. Carter, "The antibacterial activity of honey derived from Australian flora," *PLoS ONE*, vol. 6, no. 3, Article ID e18229, 2011.

[6] A. Moussa, D. Noureddine, H. S. Mohamed, M. Abdelmelek, and A. Saad, "Antibacterial activity of various honey types of Algeria against Staphylococcus aureus and Streptococcus pyogenes," *Asian Pacific Journal of Tropical Medicine*, vol. 5, no. 10, pp. 773–776, 2012.

[7] K. L. Allen, P. C. Molan, and G. M. Reid, "A survey of the antibacterial activity of some New Zealand honeys," *Journal of Pharmacy and Pharmacology*, vol. 43, no. 12, pp. 817–822, 1991.

[8] P. H. S. Kwakman, A. A. Te Velde, L. De Boer, D. Speijer, C. M. J. E. Vandenbroucke-Grauls, and S. A. J. Zaat, "How honey kills bacteria," *The FASEB Journal*, vol. 24, no. 7, pp. 2576–2582, 2010.

[9] P. H. S. Kwakman, L. De Boer, C. P. Ruyter-Spira et al., "Medical-grade honey enriched with antimicrobial peptides has enhanced activity against antibiotic-resistant pathogens," *European Journal of Clinical Microbiology & Infectious Diseases*, vol. 30, no. 2, pp. 251–257, 2011.

[10] P. C. Molan and K. L. Allen, "The effect of gamma-irradiation on the antibacterial activity of honey," *Journal of Pharmacy and Pharmacology*, vol. 48, no. 11, pp. 1206–1209, 1996.

[11] P. E. Lusby, A. Coombes, and J. M. Wilkinson, "Honey: a potent agent for wound healing?" *Journal of Wound Ostomy & Continence Nursing*, vol. 29, no. 6, pp. 295–300, 2002.

[12] M. R. Adams and Moss M. O., *Food Microbiology*, RCS Publishing, 3rd edition, 2008.

[13] M. Hellwig, J. Degen, and T. Henle, "3-Deoxygalactosone, a 'new' 1,2-dicarbonyl compound in milk products," *Journal of Agricultural and Food Chemistry*, vol. 58, no. 19, pp. 10752–10760, 2010.

[14] M. D. Mandal and S. Mandal, "Honey: its medicinal property and antibacterial activity," *Asian Pacific Journal of Tropical Biomedicine*, vol. 1, no. 2, pp. 154–160, 2011.

[15] M. Madigan, J. Martinko, K. Bender, D. Buckley, and D. Stahl, *Brock Biology of Microorganism*, Pearson, 14th edition, 2015.

[16] K. Brudzynski, "Effect of hydrogen peroxide on antibacterial activities of Canadian honeys," *Canadian Journal of Microbiology*, vol. 52, no. 12, pp. 1228–1237, 2006.

[17] L. M. Bang, C. Buntting, and P. Molan, "The effect of dilution on the rate of hydrogen peroxide production in honey and its implications for wound healing," *The Journal of Alternative and Complementary Medicine*, vol. 9, no. 2, pp. 267–273, 2003.

[18] R. Dina Jarjis, B. Thomas Crewe, and S. Henrik Matzen, "Postbariatric abdominoplasty resulting in wound infection and dehiscence—conservative treatment with medical grade honey: a case report and review of literature," *International Journal of Surgery Case Reports*, vol. 20, pp. 1–3, 2016.

[19] J. Atrott and T. Henle, "Methylglyoxal in manuka honey—correlation with antibacterial properties," *Czech Journal of Food Sciences*, vol. 27, pp. S163–S165, 2009.

[20] N. F. Brady, P. C. Molan, and C. G. Harfoot, "The sensitivity of dermatophytes to the antimicrobial activity of manuka honey and other honey," *Journal of Pharmaceutical Sciences*, vol. 2, no. 10, pp. 471–473, 1996.

[21] J. Irish, D. A. Carter, T. Shokohi, and S. E. Blair, "Honey has an antifungal effect against Candida species," *Medical Mycology*, vol. 44, no. 3, pp. 289–291, 2006.

[22] S. E. Maddocks and R. E. Jenkins, "Honey: a sweet solution to the growing problem of antimicrobial resistance?" *Future Microbiology*, vol. 8, no. 11, pp. 1419–1429, 2013.

[23] N. S. Al-Waili, "Investigating the antimicrobial activity of natural honey and its effects on the pathogenic bacterial infections of surgical wounds and conjunctiva," *Journal of Medicinal Food*, vol. 7, no. 2, pp. 210–222, 2004.

[24] A. Roberts, H. L. Brown, and R. Jenkins, "On the antibacterial effects of manuka honey: mechanistic insights," *Research and Reports in Biology*, vol. 2015, no. 6, pp. 215–224, 2015, https://www.dovepress.com/on-the-antibacterial-effects-of-manuka-honey-mechanistic-insights-peer-reviewed-article-RRB, 2017.

[25] M. Balouiri, M. Sadiki, and S. K. Ibnsouda, "Methods for *in vitro* evaluating antimicrobial activity: a review," *Journal of Pharmaceutical Analysis*, vol. 6, no. 2, pp. 71–79, 2016.

[26] P. E. Lusby, A. L. Coombes, and J. M. Wilkinson, "Bactericidal activity of different honeys against pathogenic bacteria," *Archives of Medical Research*, vol. 36, no. 5, pp. 464–467, 2005.

[27] J. P. Junker, R. A. Kamel, E. J. Caterson, and E. Eriksson, "Clinical impact upon wound healing and inflammation in moist, wet, and dry environments," *Advances in Wound Care*, vol. 2, no. 7, pp. 348–356, 2013.

[28] M. Subrahmanyam, "A prospective randomised clinical and histological study of superficial burn wound healing with honey and silver sulfadiazine," *Burns*, vol. 24, no. 2, pp. 157–161, 1998.

[29] P. C. Molan, "Re-introducing honey in the management of wounds and ulcers-theory and practice," *Ostomy Wound Management*, vol. 48, no. 11, pp. 28–40, 2002.

[30] L. Tahmaz, F. Erdemir, Y. Kibar, A. Cosar, and O. Yalcýn, "Fournier's gangrene: report of thirty-three cases and a review of the literature," *International Journal of Urology*, vol. 13, no. 7, pp. 960–967, 2006.

[31] S. Z. Hussein, K. M. Yusoff, S. Makpol, and Y. A. M. Yusof, "Does gamma irradiation affect physicochemical properties of honey?" *La Clinica Terapeutica*, vol. 165, no. 2, pp. e125–e133, 2014.

[32] J. M. Wilkinson and H. M. A. Cavanagh, "Antibacterial activity of 13 honeys against Escherichia coli and Pseudomonas aeruginosa," *Journal of Medicinal Food*, vol. 8, no. 1, pp. 100–103, 2005.

27

Dietary Habits in Patients with Chronic Spontaneous Urticaria: Evaluation of Food as Trigger of Symptoms Exacerbation

Jorge Sánchez [ID],[1,2] **Andres Sánchez,**[1,2,3] **and Ricardo Cardona**[1]

[1]*Group of Clinical and Experimental Allergy, IPS Universitaria, University of Antioquia, Medellin, Colombia*
[2]*Foundation for the Development of Medical and Biological Sciences (FUNDEMEB), Cartagena, Colombia*
[3]*Faculty of Medicine, Corporation University Rafael Nunez, Cartagena, Colombia*

Correspondence should be addressed to Jorge Sánchez; jotamsc@yahoo.com

Academic Editor: Giuseppe Stinco

Background. Many patients with chronic spontaneous urticaria (CSU) identify different foods as triggers of their symptoms and frequently make dietary restrictions without enough information. *Objective*. To explore the diet habits of CSU patients and estimate the clinical impact of the foods most frequently reported to be suspect. *Methodology*. Patients were interrogated about their clinical history of urticaria. Skin prick test and sIgE serum were done for most frequently reported foods by patients. Food challenge test was also performed. A group of healthy subjects was included to compare the dietary habits and the results of the diagnostic tests. *Results*. Patients with CSU (n 245) and healthy (n 127) subjects were included. 164 (66%) subjects from CSU group and 31 (24%) from the control group reported at least one adverse reaction with foods. Food IgE sensitization was similar in both groups (17.5% versus 16.5%, respectively). 410 food challenge tests in 164 CSU patients and 38 in 38 control subjects were performed. 1.2% in CSU group and 0.7% in control group had a positive oral challenge test. *Conclusion*. Despite the high frequency of self-report by patients, foods are uncommon triggers of CSU. Nevertheless, food challenge tests have to be offered early during medical evaluation to avoid unnecessary restrictions.

1. Introduction

Urticaria is a common cutaneous disease, where the chronic form affects around 1% of general population and has an important impact in the quality of life. Chronic spontaneous urticaria (CSU) can appear at any moment and for that reason patients associate foods, drugs, and different activities as possible triggers of their exacerbations [1, 2]. Usually, patients avoid the suspicious food, and this action has implications in their diet as well as personal and social life. In acute urticaria, food may play a causal role in some patients, but in chronic forms the role of food as a cause or trigger of CSU is not so clear.

Some studies have evaluated how often the triggers considered by the patient actually are associated with their symptoms. In a previous study, we observed that the prevalence of inducible urticaria self-reported was 75%, but the prevalence based on positive challenge tests was only 36%, indicating that a high number of patients did unnecessary restrictions [3]. Hsu ML et al. [4], observed that 32% of patients with chronic urticaria self-reported food as a possible trigger of urticaria, but after one month a restrictive diet was ineffective in 82.9% of patients. These results suggested that a self-reported evaluation is not adequate for studying some triggers of CSU. Furthermore, the GA²LEN/WAO/EAACI guidelines do not recommend any particular dietary restrictions for urticaria patients, except when a clear relationship is demonstrated [5]. However, to demonstrate "a clear relationship", challenge tests are required and most studies evaluating the prevalence of food as a cause or trigger of chronic urticaria do not include this diagnostic test.

In this study, we evaluated the role of foods as triggers of urticaria in CSU patients, taking into account not only self-reported information, but also challenge test. As a secondary objective, we evaluated the frequency of IgE sensitization to the most common reported foods reported and their possible association as causal mechanism.

2. Methodology

2.1. General Characteristics. Based on a previously described cohort (URTICA project, ClinicalTrials.gov Identifier: NCT01940393) [6], we collected data from patients older than 12 years diagnosed with CSU, which was defined as the recurrence of hives for at least 6 weeks, in whom the diagnosis had been made by an allergist or a dermatologist. The severity of the disease and quality of life were evaluated with UAS (Urticaria Activity Score) and DLQI (Dermatology Life Quality Index), respectively. The exclusion criteria included the following: use of omalizumab; systemic disease associated with the hives; use of systemic corticosteroids for three weeks before recruitment; immunodeficiency, dermatitis, and/or any other disease that could alter the oral challenge or skin test results. Patients using antihistamines were included, but they had to be suspended at least 4 days before the challenge test.

The control group consisted of healthy subjects without urticaria to compare the prevalence results of the self-reports, the frequency of IgE sensitization (atopy), and the challenge test results from the CSU group. The control group consisted of people older than 12 years, with no history of chronic urticaria in the last two years. Prior to enrollment a physician evaluated each person in the control group.

2.2. Study Design. The study aim was to explore the diet habits of CSU patients and estimate the clinical impact of the foods most frequently reported as suspect. To reach this goal, we evaluated the role of foods as triggers of urticaria exacerbation in patients with CSU using self-reported data, IgE sensitization, and challenge tests. All subjects in the CSU and control group filled out a questionnaire where they identified possible previous acute reactions to any food.

Skin prick test (SPT) and measurement of specific IgE (sIgE) by immunofluorescence were performed to 10 foods (beef, pork, chicken, shrimp, fish, milk, egg, strawberries, soybeans, and wheat) in all the subjects in both groups. These ten foods were chosen based on the results of the questionnaire about the most frequent foods associated with urticaria exacerbation in the same population. Additional foods were tested in those patients with self-reported reactions with other foods. Those foods that did not have standardized extract (e.g., sauces, "spicy foods") were directly tested by prick-by-prick and/or by oral challenge test.

The oral challenges were made with foods that each patient reported as suspect. Also, we did food challenge test to those foods that were not reported by patients but were positive in SPT or IgE serum.

2.3. IgE Sensitization Assessment. **Skin tests:** The IgE sensitization to beef, pork, chicken, shrimp, fish, milk, egg, strawberries, soybeans, and wheat was assessed by skin prick tests (SPT) according to international guidelines [7, 8]. Sensitization to mites (D. pteronyssinus, D. farinae, and B. tropicalis) and pets' dander (Cat and Dog) was also investigated. In patients with other suspicious foods than those tested, additional tests were performed with it or them.

Detection of serum IgE: Total and sIgE levels were measured in the serum using the ImmunoCAP 100 instrument (Pharmacia Diagnostic AB/Thermo Fisher, Uppsala, Sweden) according to the manufacturer's instructions. Results greater than $0.35kU_A/L$ for sIgE were considered positive.

2.4. Food Challenge Test. Patients blinded placebo controlled food challenge tests with fresh foods were performed using another food that the patient tolerated to camouflage the taste. Those patients using daily antihistamine have to suspend it for at least 4 days before the challenge test. When patients had exacerbation before the challenge test, they could go to medical office or send a photographic register to be evaluated by their medical doctor and define if they required antihistamines or not. If patients required antihistamines, a new appointment for challenge test was offered.

Patients received a portion equivalent to the expected daily intake of the food investigated [9]. Foods for challenge test were selected according to the clinical history and self-report of the patients. We also did a challenge test for those foods with a positive sensitization test (SPT or IgE serum), independently of being reported as suspicious. In patients with self-reported food trigger but negative sIgE and SPT, challenge tests were made by administering the total food serving, divided into two portions separated from one another by one hour (10% and 90% of the total serving to be administered). In cases of positive IgE and a clinical history of reaction, food administration was divided into four portions (10%, 20%, 30%, and 40%). The evaluation period after the challenge was four hours and the patients were also instructed to give notice in case of late reactions. A challenge test was considered positive when the patient showed hives or angioedema during the evaluation period. Other symptoms like wheezing, diarrhea, and vomiting were also indicative of a positive test but were recorded separately if urticaria symptoms were no present.

The oral challenge was contraindicated for those patients with a clear clinical history of anaphylactic reaction in the last 12 months within less than an hour after ingesting the suspect food and with a positive SPT or serum sIgE.

2.5. Ethical Considerations. Institutional Review Board approved this study. The work description was carried out in accordance with the Code of Ethics of the World Medical Association (Declaration of Helsinki) for experiments involving humans: Uniform. Informed consent was obtained from each subject.

2.6. Statistical Analyses. Statistical analyses were performed using IBM SPSS Statistics for Windows, Version 21.0 program (IBM Corp, Armonk, New York). The mean and SDs were reported for descriptive variables. Differences between proportions were analyzed using the Pearson chi-square test.

Univariate analysis based on logistic regression was performed for categorical variables to assess the relationship between exposure and outcome (e.g., food sensitization and positive challenge or self-report). A p value < 0.05 was considered statistically significant.

TABLE 1: Population characteristics.

Characteristics	CSU group (n 245)	Control group (n 127)	p
Age (y)	28 (14-50)	27 (15-55)	–
Age of onset (y)	25 (4-49)	NA	NA
Sex: female, n (%)	150 (61)	79 (62)	–
IgE sensitization*, n (%)	105 (42)	37 (29)	0.04
Asthma, n (%)	36 (14)	5 (3)	0.05
Rhinitis n (%)	105 (42)	50 (39)	–
DLQI score, mean + SD	15 + 3	NA	NA
UAS, mean + SD	3 + 1	NA	NA
History of food urticaria (%)	164 (66)	31 (24)	0.03
History of Drug urticaria (%)	92 (37)	30 (23)	0.04

Values are presented as % or mean. DLQI: Dermatology Life Quality Index. UAS: Urticaria Activity Score. NA: not applicable. *Sensitization to mites or pets dander. –: > 0.05.

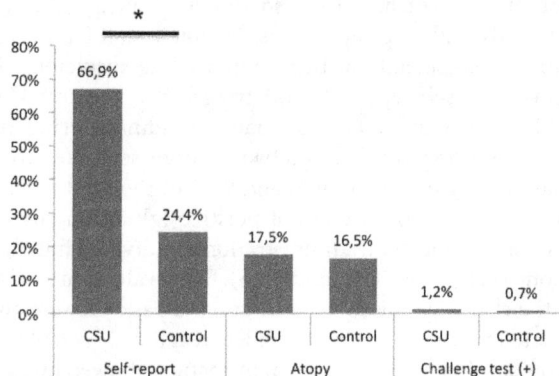

FIGURE 1: **Self-report, sensitization, and challenge test in CSU and control group.** Frequency of food sensitization and food trigger by self-report and challenge test to any food. Prevalence of Self-report, sensitization, and positive challenge test. Challenge test was done on 164 patients with CSU and 38 control subjects. The prevalence was calculated for the total number of patients in each group (CSU group 245, control group 127).

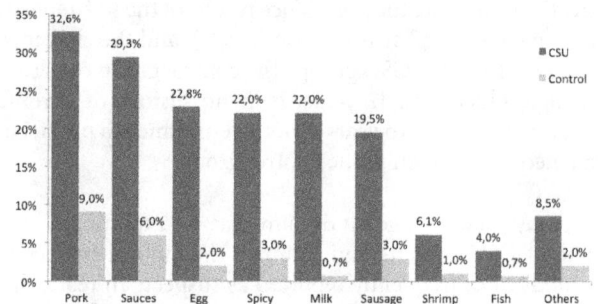

FIGURE 2: **Principal foods suspected by self-report.** Principal foods suspected by patients and control group.

3. Results

3.1. General Characteristics. A total of 245 patients with CSU (CSU group) and 127 healthy subjects (control group) participated in this study (Table 1). IgE sensitization and asthma were significantly more frequent in patients with CSU than in the control group (p < 0.05). No other differences regarding general characteristics were observed between the CSU group and the control group.

3.2. Self-Reported Food Triggered Exacerbations. One hundred sixty-four (66%) subjects from the CSU group and 31 (24%) from the control group reported at least one reaction with some food (p <0.01) (Figure 1) and 92% of them make a dietary restriction. In the group with urticaria, the patients self-reported an exacerbation of urticaria with these foods, while in the control group the symptoms that were self-reported were mainly cutaneous type pruritus, but 50% also

reported erythema and hives. According to the reports of patients and control subjects, the primary food or food products suspected of causing reactions were pork and sauces for both groups (Figure 2). At least two foods were suspected of causing reaction in 40% of the CSU and 12 of the control group. Self-reported exacerbations were always higher than sensitization or positive challenge test except for shrimp (Figure 3).

3.3. Sensitization Evaluation. Food sensitization was similar in both groups (17.5% versus 16.5%, respectively) (Figure 1). There were no significant differences regarding SPT or serum sIgE for any food. Also, there were no significant differences between sensitization and challenge tests results except for shrimp (p <0.01) (Figure 3). Self-report of reactions to shrimp was less than 10% (Figure 2), but IgE sensitization was the highest among foods tested in CSU group (12.2%) and in control group (14.1%) (Figure 3).

Self-reported reaction to pork was 32% in CSU group and 9% in control group, but sensitization to pork was present in only one patient. A group of 21 patients (8.5%) reported other foods or food products as a potential for their urticaria: 5 had positive skin tests, which represents 23% of patients with self-reported exacerbations to foods but only 2% of the total of patients in the CSU group. One of them had a

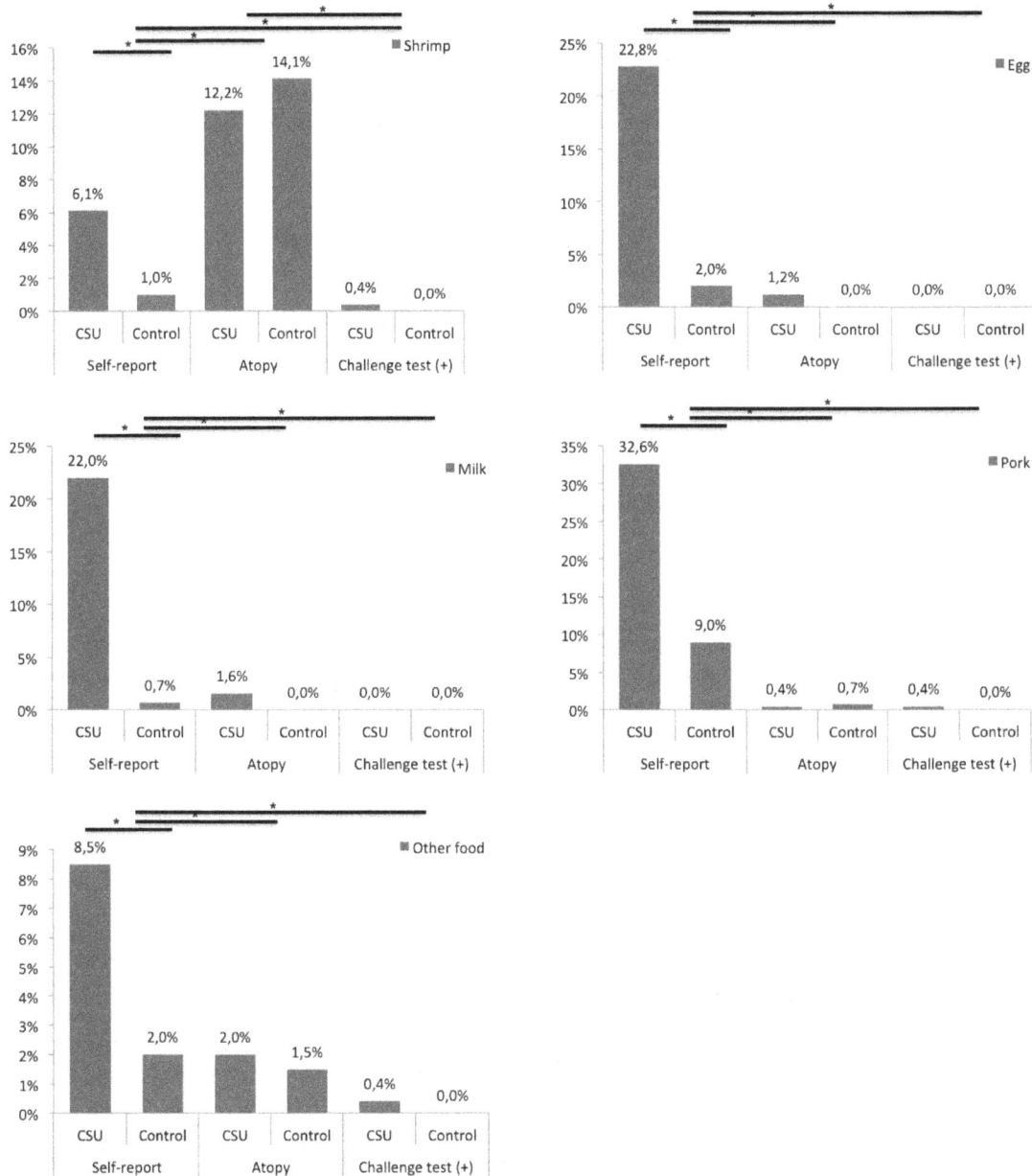

FIGURE 3: **Results of self-report, sensitization, and challenge test for the main suspect foods.** Percentages are based on the total number of patients with CSU or control group. *p <0.01.

positive challenge test with mustard. IgE sensitization and oral challenge with beef, chicken, fish, strawberries, soybeans, and wheat were negative in all subjects from CSU and control groups.

3.4. Oral Challenge Test: Relationship with IgE Sensitization and Self-Reported Triggers. A total of 448 food challenge tests were made: 410 in 164 patients and 38 in 38 control subjects, respectively. Three patients in CSU group (1 shrimp, 1 pork, 1 pineapple) with negative sensitization tests (SPT and IgE) had positive challenge tests, representing 1.2% of the patients from the CSU group (Figure 3). IgE sensitization to shrimp was frequent in both groups, but the only patient with a

positive challenge test result had negative SPT and serum IgE. Despite the high frequency of self-reported reactions with pork, only one subject (0.7%) in the control group had a positive test. This patient had a very suggestive clinical history of anaphylaxis in the last six months, so it was considered as a positive outpatient challenge and confirmation was not required for an additional challenge test.

None of the patients with self-reported exacerbations with egg, milk, sauces, spicy food, or fish in any of the groups had a positive challenge test. Of the 21 patients who reported reactions to other foods, one was sensitized and had a positive challenge test with mustard. There were no patients with positive sensitization tests or challenge test for other foods like sauces (tested in 48 from the CSU group and 4 from the control group), spicy foods (n= 54 and 4, respectively), fish (n=10 and 1, respectively), or any other food tested. None of the subjects had a positive placebo reaction. During the administration of the placebo, some subjects in the urticaria group (n 8) and the control group (n 4) manifested itching; however, none presented objective reactions, so the challenge continued with food being tolerated in all cases.

3.5. Follow-Up. Patients with a negative challenge were informed that they could consume the tested food and six months after the challenge, they were questioned about outpatient consumption. Sixty-four percent of the patients had consumed the food again and only 2 patients reported having a reaction of pruritus without hives or angioedema. Among the 36% of the patients who reported not having consumed the food, 18% did not do it out of fear, 10% did not have the opportunity to consume it again, and 8% did not want it because they did not like its taste.

4. Discussion

In CSU it is common for patients to associate the onset of symptoms with different activities [3], medications [1], or foods [2, 10] that they were performing or consuming near the time of the reaction. Similarly to what we had previously reported for inducible urticaria [3], in this study, we found that in more than 95% of patients with self-reported foods reactions the food was not related to the onset of symptoms. Additionally, over 80% of these patients were carrying out unnecessary dietary restrictions that might be detrimental to their health.

Most of the guidelines discourage food as a cause of chronic urticaria; however, it is common that patients associate the consumption of some food with worsening of the condition or as the cause of it, yet few studies have been conducted to demonstrate or discard this association. The self-reported prevalence of food as a trigger of CSU is about 13 to 80% [10–13] with different foods considered suspect according to the diet and social customs of each population. In our study, we observed a four times higher self-report of food exacerbation in CSU patients than in the control group. Most of the suspected foods corresponded to common foods in the diet of the population like pork, egg, milk, or fish but there were negatives for sIgE and challenge in most of the cases, confirming the low relevance of foods in the CSU. We do not know for sure the reasons for the high self-report. One possible explanation is the lack of information about the disease that patients receive from primary care physicians, which reflects the need for greater disclosure of international urticarial guidelines among first-level care physicians, to avoid these errors. Another hypothesis that does not exclude the first one is that the patient identifies the last action he performs as a possible trigger for his illness, and because the urticaria has a spontaneous appearance, it can frequently occur around the meals.

Similar to our results, some studies using diet restrictions have shown that foods are not relevant in CSU and diet restrictions are ineffective [4, 10]. Nevertheless, other studies with diet restrictions [11–13] observed that 17% to 73% of patients with CSU achieve complete or significant remission of symptoms after restriction diets, which highlights the importance of the oral challenge to clear the patients' fears and show the real impact of foods in CSU [4, 14].

The use of the basophil activation test, SPT, and sIgE serum for the diagnosis of urticaria triggered by food had conflicting results [15, 16], most of them showing a low sensitivity and suggesting that these tests do not replace the food challenge. When we compared CSU and control group, we observed a similar frequency of food sensitization (17.5% versus 16.5%). However, in the self-report, most of the control subjects reported mild gastrointestinal and skin reactions, which were not reproduced in the provocation tests, which suggests that these reactions were not allergic. Compared to other foods, the higher IgE sensitization to shrimp found in our patients may be because of the fact that the sensitization to mites is prevalent in our environment and there is a high cross-reactivity between some proteins of these two species [17–19]. This is supported by the fact that 30% of patients with IgE sensitization to shrimp had not previously consumed it and practically all subjects with atopy to shrimp were also sensitized to mites. Because none of the patients with IgE sensitization to shrimp had a positive challenge to it, we can assume that in most cases this sensitization results from cross-reactivity and therefore is not clinically relevant for patients with urticaria. In Latin America and our population, sensitization to pollen grains is low (<10%) [20]. Therefore, despite the high frequency of atopy and allergic respiratory diseases in the two study groups, pollen-food allergy syndrome does not seem to be an aggravating factor in urticaria.

"Pseudoallergens" are substances that induce hypersensitive/intolerance reactions that are similar to true allergic reactions. They include food additives, vasoactive substances such as histamine, and some natural substances in fruits, vegetables, and spices. Some studies suggest that eliminating pseudoallergens from the diet can reduce symptom severity and improve patient quality of life. M Magerl et al., from 140 subjects, found that one of each three subjects made a substantial reduction in their medication without experiencing worse symptoms or quality of life after pseudoallergen-free diet [21]. In our study, we did not specifically evaluate food additives or "pseudoallergens". It cannot be ruled out that in some patients foods with "pseudoallergens" may be the cause of urticaria or at least act as triggers. However, we tested the most frequent foods referred by patients and evaluated sIgE sensitization and their clinical relevance. Also, before entering the study, our patients had observed restriction diets on suspected foods without observing a significant improvement (data not shown).

One of the strengths of our study is that we conducted more than 400 challenge tests in 245 patients and 127 control subjects and we did a prospective follow-up to evaluate ambulatory tolerance to tested foods, which makes the results of the study quite reliable. During the follow-up, we observed that 18% of the patients did not eat the food out of fear even with a negative challenge test and medical support, which shows how this disease can have a significant impact on patients.

In conclusion, food challenge tests have to be offered early during the medical evaluation to avoid unnecessary avoidance of foods, as they are uncommon triggers of CSU.

Acknowledgments

This study was sponsored by the Clinical and Experimental Allergy Group of the University of Antioquia (Medellin, Colombia).

References

[1] M. Sánchez-Borges, F. Caballero-Fonseca, and A. Capriles-Hulett, "Cofactors and comorbidities in patients with aspirin/NSAID hypersensitivity," *Allergologia et Immunopathologia*, vol. 45, no. 6, pp. 573–578, 2017.

[2] S. F. Thomsen, E. C. Pritzier, C. D. Anderson et al., "Chronic urticaria in the real-life clinical practice setting in Sweden, Norway and Denmark: baseline results from the non-interventional multicentre AWARE study," *Journal of the European Academy of Dermatology and Venereology*, vol. 31, no. 6, pp. 1048–1055, 2017.

[3] J. Sánchez, E. Amaya, A. Acevedo, A. Celis, D. Caraballo, and R. Cardona, "Prevalence of inducible urticaria in patients with chronic spontaneous urticaria: associated risk factors," *Journal of Allergy and Clinical Immunology: In Practice*, vol. 5, no. 2, pp. 464–470, 2017.

[4] M.-L. Hsu and L.-F. Li, "Prevalence of food avoidance and food allergy in Chinese patients with chronic urticaria," *British Journal of Dermatology*, vol. 166, no. 4, pp. 747–752, 2012.

[5] T. Zuberbier, W. Aberer, R. Asero, C. Bindslev-Jensen, Z. Brzoza, G. W. Canonica et al., "The EAACI/GA(2) LEN/EDF/WAO Guideline for the definition, classification, diagnosis, and management of urticaria: the revision and update," *Allergy*, vol. 69, no. 7, pp. 868–887, 2013.

[6] J. Sánchez, J. Zakzuk, and R. Cardona, "Prediction of the efficacy of antihistamines in chronic spontaneous urticaria based on initial suppression of the histamine-induced wheal," *Journal of Investigational Allergology and Clinical Immunology*, vol. 26, no. 3, pp. 177–184, 2016.

[7] G. J. Burbach, L. M. Heinzerling, G. Edenharter et al., "GA2LEN skin test study II: Clinical relevance of inhalant allergen sensitizations in Europe," *Allergy: European Journal of Allergy and Clinical Immunology*, vol. 64, no. 10, pp. 1507–1515, 2009.

[8] L. M. Heinzerling, G. J. Burbach, G. Edenharter et al., "GA(2)LEN skin test study I: GA(2)LEN harmonization of skin prick testing: novel sensitization patterns for inhalant allergens in Europe," *Allergy*, vol. 64, no. 10, pp. 1498–1506, 2009.

[9] H. A. Sampson, R. Gerth Van Wijk, C. Bindslev-Jensen et al., "Standardizing double-blind, placebo-controlled oral food challenges: American Academy of Allergy, Asthma & Immunology-European Academy of Allergy and Clinical Immunology PRACTALL consensus report," *The Journal of Allergy and Clinical Immunology*, vol. 130, no. 6, pp. 1260–1274, 2012.

[10] B. Y. Chung, Y. S. Cho, H. O. Kim, and C. W. Park, "Food allergy in Korean patients with chronic urticaria," *Annals of Dermatology*, vol. 28, no. 5, pp. 562–568, 2016.

[11] T. Zuberbier, S. Chantraine-Hess, K. Hartmann, and B. M. Czarnetzki, "Pseudoallergen-free diet in the treatment of chronic urticaria. A prospective study," *Acta Dermato-Venereologica*, vol. 75, no. 6, pp. 484–487, 1995.

[12] B. Bunselmeyer, H. J. Laubach, M. Schiller, M. Stanke, T. A. Luger, and R. Brehler, "Incremental build-up food challenge - A new diagnostic approach to evaluate pseudoallergic reactions in chronic urticaria: A pilot study - Stepwise food challenge in chronic urticaria," *Clinical & Experimental Allergy*, vol. 39, no. 1, pp. 116–126, 2009.

[13] G. Malanin and K. Kalimo, "The results of skin testing with food additives and the effect of an elimination diet in chronic and recurrent urticaria and recurrent angioedema," *Clinical & Experimental Allergy*, vol. 19, no. 5, pp. 539–543, 1989.

[14] K. Kulthanan, S. Jiamton, N.-O. Rutnin, M. Insawang, and S. Pinkaew, "Prevalence and relevance of the positivity of skin prick testing in patients with chronic urticaria," *The Journal of Dermatology*, vol. 35, no. 6, pp. 330–335, 2008.

[15] S. Thaiwat, A. Nakakes, and A. Sangasapaviliya, "The effect of food avoidance in adult patients with chronic idiopathic urticaria," *Journal of the Medical Association of Thailand*, vol. 98, no. 12, pp. 1162–1168, 2015.

[16] M. Kang, W. Song, H. Park et al., "Basophil activation test with food additives in chronic urticaria patients," *Clinical Nutrition Research*, vol. 3, no. 1, pp. 9–16, 2014.

[17] R. E. Rossi, G. Monasterolo, C. Incorvaia et al., "Lack of neo-sensitization to Pen a 1 in patients treated with mite sublingual immunotherapy," *Clinical and Molecular Allergy*, vol. 8, article 4, 2010.

[18] A. Yang, L. Arruda, A. Santos et al., "Cross-reactivity Between Mite And Shrimp: the effect of immunotherapy with dust mite extract," *The Journal of Allergy and Clinical Immunology*, vol. 125, no. 2, article AB35, 2010.

[19] L. Caraballo, J. Zakzuk, B. W. Lee et al., "Particularities of allergy in the Tropics," *World Allergy Organization Journal*, vol. 9, no. 1, 2016.

[20] J. Sánchez and A. Sánchez, "Epidemiology of food allergy in Latin America," *Allergologia et Immunopathologia*, vol. 43, no. 2, pp. 185–195, 2015.

[21] M. Magerl, D. Pisarevskaja, R. Scheufele, T. Zuberbier, and M. Maurer, "Effects of a pseudoallergen-free diet on chronic spontaneous urticaria: A prospective trial," *Allergy: European Journal of Allergy and Clinical Immunology*, vol. 65, no. 1, pp. 78–83, 2010.

28

Comparison of the Morphological and Physical Properties of Different Absorbent Wound Dressings

Sukhontha Hasatsri ⓘ, Anuphap Pitiratanaworanat, Suwit Swangwit, Chadaporn Boochakul, and Chamaipond Tragoonsupachai

Department of Pharmacy Practice, Faculty of Pharmacy, Rangsit University, Pathum Thani, Thailand

Correspondence should be addressed to Sukhontha Hasatsri; sukhontha.h@rsu.ac.th

Academic Editor: Markus Stucker

Good quality wound dressings should have exceptional properties for usage, such as being able to remove excess wound exudates, having rapid dehydration, and providing optimal water vapour permeability. This study evaluated and compared the morphological and physical properties of six different commercially absorbent wound dressings in Thailand: two hydrocolloids, two alginates, and two foams. These wound dressings are available in a variety of components and structures, some of which have a multilayer structure. The results showed that the calcium sodium alginate dressings had better absorption properties than the calcium alginate dressings, hydrocolloid dressings, hydrocolloid with foam layer dressings, foam with polyurethane film layer dressings, and foam with hydrogel and polyurethane film layer dressings. Furthermore, the calcium sodium alginate dressings had the highest rate of dehydration and provided an optimal water vapour transmission rate. However, the calcium sodium alginate dressings could not retain the original structure after being submerged with a wound exudate.

1. Introduction

The selection of a wound dressing is usually based on a wound's characteristics [1, 2]. In addition, for a wound dressing to be of good quality, it needs to have specific properties including the ability to maintain a moist environment, absorb exudate, minimise maceration to the edges of the wound, permit exchanges of bodily gas, be easy to remove, and minimise pain from the wound [3, 4]. Wounds with high exudate require absorbent wound dressings with a high absorption capacity and rapid dehydration to avoid maceration [4]. In addition, wound dressings with optimal gas exchange between the exterior and interior of the dressing or an optimal water vapour transmission rate (WVTR) are able to maintain an optimal environment for the wound to heal [5]. The dispersion of a wound dressing can cause trauma during removal of the dressing because it adheres, and as nerve endings are exposed, that can be painful. Therefore, the ideal wound dressings should minimise pain and trauma to the wound [6]. Absorbent wound dressings, commonly used in wound care, can be categorized into three types:

hydrocolloids, alginates, and foams. However, films and hydrogels are nonabsorbent types of dressings [4, 7, 8]. This study focused on commercially available absorbent wound dressings in Thailand that were categorized into three groups: two hydrocolloids, two alginates, and two foams in which some of them had a multilayer structure. The wound dressings were evaluated and compared *in vitro*.

2. Materials and Methods

2.1. Materials. A number of materials were used in this study. These included hydrocolloid dressing (Nexcare™) manufactured by the 3 M Company, Minnesota, United States of America; hydrocolloid with a foam layer dressing (Duo-DERM®CGF™) produced by ConvaTec Inc., New Jersey, United States of America; calcium alginate dressing (Algisite®M) manufactured by Smith and Nephew Public Limited Company, London, United Kingdom; calcium sodium alginate dressing (Kaltostat®) made by ConvaTec Inc., Deeside, United Kingdom; foam with a polyurethane film layer dressing (Allevyn®) manufactured by Smith and Nephew Public

Limited Company, London, United Kingdom; and foam with a hydrogel and polyurethane film layer dressing (Askina®) produced by B. Braun Hospicare Ltd., County Sligo, Ireland. Sodium chloride and calcium chloride dihydrate were analytically graded without further purification.

2.2. Morphological Properties. The morphology of each dressing was assessed with a scanning electron microscope (SEM, JSM-6610 LV, JEOL) with upper (50x), lower (50x), and cross-sectional (15x) images being recorded at different magnifications. The pore size of the dressing was measured using ImageJ® software and represented in a mean ± standard deviation.

2.3. Absorption Properties. The absorption properties of the dressing were examined using BS EN 13726-1: 2002, Part 1: the aspects of absorbency, Section 3.2: free swell absorptive capacities with slight modifications [9]. A dressing (2 cm × 2 cm) was prepared. A test solution (8.298 g of NaCl (0.142 mol/L) and 0.367 g of $CaCl_2 2H_2O$ (0.0025 mol/L) were added to one litre of deionised water) represented a pseudo-wound exudate. The dressing was immersed in the test solution and then incubated at 37°C. At different periods, the dressing was removed and weighed. The experiments were performed in triplicate, and the weight increase was represented in a percentage and mean ± standard deviation.

2.4. Dehydration Properties. The dressing (2 cm × 2 cm) was immersed in the test solution for 30 minutes. After that, the dressing was removed, weighed, and incubated in an oven at 37°C. At different periods, the dressing was weighed. The experiments were performed in triplicate, and the dehydration rate was represented in a mean ± standard deviation [10].

2.5. Water Vapour Transmission Rate. The water vapour transmission rate (WVTR) of the dressing was examined using BS EN 13726-2: 2002, Part 2: the moisture vapour transmission rate of permeable film dressings with slight modifications [11]. The dressing (5 cm × 5 cm) was prepared, then a bottle of the test solution was covered with the dressing. The positive control was the bottle of the test solution that had no cover, and the negative control was the bottle of the test solution covered with a paraffin film. All of them were incubated in an oven at 37°C. At different periods, they were weighed. The experiments were performed in triplicate, and the WVTR was represented in a mean ± standard deviation.

2.6. Dispersion Characteristics. The dispersion characteristics of the dressing were examined using BS EN 137262: 2002, Part 1: the aspects of absorbency, Section 3.6: dispersion characteristics with slight modifications [12]. The dressing (2 cm × 2 cm) was immersed in the test solution and shaken for 60 seconds at 100 revolutions per minute. After that, the integrity of the dressing was visually established. The absorbance of the collected test solution was measured by using a UV-spectrophotometer at 200–400 nm.

3. Results and Discussion

3.1. Morphological Properties. Upper, lower, and cross-sectional images of the wound dressings are shown in Figure 1. These results show that the thickness of the foam with a polyurethane film dressing was the highest. A wound contact surface (lower image) of foam with a hydrogel and polyurethane film layer dressing showed a greater spread pore structure than foam with a polyurethane film layer dressing. The pore size of hydrocolloid with a foam layer dressing, foam with a polyurethane film dressing, and foam with a hydrogel and polyurethane film layer dressing were 600.18 ± 95.40, 297.88 ± 26.51, and 568.42 ± 78.63 μm, respectively. However, the number of pores of foam with a polyurethane film dressing was higher when compared with the other dressings. In addition, cell attachment, migration, and proliferation are an important process for the healing of a wound and an appropriate pore size range for these processes is 90–400 μm; cells cannot migrate, if pores are too small and cells cannot attach, if there is not enough surface area [13, 14]. Therefore, the foam with a polyurethane film dressing displayed an appropriate structure for the wound to heal. The multilayer structure of hydrocolloid with a foam layer dressing and foam with a hydrogel and polyurethane film layer dressing were clearly identified. Both alginate dressings showed a fibrous structure. The contrasting structures with or without using different components within the wound dressing affected the various properties.

3.2. Absorption Properties. This was the first study to demonstrate the absorption characteristics of a wound dressing during a 12-hour period. The absorption properties of the wound dressing are shown in Figure 2. The calcium sodium alginate dressing had the highest absorption capacity and after 4 hours, it degraded. However, the calcium alginate dressing degraded after 1 hour due to the difference in the chemical structure. The sodium ions in an alginate dressing stimulate the gel formation resulting in a high absorption capacity [15]. The calcium sodium alginate dressing showed a slow degradation probably because of the high glucuronic acid content [6, 15]. The researchers found that the number of pores was an important factor affecting the absorption capacity among the foam dressings (Figure 1). The absorption capacity of foam with a polyurethane film layer dressing was higher when compared to other foam dressings and was almost equivalent to a calcium alginate dressing. Both of the hydrocolloid dressings had a low absorption capacity and absorbed exudates slowly. Interestingly, the absorption capacity of hydrocolloid with a foam layer dressing was lower when compared with the hydrocolloid dressings. This indicated that the multilayer structure was not usually associated with increasing absorption properties.

3.3. Dehydration Properties. The dehydration properties of the wound dressings are shown in Figure 3. The alginate dressings had the highest dehydration rate. The foam with a polyurethane film layer dressing demonstrated a moderate rate of dehydration while the dehydration rate of foam

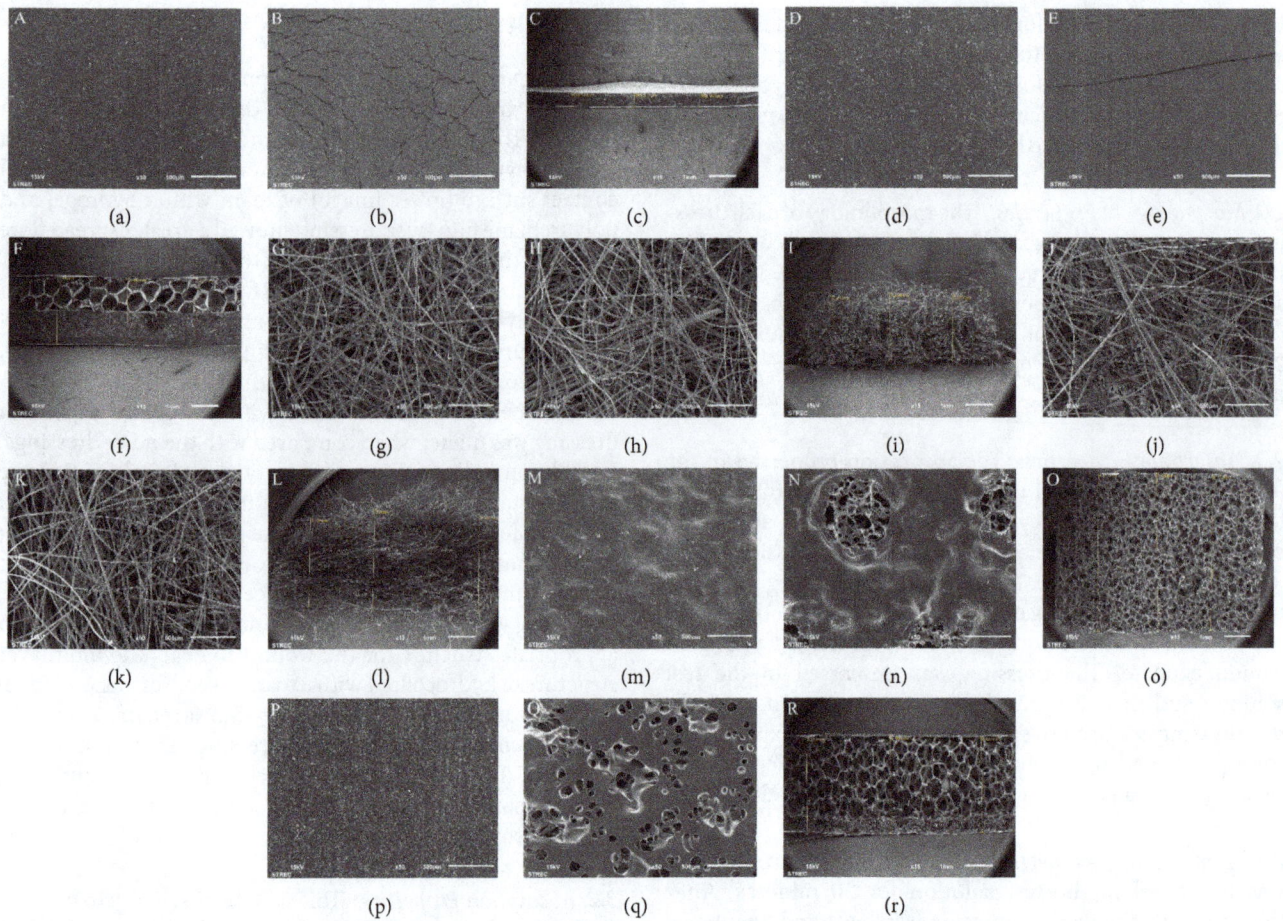

FIGURE 1: SEM photograph of (a) the upper surface, (b) lower surface, and (c) cross section of a hydrocolloid dressing; (d) the upper surface, (e) lower surface, and (f) cross section of hydrocolloid with a foam layer dressing; (g) the upper surface, (h) lower surface, and (I) cross section of a calcium alginate dressing; (j) the upper surface, (k) lower surface, and (l) cross section of a calcium sodium alginate dressing; (m) the upper surface, (n) lower surface, and (o) cross section of foam with a polyurethane film layer dressing; (p) the upper surface, (q) lower surface, and (r) cross section of foam with a hydrogel and polyurethane film layer dressing.

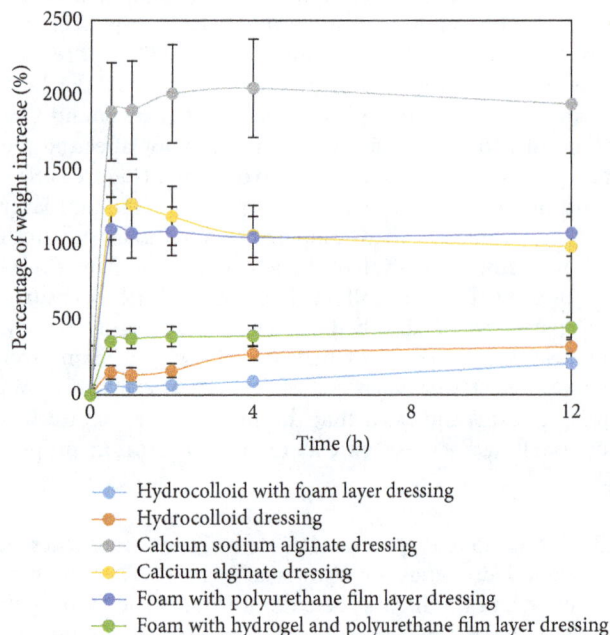

FIGURE 2: Absorption properties.

with a hydrogel and polyurethane film layer dressing was lower when compared to foam with a polyurethane film layer dressing. This may cause maceration because it has a low-to-moderate absorption capacity, which would interfere with the wound's healing process [7]. The wound dressing should have a balance between the absorption capacity and dehydration rate to prevent maceration. The hydrocolloid dressing had a high dehydration rate in the first 30 minutes, then it decreased dramatically. Hydrocolloid with a foam layer dressing also had a low dehydration rate. However, both of the hydrocolloid dressings absorbed exudate slowly resulting in nonmaceration.

3.4. Water Vapour Transmission Rate.

The water vapour transmission rate (WVTR) of the wound dressings is shown in Figure 4. One of the important properties of an ideal wound dressing would allow permeable water vapour to avoid the accumulation of the wound exudates [5, 6]. These results showed that the hydrocolloid dressings could not allow for permeable water vapour whereas other dressings showed the appropriate properties, especially the alginate dressings. Therefore, if an innovative hydrocolloid dressing

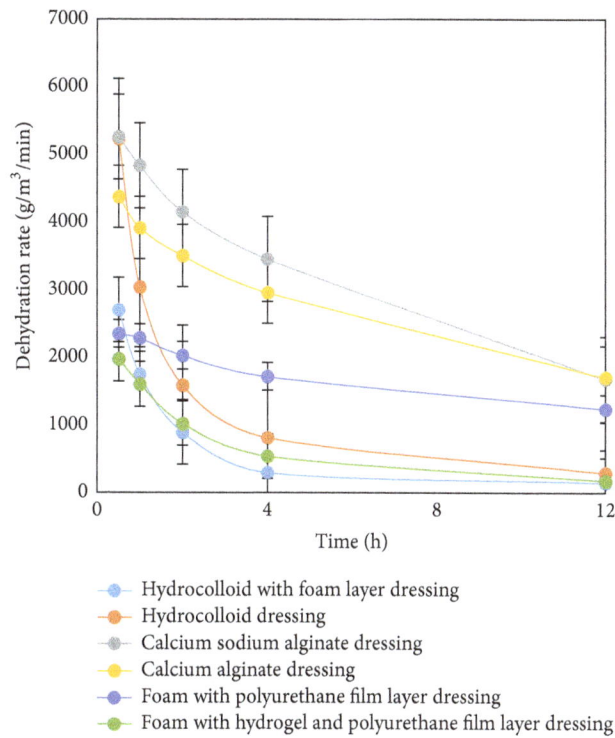

FIGURE 3: Dehydration properties.

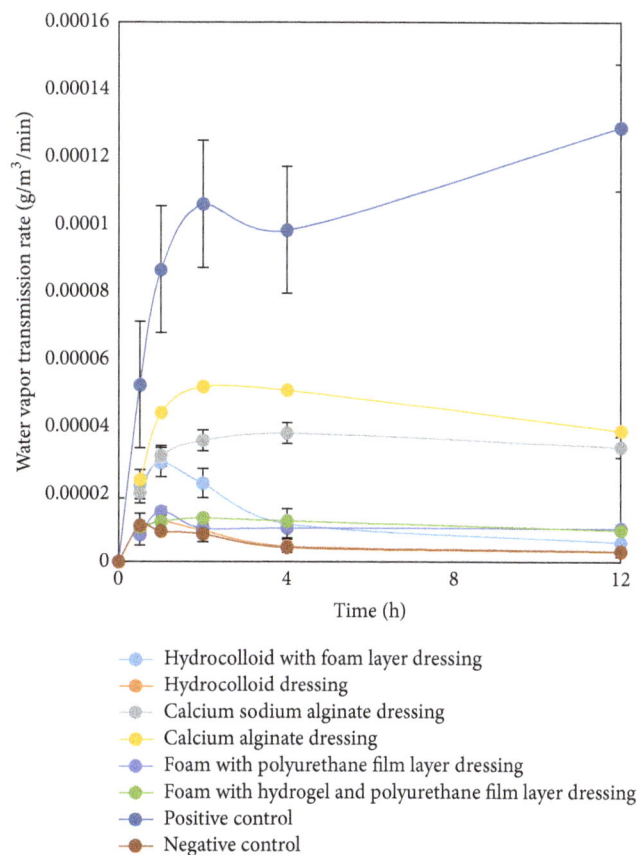

FIGURE 4: Water vapour transmission rate.

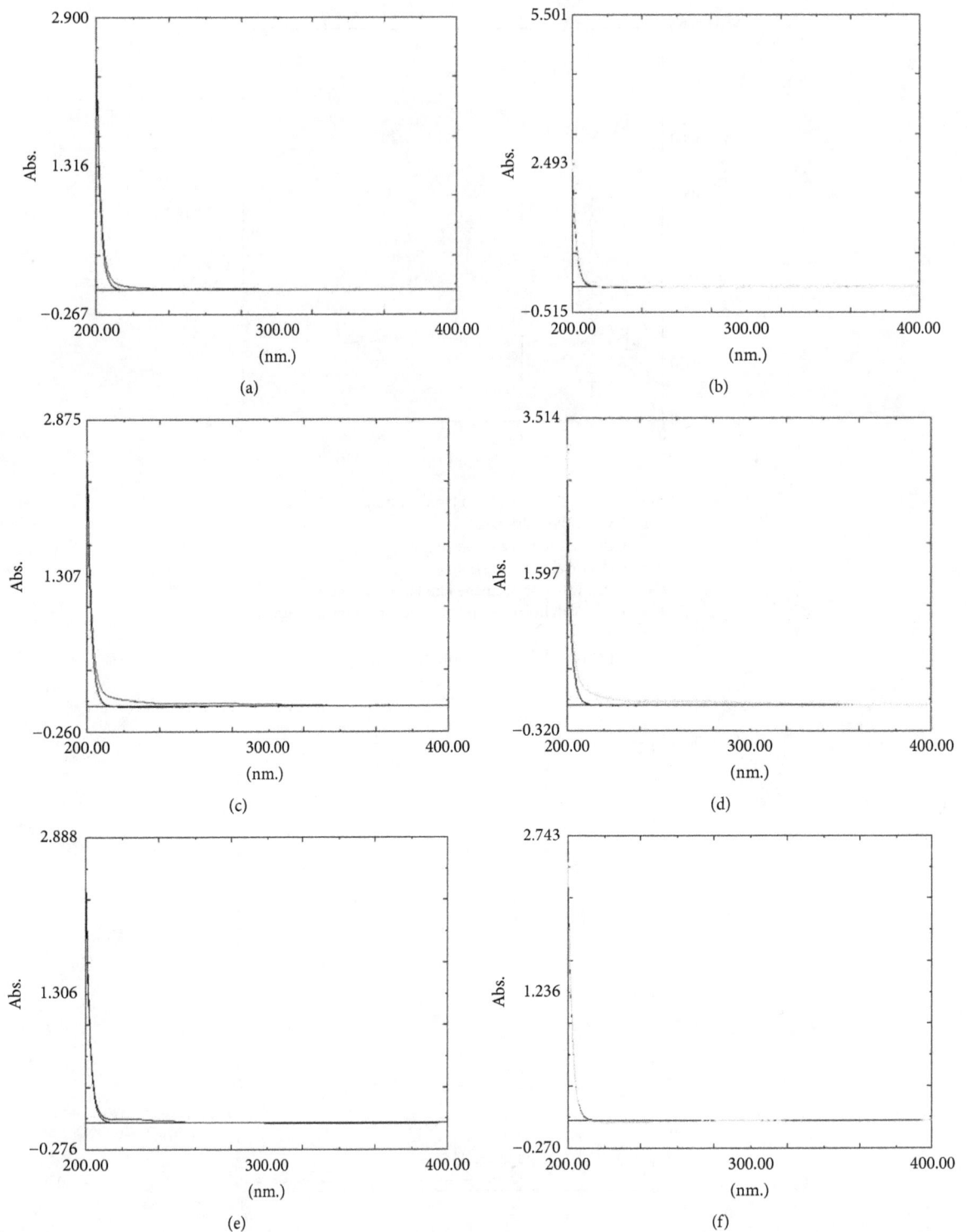

FIGURE 5: Dispersion characteristics compared with a pseudo-wound exudate: (a) hydrocolloid with a foam layer dressing, (b) hydrocolloid dressing, (c) calcium sodium alginate dressing, (d) calcium alginate dressing, (e) foam with a polyurethane film layer dressing, and (f) foam with a hydrogel and polyurethane film layer dressing.

is to be developed with these properties, it would require creating a multilayer structure.

3.5. *Dispersion Characteristics.* The dispersion characteristics of the wound dressings are shown in Figure 5. The dispersions

were shown visually from both alginate dressings resulting in the difficulty of removing the dressing. In addition, the spectra of the pseudo-wound exudate after being submerged with the alginate dressings were not quite similar to those of the pseudo-wound exudate, but other wound dressings were not dispersed in a pseudo-wound exudate. The wound dressing should retain the original structure after being submerged with a wound exudate for painless removal.

4. Conclusions

Calcium sodium alginate dressings demonstrate the highest quality among absorbent wound dressings. However, the integrity of alginate dressings should be taken into consideration and further research should be undertaken.

Abbreviations

WVTR: Water vapour transmission rate
SEM: Scanning electron microscope.

Acknowledgments

This work was supported by the Faculty of Pharmacy, Rangsit University, Thailand.

References

[1] M. Bennett-Marsden, "How to select a wound dressing," *Clinical Pharmacist*, vol. 2, no. 11, pp. 363–365, 2010.

[2] S. Baranoski, "Wound & skin care: Choosing a wound dressing, part 1," *Nursing*, vol. 38, no. 1, pp. 60-61, 2008.

[3] N. F. Watson and W. Hodgkin, "Wound dressings," *Surgery (Oxford)*, vol. 23, no. 2, pp. 52–55, 2005.

[4] K. C. Broussard and J. G. Powers, "Wound dressings: Selecting the most appropriate type," *American Journal of Clinical Dermatology*, vol. 14, no. 6, pp. 449–459, 2013.

[5] R. Xu, H. Xia, W. He et al., "Controlled water vapor transmission rate promotes wound-healing via wound re-epithelialization and contraction enhancement," *Scientific Reports*, vol. 6, no. 1, 2016.

[6] V. Jones, J. E. Grey, and K. G. Harding, "ABC of wound healing: wound dressings," *British Medical Journal*, vol. 332, no. 7544, pp. 777–780, 2006.

[7] S. Baranoski and E. A. Ayello, *Wound care essentials: practice principles*, Wolters Kluwer, Philadelphia, 2016.

[8] D. Weir, "Top tips for wound dressing selection," *Wounds International*, vol. 3, no. 4, pp. 18–22, 2012.

[9] British Standards Institution, *Test methods for primary wound dressings. Part 1; Aspects of absorbency. Section 3.2- Free Swell Absorptive capacities. BS EN 13726-1*, 2002.

[10] D. Parsons, P. G. Bowler, V. Myles, and S. Jones, "Silver antimicrobial dressings in wound management: A comparison of antibacterial, physical, and chemical characteristics," *Wounds*, vol. 17, no. 8, pp. 222–232, 2005.

[11] British Standards Institution, *Test methods for primary wound dressings. Part 2; Moisture vapour transmission rate of permeable film dressings BS EN 13726-2*, 2002.

[12] British Standards Institution, *Test methods for primary wound dressings. Part 1; Aspects of absorbency. Section 3.6 - Dispersion characteristics. BS EN 13726-1*, 2002.

[13] S. P. Miguel, M. P. Ribeiro, H. Brancal, P. Coutinho, and I. J. Correia, "Thermoresponsive chitosan-agarose hydrogel for skin regeneration," *Carbohydrate Polymers*, vol. 111, pp. 366–373, 2014.

[14] F. Han, Y. Dong, Z. Su, R. Yin, A. Song, and S. Li, "Preparation, characteristics and assessment of a novel gelatin-chitosan sponge scaffold as skin tissue engineering material," *International Journal of Pharmaceutics*, vol. 476, no. 1, pp. 124–133, 2014.

[15] S. Thomas, "Alginate dressings Do they influence wound healing?" *Journal of Wound Care*, vol. 9, no. 2, pp. 1–5, 2000.

29

A Real-Life Based Evaluation of the Effectiveness of Antibacterial Fabrics in Treating Atopic Dermatitis

Dirk Höfer (ID)

Hohenstein Institute for Textile Innovation, Schlosssteige 1, 74357 Bönnigheim, Germany

Correspondence should be addressed to Dirk Höfer; d.hoefer@hohenstein.de

Academic Editor: E. Helen Kemp

Background. Antibacterial clothes are classified as a complementary treatment in line with antisepsis, although meta-studies are unable to find significant improvements of eczemas. *Methods.* The antibacterial effectiveness of conventional AD clothes was compared across each other by (i) standard suspension tests for the appraisal of antibacterial products and (ii) a real-life setup of affected AD skin using *S. aureus* colonised artificial skin, to assess if functional clothes are effective under practical wear conditions. Additionally, the interaction of the fibre types with a moisturising cream was evaluated during a real wearing situation and after domestic laundry. *Results.* In the real-life setup simulating dry skin microenvironment, all samples failed to reduce *S. aureus*. Silver and zinc-fabrics showed a slight activity only under unrealistic moist conditions. When using standard suspension tests, samples differed considerably in their antibacterial effectiveness, where silver and zinc endowed fibres outperformed AEGIS endowed silk fabrics. Garments absorbed the cream dependent on the particular fibre types. Furthermore, domestic laundry was unable to completely remove the cream. *Conclusion.* Considerable differences in the antibacterial effectiveness of conventional AD clothes were revealed. Under practical (dry) wear conditions, garments were unable to modify skin colonization with *S. aureus*, although effectiveness can be triggered by wetting the garments. Remnants of moisturising cream remain on the fibres after laundry.

1. Introduction

Atopic dermatitis (AD) is a chronic, recurrent inflammatory skin disease with a significant social and economic burden. It has an estimated prevalence of up to 20 % in children and 2 % in adults [1, 2] and a considerable impact on the patient's quality of life, depending on the severity of the disease. AD is a multifactorial disease that is influenced by inheritance as well as by a variety of environmental factors. Its pathophysiology comprises immunological deregulations such as Th1/Th2 dysbalance and interleukin 31 as a key pruritic skin factor, leading to defects in skin barrier function like reduced water retention [3, 4]. The complex network of immunological deregulations may also explain the high rate of cutaneous colonization with *Staphylococcus aureus* (up to 90% in moderate to severe eczema) and *Staphylococcus epidermidis* in AD [5–7]. Only *S. aureus* is able to produce virulence factors such as super-antigens and therefore exacerbates the skin inflammation [8]. However, dysbiosis in skin microbiome of AD patients does not only implicate

Staphylococcus species, but also implicate microbes such as *Cutibacterium spp.* and *Malassezia* [9].

Clothing plays a pivotal role as a provoking factor of AD. Therefore, patients carefully choose smooth clothing and avoid irritating fabrics and fibres like wool to prevent primary skin irritation [10, 11]. This insight led to the development of functional textiles. However, whereas some fabrics such as cotton and silk garments tend to reduce scratching by smooth fibre types, a subset of garments have been specifically designed, claiming to reduce the intensity of the eczemas by modulating the skin staphylococcal profile via an antibacterial activity [12, 13]. Some antibacterial clothes therefore use the deposition or incorporation of metallic silver or silver compounds in or onto synthetic fibres [14], whereas others use zinc or quaternary ammonium as antibacterial agents [15, 16]. Subsequently, a number of clinical trials (randomized controlled or observational) were conducted using antibacterial clothes for AD treatment, most of which claimed skin improvements in SCORAD, fewer symptoms, or reduced itching. However, a systematic meta-analysis study stated that these trials are of low quality of supporting evidence regarding the effectiveness in AD symptoms and severity: The test designs were unable to guarantee randomization of the test subjects, showed a small sample size, used different active agents in the respective clothes, or continued comedication with topical glucocorticoids, calcineurin inhibitors, or moisturising creams during the trial [17]. The meta-analysis study concluded that recommendation for the use of functional textiles in AD treatment is weak and that more studies with better methodology and longer follow-up are needed. Although, in the considered RCTs, AD patients mostly assessed functional clothes positively, it was unclear if this vote can be assigned to either the antibacterial effect, the use of smooth fibres, or, for example, a combination of both traits. In contrast to this, a Cochrane review on interventions to reduce S. aureus in the management of AD stated that topical antibiotics as well as antiseptics (including one trial using silver textiles) showed no significant improvements in eczema [18], a finding that was supported by a recent health technology assessment, which studied the effectiveness of oral and topical antibiotics [19].

Against this background, it is not surprising that medical guidelines pertaining to AD emphasize that antibacterial clothes could at least "potentially improve disease severity" in patients prone to noncommensal bacteria colonisation and skin barrier impairment [20]. Furthermore, health technology assessments merely summarized the effect of antibacterial clothes "to be considered as a complementary treatment." In this situation, a situation full of contrasts, it might be helpful to study the effectiveness with a practical in vitro approach, for example, by using a S. aureus-affected skin model, in order to assess whether antibacterial effects of functional clothes on dystopic skin can be substantiated on a laboratory scale.

Besides clothing, the use of moisturisers is emphasized by healthcare professionals and the guidelines as a basic part in the treatment of AD. Moisturisation is suggested to enhance the healing of eczemas and to prolong the clinical improvement after discontinuation of anti-inflammatory therapy, thereby reducing the need for additional treatment, including topical corticosteroids [21–23]. Up to now, there is no data available if and how functional clothes and fibre types interfere with moisturisers. For instance, the presumed antibacterial effect of functional clothes might actually be disturbed by the simultaneous use of moisturising creams. On the other hand, cream remnants might cling to the clothes, mitigating the severity of eczemas.

In this respect, this research study conducted controlled in vitro tests: First, to compare the antibacterial effectiveness of five conventional functional clothes for AD treatment by quantitative international standard suspension tests. Second, as these normative approaches are not an accurate reflection of the environmental conditions under which AD garments are worn, a real-life setup of affected AD skin was used, based on artificial skin inoculated with S. aureus (i.e., a practical wear simulation of dysbiotic skin), to compare the clothes antibacterial activity in vitro. Finally, the interaction of the fibre types with a lipid-containing moisturising cream was evaluated during a real wearing situation and after domestic laundry.

2. Material and Methods

2.1. Fabric Characterisation. To objectively measure the potential antibacterial efficacy of antibacterial fabrics against a S. aureus strain, 5 commercial clothes were enrolled that have documented clinical benefits in treating atopic dermatitis in published reports: Sample #1 (Lyo-Zinc): Benevit Zinc+ (Benevit Van Clewe, Dingden, Germany) which consists of 74% lyocell, 19% SmartCell sensitive fibre, and 7% spandex [16]. Sample #2 (Silk-Aegis): Microair Dermasilk, a pure form of silk consisting exclusively of fibroin and containing a finish of AEGIS AEM 5772/5, an insoluble colorless, odorless ammonium as antibacterial agent [5, 13]. Sample #3 (PA-Silver): Padycare (Texamed, Ismaning, Germany), a micromesh material of 82% polyamide, 18% lycra with woven silver filaments with a silver content of 20% in total (130 g/m^2) [12]. Sample #4 (Smart-Zinc): Smartcel sensitive consisting of 70% Supima cotton, 18% lyocell, and 12% elasthane [24]. Sample #5 (Modal-Silver): Binamed made of 79% modal, 14% silver yarn, and 7% lycra (210 g/m^2).

Published reports were analysed comprising randomised controlled trials (RCTs) and observational and case-studies (with a cohort or case-control design) that compared the effects of patients with a clinical diagnosis of atopic dermatitis, irrespective of the age of the patients. Data was extracted exclusively with respect to the preclinical characterisation of the devices, especially, if standardised tests have been run to evaluate the antibacterial effectiveness.

2.2. Determination of Antibacterial Activity via Standards. The antibacterial activities of all textile samples were evaluated with the suspension test according to the standard ISO 20743:2007 "Textiles-determination of antibacterial activity of antibacterial finished products." All tests were run in triplicate. The determination of the antibacterial activity was performed by the absorption method, in which a test bacterial suspension is inoculated directly onto samples. In brief, textile swatches were inoculated with a starting suspension of 10^7 of Staphylococcus aureus (American Type Culture Collection 6538) obtained from the Deutsche Sammlung von Mikroorganismen und Zellkulturen (DSMZ, Braunschweig, Germany; since the resident skin microflora does not include gram-negative germs, we did not investigate the effect of the samples towards Klebsiella pneumoniae, another test germ of the standard). After 6 h, 18h, and 24 h of incubation at 37°C, the colony plate count method was used for the enumeration of bacteria colony forming units (CFUs; detection level < 20 cfu/sample). The specific antibacterial activity A was determined by inoculating a negative control PES fabric but without the antibacterial activity. The efficiency of the activity was then calculated by the following equation:

$$A = (\log_{10}C_t - \log_{10}C_{0h}) - (\log_{10}T_t - \log_{10}T_{0h}) \quad (1)$$

where C = control material, T = sample, and t = time point.

The antibacterial effectiveness of the Silk-Aegis and Smart-Zinc samples was further evaluated with the dynamic shake flask test ASTM E2149-01 as recommended by published data [25]. Therefore, 1 gram of the textile was cut in small pieces and the whole amount was inserted in sterile flasks containing 50 ml of shake-flask buffer. Each flask was inoculated with a final concentration of 1-6 x 10^7 CFU/ml of *S. aureus* and 1 ml of suspension was taken and used to assess the initial load of microorganism (defined as T0 load and expressed as CFU/ml). Flasks were then incubated under gentle shaking aerobic conditions for up to 24 hours at 37°C. At the end of incubation (6h, 18 h, or 24 h), 1 ml of the *S. aureus* was plated onto agar plates as described above. The antimicrobial activity of the Silk-Aegis and Smart-Zinc samples was evaluated according to the formula below [26, 27], where B represents the number of bacteria for blank (PES negative) and A is the number of bacteria for the samples after contact time:

$$\text{average microbial growth reduction, log} \qquad (2)$$
$$= (\log B - \log A).$$

where A = cfu in the tested sample after x hour, B = cfu estimated in the starting suspension before the addition of the sample (0 h).

The general assessment criteria follow a definition by the ISO 20743 in that a growth reduction efficacy of <0.5 corresponds to no antibacterial activity, whereas ≥0.5 to <1 corresponds to slight, ≥1 to <3 to significant, and a growth reduction of ≥3 indicates a strong antibacterial activity, respectively. Standard ASTM: E2149 – 01 does not quote any criteria to define the level of antibacterial properties.

2.3. Real-Life Setup of Affected AD Skin.

To simulate *S. aureus* affected human AD skin and to evaluate bacterial reduction during garment contact, a real-life setup of fabrics worn on inoculated artificial AD skin was developed. The test was designed to reflect normal conditions of use in terms of humidity, temperature, and contact frequency. In principle the setup followed the disc carrier test published by Ebert et al. [28]. As a replacement of metal disks, the standardized artificial skin VITRO-SKIN® N-19 (IMS Inc) was used. Pieces of VITRO-SKIN® N-19 were cut into squares of 3 cm² and placed in chambers with 15% glycerine for 18 h in order to achieve humidity. 50 μl of 1 x 10^8 CFU/ml of a starting suspension of *S. aureus* in tryptone-NaCl were inoculated at 0 h on the artificial skin with a sterile glass spatula to gently spread the suspension, which was then dried for a short time and then covered with either antibacterial samples or nonantibacterial control textile swatches. The tests were run in triplicate either in dry (50% relative humidity at 30°C) or wet conditions. For the latter, all samples were prewetted prior to the contact with the skin for 1 min with PBS Phosphate-Buffered Saline (containing 137mM NaCl, 2.7mM KCl, and 10mM phosphate, pH 7.4) to allow the samples to be completely wetted with the solution and to become saturated with it. It was ensured that all textile samples had a close fit to the skin by placing a glass slide on top of each sample so that they were permanently covering the artificial skin. In addition, the relative water content of all samples was measured under standard climate prior and after wetting the samples in PBS for 1 min.

The antibacterial activity of the textile swatches against *S. aureus* was analysed quantitatively on the artificial skin over a contact period of up to 18 h and assessed against the internal positive control Biatin AG® (Coloplast GmbH, Hamburg, Germany), a conventional foam dressing containing homogeneously distributed silver which continuously releases silver. A PES material without antibacterial activity served as negative control. If a significant germ reduction appeared within this wearing/exposure period, the textile was regarded as effective with respect to effects towards the human skin flora. Bacterial solutions were collected from the artificial skin immediately after the exposure times (1 h, 4h, and 18 h). For that, the remaining flora was collected by elution of the skin with 2 mL of sterile NaCl with 0.2% Tween 80. 100 μL was plated on agar medium. Plates were incubated at 36°C under aerobic conditions and inspected after 2 days. The number of colony forming units (CFUs)/200μl was determined using a colony counter (IUL Instruments GmbH, Koenigswinter, Germany). The efficiency of the activity was then calculated analogous to the ISO 20743.

2.4. Emollient Application and Wear.

The reference moisturising cream for the emollient application used in this study was Linola Fett (Dr. Wolff, Bielefeld, Germany), a W/O emulsion with a lipid content of 60%. Linola Fett contains unsaturated fatty acids (including linoleic acid) which are needed for the barrier function in healthy skin and is prescribed for patients suffering from AD. According to the instructions of the manufacturer, the upper arms of a test person, which was checked for absence of any *S. aureus* colonization, were creamed after taking a shower with a recommended quantity of cream (2 cm per 130 cm² of skin). Then 8 cm x 8 cm textile swatches were placed over the skin area fixed with a loose sleeve. After 4 h, the specimens were removed and further processed to either gravimetric lipid determination, domestic laundry, or the experimental model of inoculated AD skin.

2.5. Domestic Laundry and Gravimetric Lipid Determination.

In order to exclude cross contamination with lipids, standardised small-scale laundry laboratory tests were conducted. Laundry was carried out in a Linitest according to ISO-105-C06-A1S with some modifications for temperature and detergent concentration, according to the fabric manufacturer's specifications for care instructions of each sample, that is, at either 30°C or 60°C, for 30 min. As detergent solution, the standard IEC detergent was used (4.0 g/l; 150 ml per sample). Disinfectants, chlorine-based products as well as fabric softeners, and ballast load were omitted. After laundry, all specimens were rinsed twofold with H_2O for 2 min and finally air-dried. For the gravimetric lipid determination, all specimens were subjected into a round bottom flask after the wearing period. Following this, 250 ml of hexane was added and the bottom flask attached to a Soxhlet extraction apparatus. After 3 h extraction, the amount of lipid was recovered and its percentage in the original sample was calculated gravimetrically:

Mass of lipid = (weight of the flask + boiling chips

TABLE 1: Time-trend comparison of antibacterial effectiveness of conventional AD clothes against *S. aureus* according to the standards ISO 20743 and ASTM E 2149-01. Results depicted as log 10 reduction factors, means of triplicates with SDs. The ISO setup revealed a strong antibacterial effect for the silver-polyamide and the zinc-containing lyocell fabrics. The weakest activity was obtained with the Silk-Aegis sample. Right side: Evaluation of the antibacterial activity of the Silk-Aegis sample via ASTM test. Note failure of activity for the silk garment.

| | ISO EN | 20743 | | ASTM E | 2149-01 | |
| | Microbial [log cfu] | Activity | A | Microbial [log cfu/ml] | growth | reduction |
	6 h	18 h	24 h	6 h	18 h	24 h
PES negative	0 ± 0.1	0 ± 0.1	0 ± 0.1	0 ± 0.1	0 ± 0.1	0 ± 0.1
PES positive	5.89 ± 0.1	6.29 ± 0.2	6.37 ± 0.2			
Lyo-Zinc	5.89 ± 0.1	6.29 ± 0.2	6.37 ± 0.2			
Silk-Aegis	2.23 ± 0.1	1.64 ± 0.1	1.54 ± 0.1	-0.03 ± 0.1	0.36 ± 0.1	-0.23 ± 0.1
PA-Silver	5.89 ± 0.1	6.29 ± 0.2	6.37 ± 0.2			
Smart-Zinc	3.96 ± 0.2	4.22 ± 0.2	3.54 ± 0.1	0.92 ± 0.2	6.53 ± 0.1	6.02 ± 0.1
Modal-Silver	4.12 ± 0.1	3.73 ± 0.1	3.91 ± 0.2			

+ extracted oil) − (weight of the flask

+ boiling chips).

$$\text{The lipid content } (\%) = \frac{\text{mass of lipid extracted (g)}}{\text{sample weight (g)}}$$

$\times 100.$

(3)

3. Results

For the five selected antibacterial clothes, a total of ten clinical studies concerning treatment of AD were found [5, 12, 13, 15, 16, 29–33]. These reports investigated as main endpoint the colonisation with *S. aureus* by swabbing the skin at affected skin sites of AD patients before and after the application of the clothes. All studies, except one [16], excluded a basic verification of the devices according to international standards to prove their antibacterial effectiveness in vitro. Thus, a lack of data was found concerning the comparability or equivalence of the products in terms of their antibacterial effectiveness as well as the clinical evaluation of the products on the basis of the current state of the art. However, all studies claimed mitigating effects of clothes in AD due to the respective antibacterial agents. Four studies continued comedication with topical glucocorticoids, calcineurin inhibitors, or moisturising creams during the trials.

In order to evaluate the antimicrobial effectiveness of each sample and to compare the results with the other conventional devices, the antibacterial activity of all samples was evaluated using the international standard ISO 20743 in a time-trend comparison. In these suspension tests, the five samples considerably differed in their respective antibacterial activity. As expected, an internal silver-containing antibacterial PES material, used for validation over time, resulted in constant 6-log-step reduction of *S. aureus* over 24 h. According to the standard method ISO 20743, Lyo-Zinc and PA-Silver exhibited strong antibacterial activities of almost 6 log steps within the first 6 h and kept it at constant levels at least for 24 h. In contrast to this, Smart-Zinc started with a

lesser antibacterial activity of 4 log steps at 6 h that was kept at constant level within the next 18 h. The biocidal activity of Modal-Zinc corresponded with Smart-Zinc of showing a significant activity at 6 h and keeping it constant over 18 h and 24 h (Table 1, left side). With an approximately 1.6-log-step reduction, the non-silver or zinc containing Silk-Aegis sample displayed a much weaker antibacterial activity following the ISO 20743 protocol. Interestingly, this sample failed to exhibit a microbial reduction in the shake flask test ASTM E 2149-01 over the entire period, although the shake flask test is recommended for the respective biocide AEGIS. In contrast to that, the Smart-Zinc sample showed a strong activity, which was even slightly higher in the ASTM setup compared to the ISO standard (Table 1, right side).

As quantitative suspension tests are not an accurate reflection of the environmental conditions under which AD garments are worn on a patient's skin, a real-life setup of affected AD skin was used, based on artificial skin inoculated with *S. aureus*, to assess the effectiveness of antibacterial textiles in vitro towards a dysbiotic human skin flora. In contrast to the ISO and ASTM methods, in this setup none of the samples displayed a significant antibacterial effect over a time period of 4 h and 18 h when the clothes were worn at 50 % relative humidity at dry skin environment and in close contact on the artificial skin (see Table 2). However, when the samples were wetted to their individual water absorption capacity and left on the skin for 18 h, the zinc-containing fabrics (Lyo-Zinc and Smart-Zinc) displayed considerable stronger antibacterial activities than the silver-containing samples made of modal and polyamide. Although the wearing of wetted AD clothes is unrealistic in real life for AD patients, we explored in this setup the onset of the antibacterial action towards the *S. aureus* colonised skin. The positive control of wetted Biatain Ag reduced the inoculum after 1 h to about 1.42 log steps and after 4 h to about 4 log steps. Besides Biatain Ag, none of the other samples exerted a significant activity over 1 h under wet wearing conditions. The wetted PA-Silver sample at least showed a 2-log-step reduction after 4 h of application.

Fabrics were further evaluated for their respective lipid absorption capacity after a 4 h wear period with the reference moisturising cream. The Silk-Aegis fabric absorbed

TABLE 2: Comparison of antibacterial activity of conventional AD fabrics subjected to the *S. aureus* inoculated artificial skin. Results depicted as log 10 reduction factors, means of triplicates with SDs. The zinc-containing samples displayed considerable stronger antibacterial activities after 18 h followed by the silver-containing samples, but only when the samples were prewetted to their individual water absorption capacity. No short-term effect (1 h) of wetted samples on colonized skin was observed.

	Water absorption [g/swatch]	Real-Life Microbial 1 h wet	Setup of Growth 4h wet	affected Activity 4 h dry	AD skin [log cfu] 18 h wet	18 h dry
Biatain Ag	5.70	1.42 ± 0.1	3.96 ± 0.1	0.85 ± 0.1	3.13 ± 0.1	2.65 ± 0.1
PES negative	0.41	0 ± 0.1	0 ± 0.1	0 ± 0.1	0 ± 0.1	0 ± 0.1
PES positive	0.46	0.15 ± 0.1	0.21 ± 0.2	0.50 ± 0.1	0.15 ± 0.2	0.17 ± 0.2
Lyo-Zinc	0.68	0.11 ± 0.1	0.62 ± 0.2	0.39 ± 0.2	2.99 ± 0.2	-0.67 ± 0.1
Silk-Aegis	0.14	-0.2 ± 0.1	-0.22 ± 0.1	-0.16 ± 0.1	-0.19 ± 0.1	-1.33 ± 0.2
PA-Silver	0.07	0.14 ± 0.1	2.09 ± 0.2	0.47 ± 0.2	1.75 ± 0.2	-0.58 ± 0.2
Smart-Zinc	0.64	0.11 ± 0.2	0.50 ± 0.2	0.31 ± 0.1	2.02 ± 0.2	-0.65 ± 0.1
Modal-Silver	1.23	0.25 ± 0.1	0.93 ± 0.1	0.43 ± 0.2	1.51 ± 0.2	-0.56 ± 0.1

TABLE 3: Lipid absorption values of five AD fabrics after wearing a moisturising cream for 4 h and after laundry. All values are means of triplicates and shown in mgr/gr of textile swatch.

	Lyo-Zinc	Silk-Aegis	PA-Silver	Smart-Zinc	Modal-Silver
After wear	171	310	196	173	125
After laundry	168	260	46	74	48

the cream slightly to more than 30% of its own weight (310 mgr of cream/gr fabric), whereas the Lyo-Zinc sample, PA-Silver, Smart-Zinc, and Modal-Silver samples showed a rather fibre independent uptake of the moisturising cream. After laundering of the fabrics, there was still a considerable lipid load present on all samples (see Table 3). Washing at 30°C did not remove the moisturising cream and left a considerable quantity on the samples, whereas washing at 60°C reduced the lipid load to about 5%.

4. Discussion

To the best of the author's knowledge, no in vitro study has been done across different garments to compare the effectiveness of conventional antibacterial clothes in AD treatment. All RCTs and observational studies used for the analysis therein [5, 12, 13, 15, 16, 29–33] excluded a basic verification of the respective fabrics according to international standards to determine the antibacterial activity of the textile product [25]. Products thus were unfortunately not comparable to each other across the studies. However, all trials claimed mitigating skin effects to the respective antibacterial agents, like SCORAD improvement or reduced *S. aureus* colonisation at affected skin sites, although no sample was subjected to a comparative in vitro approach to prove the claimed biotic action.

This research first compared the effectiveness of functional AD clothes by quantitative suspension standard tests to prove the antibacterial activity of the conventional fabrics quantitatively. The fabrics differed considerably in their antibacterial properties. The silk-based sample endowed with the biocide AEGIS showed only a weak activity according to the standard ISO 20743 and even failed when using the

recommended dynamic shake flask test ASTM E2149-01 [25]. These results are in close correlation with previous in vivo findings by Ricci et al. [15], who were unable to demonstrate that silk fabrics coated with AEGIS AEM 5572/5 have an antibacterial activity by counting bacteria of the antecubital area of AD patients. However, the authors (and other studies using this kind of silk material) referred to an in vitro activity of the silk fabric which goes back to a single industry-led research in 1978 [34]. In case of standard ISO 20743, the antibacterial effectiveness of the silver-coated polyamide and the zinc-containing lyocell fibre performed best among the samples, whereas the silver-containing modal fibre and the cotton/lyocell samples displayed somewhat weaker antibacterial activities over 24 hours. Thus, to a certain extent, the zinc-containing sample confirmed its antibacterial activity in vitro, as shown for this material by Wiegand et al. [16], albeit the present study found markedly lower reduction values.

A first reason for the different performances by the samples is explained by the technical setup of the normative ISO and ASTM approaches. It is generally accepted that standard tests favour outcomes of antibacterial activities by creating favourable moist and warm conditions. That is why Kramer et al. in 2006 already encouraged further development of international standards for the in vitro testing and preclinical evaluation of efficacy and tolerance of hygienic AD clothes [26]. In their view, the mere product claim does not indicate a true effect and should be demonstrated independently for each device. Following the idea of Kramer, this research therefore simulated a real-life wear setup in vitro, using artificial skin colonised with *S. aureus*, to evaluate and compare the advantages of the antibacterial properties for the intended use of correcting a dysbiotic AD skin. The real-life setup proved to be a useful and easy-to-apply method to evaluate the antibacterial effectiveness of antimicrobial clothes in direct contact to skin. The test reflected normal conditions of use in terms of humidity (50% rH), temperature (30°C), and contact frequency. Furthermore, the test method allowed a more realistic assessment simulating conditions on the AD skin, that is, an evaluation of the staphylococcal profile under different environmental wear conditions. It also imposed more stringent requirements on antibacterial effectiveness over time than a quantitative standard suspension test, since contact between the garment and the test organism suspension to which the fabric is exposed is less intense on the artificial skin than during a suspension test, where samples are soaked with the inoculum. Furthermore, the normative approaches use test conditions with significant amount of liquid to allow diffusion of the incorporated agents to test organisms at planktonic and dynamic conditions and also provide optimum temperature conditions for the microbial growth.

In contrast to the ISO and ASTM methods, in the real-life setup none of the samples displayed a significant antibacterial activity after a wear period of 4 h and 18 h when the clothes were worn at a realistic skin microenvironment, that is, relative humidity of 50% and in close contact with the inoculated skin. In terms of the dermatological point of view, wearing of wetted AD clothes is unrealistic in real life that would hardly be tolerated by AD patients. Despite this fact, when the samples nevertheless were wetted to their individual water absorption capacity and left on the skin for 18 h, the zinc-containing fabrics (Lyo-Zinc and Smart Zinc) displayed stronger antibacterial activities than the silver-containing samples made of modal and polyamide. This observation supports the fact that moisture is needed to release a sufficient amount of contact biocide from antibacterial fibres. That is why the standard ISO 20743 is assessed to often overestimate antibacterial properties and to seem unsuitable to evaluate devices for practical applications. The poor antibacterial effectiveness of the samples in the real-life setup subjected to the dry skin microenvironment is corroborated by a previous placebo-controlled side-by-side study [35], in which 60 healthy human volunteers wore either of the functional clothes (silver-finished or silver-doped) of similar structure and with strong antibacterial activity according to standard methods for six weeks. In this field trial, the antibacterial halves did not disturb the skin microbiome in either germ number or composition and thus displayed no adverse effects on the ecological balance of the healthy human skin microflora. In the real-life setup simulating an affected skin, even under wet wearing conditions none of the samples exerted a significant antibacterial activity after 1 h; the PA-Silver fabric was merely effective after 4 h.

To the best of the author's knowledge, none of the RCTs and observational studies on functional clothes discussed the mechanisms of the presumed effect of silver or other biocides towards a selective eradication of S. aureus on dysbiotic skin. Daeschlein et al. carried out a trial with AD patients that wore silver-containing antibacterial fabrics for one week, to see whether silver impregnation prevents the bacterial growth within the textile [36]. Unexpectedly, this group found high residual contaminations of S. aureus despite silver exposure present on the fabrics after a wear period of at least 2 days. Their finding supports the view that a selective eradication of S. aureus by antibacterial clothes is highly unlikely.

Against the background that many in vivo RCT trials at affected AD skin sites of patients observed a bacterial shift to a reduced S. aureus colonization of functional clothes and on the basis of the work presented here, it cannot be ruled out that the bacterial shift may result by a nonantibacterial mechanism of action, that is, secondary effects. For example, Nakatsuji et al. recently showed that the reintroduction of human skin commensal bacteria like S. epidermidis to human subjects with AD protects effectively against a S. aureus colonisation, most probably by secretion of antimicrobial peptides AMPs [37]. This finding demonstrates a possible self-regulating role of the skins microbiome and concurrently opens up a new therapeutic field in which probiotics like Extracellular serine protease (Esp)-secreting S. epidermidis could improve AD symptoms. Furthermore, modulation of the skin microbiome by antimicrobial clothes might alternatively result through the enhancement of the activity of topic pharmaceuticals, that is, by prolonging the pharmaceutical effect [27] or simply by reducing scratching effect and itching, as known from woollen clothes [11], rather than by an intrinsic antibacterial activity. This view is supported by the observation within this study that the silk sample displayed no antibacterial effect at all, but absorbed a significantly greater quantity of the moisturising cream. The drug prolongation effect might be an additional reason for the observed SCORAD improvements observed in many trials conducted with silk fabrics [5]. However, a RCT with over 300 affected children run by Thomas et al. concluded that the addition of silk garments to standard AD care is unlikely to improve AD severity, or even to be cost-effective compared with the standard care alone, for children with moderate or severe AD [38].

Finally, the fibre type might as well have an influence on the dysbiotic skin. Callewaert et al. found that, depending on the fibre, a selective bacterial enrichment takes place, resulting in another textile microbiome as compared to the autochthonous skin microbiome [39]. Accordingly, the researchers observed no bacterial enrichment on viscose, but an enrichment of Staphylococcus epidermidis spp. and Micrococci on both cotton and polyester textiles. Other authors reviewed that different textile components are associated with different effects on the skin [10, 11]. Silver-coated cotton, for example, seemed to be more effective in decreasing lesion severity, while silk fabrics appeared to be more likely to alleviate pruritus and symptoms. Silk clothes may affect overall disease status by improving comfort and reducing itch sensation or by cooling the AD skin. It is noteworthy that all man-made fibres of the selected functional clothes in this study were optimized in terms of skin friction: They have round cross sections and smooth fibre surfaces with excellent comfort and thermoregulatory properties, which, by their structures, diminish the physical movements and by this way disrupt the itch-and-scratch cycles. The same holds true for the natural silk filament. Therefore, more studies are needed to better understand the interactions of functional fabrics with the skin microbiome of healthy and affected subjects and to better understand why these clothes mitigate disease severity, symptoms, and quality of life [17].

Emollients are the mainstay of maintenance of AD therapy [40]. Therefore, it has to be taken into account that in the daily routine there is a steady contact of functional clothes with topical medications. In this study, the AD clothes also differed in their absorption capacity to the moisturising cream, most probably according to the physicochemical nature of the respective fibre types. Thus, the data affirmed the importance of the interactions of fabrics and emollients in the management of AD. For moisturising creams contain also other excipients, such as emulsifiers, pH-adjusters, chelators, and preservatives, these excipients—but also moisturisers like urea, or pharmaceuticals like glucocorticoids or calcineurin inhibitors—might as well interfere with the microbiome. It was also found that laundry according to care instructions of the manufacturers was unable to eliminate the lipids. In daily practice this might lead to an accumulation of lipids over laundry cycles that at least contributes to the skin care. Only one study so far, of Daeschlein et al., examined the effect of washing of AD clothes. The group investigated whether silver impregnation of fibres at least prevents bacterial growth within the textile [36]. Unexpectedly, they found high residual contaminations despite silver exposure. The authors concluded that the risk of a recontamination source of *S. aureus* could be eliminated by machine-based washing at 60°C using conventional washing powder. However, although 60°C safely eliminates germs in contaminated clothes, it could be ineffective in removing the remnants of a lipid-based moisturising cream.

5. Conclusion

In this research, the antibacterial effectiveness of five conventional functional clothes for AD treatment was compared. In a real-life setup simulating practical wear conditions of a dry skin microenvironment, AD clothes were unable to modify the skin colonisation with *S. aureus*. Although effectiveness can be triggered by wetting the garments, this is however contraindicated for AD patients in their everyday life. When using normative suspension tests, samples showed some antibacterial activities. Garments absorbed moisturising cream dependent on the respective fibre type and remnants of cream still remained on the fibres after laundry. More studies are needed to better understand the interactions of functional fabrics with the skin microbiome of healthy and affected subjects.

Acknowledgments

The author gratefully thanks Nadja Berner-Dannenmann from the Hohenstein Institute for technical assistance. The study received no financial support.

References

[1] J. A. Odhiambo, H. C. Williams, T. O. Clayton, C. F. Robertson, and M. I. Asher, "Global variations in prevalence of eczema symptoms in children from ISAAC Phase Three," *The Journal of Allergy and Clinical Immunology*, vol. 124, no. 6, pp. 1251–1258.e23, 2009.

[2] E. Eller, H. F. Kjaer, A. Høst, K. E. Andersen, and C. Bindslev-Jensen, "Development of atopic dermatitis in the DARC birth cohort," *Pediatric Allergy and Immunology*, vol. 21, no. 2, pp. 307–314, 2010.

[3] U. Raap, S. Weißmantel, M. Gehring, A. M. Eisenberg, A. Kapp, and R. Fölster-Holst, "IL-31 significantly correlates with disease activity and Th2 cytokine levels in children with atopic dermatitis," *Pediatric Allergy and Immunology*, vol. 23, no. 3, pp. 285–288, 2012.

[4] E. Sonkoly, A. Muller, A. I. Lauerma et al., "IL-31: a new link between T cells and pruritus in atopic skin inflammation," *The Journal of Allergy and Clinical Immunology*, vol. 117, no. 2, pp. 411–417, 2006.

[5] G. Ricci, A. Patrizi, B. Bendandi, G. Menna, E. Varotti, and M. Masi, "Clinical effectiveness of a silk fabric in the treatment of atopic dermatitis," *British Journal of Dermatology*, vol. 150, no. 1, pp. 127–131, 2004.

[6] M. Niebuhr and T. Werfel, "Innate immunity, allergy and atopic dermatitis," *Current Opinion in Allergy and Clinical Immunology*, vol. 10, no. 5, pp. 463–468, 2010.

[7] A. De Benedetto, R. Agnihothri, L. Y. McGirt, L. G. Bankova, and L. A. Beck, "Atopic dermatitis: a disease caused by innate immune defects?" *Journal of Investigative Dermatology*, vol. 129, no. 1, pp. 14–30, 2009.

[8] T. M. Zollner, T. A. Wichelhaus, A. Hartung et al., "Colonization with superantigen-producing Staphylococcus aureus is associated with increased severity of atopic dermatitis," *Clinical & Experimental Allergy*, vol. 30, no. 7, pp. 994–1000, 2000.

[9] R. D. Bjerre, J. Bandier, L. Skov, L. Engstrand, and J. D. Johansen, "The role of the skin microbiome in atopic dermatitis: a systematic review," *British Journal of Dermatology*, vol. 177, no. 5, pp. 1272–1278, 2017.

[10] W. E. Love and S. T. Nedorost, "Fabric preferences of atopic dermatitis patients," *Dermatitis*, vol. 20, no. 1, pp. 29–33, 2009.

[11] M. Mobolaji-Lawal and S. Nedorost, "The Role of Textiles in Dermatitis: An Update," *Current Allergy and Asthma Reports*, vol. 15, no. 4, article no. 17, 2015.

[12] A. Gauger, M. Mempel, A. Schekatz, T. Schäfer, J. Ring, and D. Abeck, "Silver-coated textiles reduce Staphylococcus aureus colonization in patients with atopic eczema," *Dermatology*, vol. 207, no. 1, pp. 15–21, 2003.

[13] G. Stinco, F. Piccirillo, and F. Valent, "A randomized double-blind study to investigate the clinical efficacy of adding a non-migrating antimicrobial to a special silk fabric in the treatment of atopic dermatitis," *Dermatology*, vol. 217, no. 3, pp. 191–195, 2008.

[14] U. Hipler and P. Elsner, *Silver-coated textiles in the therapy of atopic eczema. Biofunctional Textiles and the Skin*, vol. 33, Karger Publishers, 2006.

[15] G. Ricci, A. Patrizi, P. Mandrioli et al., "Evaluation of the antibacterial activity of a special silk textile in the treatment of atopic dermatitis," *Dermatology*, vol. 213, no. 3, pp. 224–227, 2006.

[16] C. Wiegand, U. C. Hipler, S. Boldt, J. Strehle, and U. Wollina, "Skin-protective effects of a zinc oxide-functionalized textile and its relevance for atopic dermatitis," *Clinical, Cosmetic and Investigational Dermatology*, vol. 6, pp. 115–121, 2013.

[17] C. Lopes, D. Silva, L. Delgado, O. Correia, and A. Moreira, "Functional textiles for atopic dermatitis: a systematic review and meta-analysis," *Pediatric Allergy and Immunology*, vol. 24, no. 6, pp. 603–613, 2013.

[18] A. J. Birnie, F. J. Bath-Hextall, J. C. Ravenscroft et al., "Interventions to reduce Staphylococcus aureus in the management of atopic eczema," *Cochrane Database Syst Rev*, 2008.

[19] N. A. Francis, M. J. Ridd, E. Thomas-Jones et al., "A randomised placebo-controlled trial of oral and topical antibiotics for children with clinically infected eczema in the community: the ChildRen with Eczema, Antibiotic Management (CREAM) study," *Health Technology Assessment*, vol. 20, no. 19, pp. 1–84, 2016.

[20] J. M. Hanifin, K. D. Cooper, V. C. Ho et al., "Guidelines of care for atopic dermatitis," *Journal of the American Academy of Dermatology*, vol. 50, no. 3, pp. 391–404, 2004.

[21] A. W. Lucky, A. D. Leach, P. Laskarzewski, and H. Wenck, "Use of an emollient as a steroid-sparing agent in the treatment of mild to moderate atopic dermatitis in children," *Pediatric Dermatology*, vol. 14, no. 4, pp. 321–324, 1997.

[22] J. Szczepanowska, A. Reich, and J. C. Szepietowski, "Emollients improve treatment results with topical corticosteroids in childhood atopic dermatitis: A randomized comparative study," *Pediatric Allergy and Immunology*, vol. 19, no. 7, pp. 614–618, 2008.

[23] S. Reitamo, T. Langeland, M. Berg et al., "Comparison of moisturizing creams for the prevention of atopic dermatitis relapse: a randomized double-blind controlled multicentre clinical trial," *Acta dermato-venereologica*, vol. 95, no. 5, pp. 587–592, 2015.

[24] "Silver-loaded cellulose fibers with antibacterial and antifungal activity in vitro and in vivo on patients with atopic dermatitis," in *Proceedings of the 5th World Textile Conference AUTEX*, J. Fluhr, D. Kowatzki, A. Bauer et al., Eds., 2005.

[25] E. Pinho, L. Magalhães, M. Henriques, and R. Oliveira, "Antimicrobial activity assessment of textiles: Standard methods comparison," *Annals of Microbiology*, vol. 61, no. 3, pp. 493–498, 2011.

[26] A. Kramer, P. Guggenbichler, P. Heldt et al., "Hygienic relevance and risk assessment of antimicrobial-impregnated textiles," *Biofunctional Textiles and the Skin*, vol. 33, pp. 78–109, 2006.

[27] S. E. Baron, S. N. Cohen, and C. B. Archer, "Guidance on the diagnosis and clinical management of atopic eczema," *Clinical and Experimental Dermatology*, vol. 37, no. 1, pp. 7–12, 2012.

[28] M. Ebert, O. Assadian, N.-O. Hübner, T. Koburger, and A. Kramer, "Antimicrobial efficacy of the silver wound dressing Biatain Ag in a disc carrier test simulating wound secretion," *Skin Pharmacology and Physiology*, vol. 24, no. 6, pp. 337–341, 2011.

[29] A. Gauger, S. Fischer, M. Mempel et al., "Efficacy and functionality of silver-coated textiles in patients with atopic eczema," *Journal of the European Academy of Dermatology and Venereology*, vol. 20, no. 5, pp. 534–541, 2006.

[30] M. Juenger, A. Ladwig, S. Staecker et al., "Efficacy and safety of silver textile in the treatment of atopic dermatitis (AD)," *Current Medical Research and Opinion*, vol. 22, no. 4, pp. 739–750, 2006.

[31] D. Y. Koller, G. Halmerbauer, A. Böck, and G. Engstler, "Action of a silk fabric treated with AEGIS in children with atopic dermatitis: a 3-month trial," *Pediatric Allergy and Immunology*, vol. 18, no. 4, pp. 335–338, 2007.

[32] K. Y. Park, W. S. Jang, G. W. Yang et al., "A pilot study of silver-loaded cellulose fabric with incorporated seaweed for the treatment of atopic dermatitis," *Clinical and Experimental Dermatology*, vol. 37, no. 5, pp. 512–515, 2012.

[33] G. Senti, L. S. Steinmann, B. Fischer et al., "Antimicrobial silk clothing in the treatment of atopic dermatitis proves comparable to topical corticosteroid treatment," *Dermatology*, vol. 213, no. 3, pp. 228–233, 2006.

[34] R. L. Gettings and B. L. Triplett, "A new durable antimicrobial finish for textiles," *Book of Papers: American Association of Textile Chemists and Colorists?* pp. 259–261, 1978.

[35] D. Hoefer and T. R. Hammer, "Antimicrobial Active Clothes Display No Adverse Effects on the Ecological Balance of the Healthy Human Skin Microflora," *ISRN Dermatology*, vol. 2011, Article ID 369603, 8 pages, 2011.

[36] G. Daeschlein, O. Assadian, A. Arnold, H. Haase, A. Kramer, and M. Jünger, "Bacterial burden of worn therapeutic silver textiles for neurodermitis patients and evaluation of efficacy of washing," *Skin Pharmacology and Physiology*, vol. 23, no. 2, pp. 86–90, 2010.

[37] T. Nakatsuji, T. H. Chen, S. Narala et al., "Antimicrobials from human skin commensal bacteria protect against Staphylococcus aureus and are deficient in atopic dermatitis," *Science Translational Medicine*, vol. 9, no. 378, 2017.

[38] K. S. Thomas, L. E. Bradshaw, T. H. Sach et al., "Randomised controlled trial of silk therapeutic garments for the management of atopic eczema in children: the CLOTHES trial," *Health Technology Assessment*, vol. 21, no. 16, pp. 1–260, 2017.

[39] C. Callewaert, E. De Maeseneire, F.-M. Kerckhof, A. Verliefde, T. Van de Wiele, and N. Boon, "Microbial odor profile of polyester and cotton clothes after a fitness session," *Applied and Environmental Microbiology*, vol. 80, no. 21, pp. 6611–6619, 2014.

[40] E. L. Simpson, T. M. Berry, P. A. Brown, and J. M. Hanifin, "A pilot study of emollient therapy for the primary prevention of atopic dermatitis," *Journal of the American Academy of Dermatology*, vol. 63, no. 4, pp. 587–593, 2010.

Permissions

List of Contributors

Faisel Abu-Duhier
Prince Fahd Bin Sultan Research Chair, Department of Medical Lab Technology, Faculty of Applied Medical Science, Prince Fahd Research Chair, University of Tabuk, Tabuk, Saudi Arabia

Vivetha Pooranachandran, Johnathan Cooper-Knock and Paul R. Heath
Department of Neuroscience, SITraN,The Medical School, University of Sheffield, Sheffield S10 2RX, UK

Andrew J. G. McDonagh
Department of Dermatology, Royal Hallamshire Hospital, Sheffield S10 2JF, UK

Andrew G. Messenger
Department of Infection, Immunity and Cardiovascular Disease,The Medical School, University of Sheffield, Sheffield S10 2RX, UK

Rachid Tazi-Ahnini
Department of Infection, Immunity and Cardiovascular Disease,The Medical School, University of Sheffield, Sheffield S10 2RX, UK
Laboratory of Medical Biotechnology (MedBiotech), Rabat Medical School and Pharmacy, University Mohammed V Rabat,Rabat, Morocco

Youssef Bakri
Biology Department, Faculty of Science, University Mohammed V Rabat, Rabat, Morocco

Naveen Kumar, Satheesha Nayak Badagabettu and Ashwini Aithal Padur
Department of Anatomy, Melaka Manipal Medical College, Manipal Academy of Higher Education, Manipal Campus, Manipal 576104, India

Pramod Kumar
King Fahad Central Hospital, Jazan 82666, Saudi Arabia

Melissa Glenda Lewis
Indian Institute of Public Health Hyderabad (IIPHH), Madhapur, Hyderabad 500033, India

Murali Adiga
Department of Physiology, Kasturba Medical College, Manipal, Manipal Academy of Higher Education, Manipal 576104, India

Nasrin Saki and Shahla Hosseinpoor
Molecular Dermatology Research Center, Shiraz University of Medical Sciences, Shiraz, Iran
Dermatology Department, Shiraz University of Medical Sciences, Shiraz, Iran

Alireza Heiran, Ali Mohammadi and Mehdi Zeraatpishe
Student Research Committee, Shiraz University of Medical Sciences, Shiraz, Iran

Teuku Alamsyah, Mutia Yusuf and Said Devi Elvin
Health Polytech Facility of Health Minister, Department of Nursing, Banda Aceh 23245, Indonesia

Said Usman
Medicine Faculty, Syiah Kuala University, Banda Aceh 23245, Indonesia

Saori Masaki and Shinichi Imafuku
Department of Dermatology, Fukuoka University School of Medicine, Fukuoka, Japan

Kotaro Ito
Department of Dermatology, Fukuoka University School of Medicine, Fukuoka, Japan
Ito Dermatology Clinic, Oita, Japan

Manabu Hamada
Hamada Dermatology Clinic, Fukuoka, Japan

Tetsuo Tokunaga
Tokunaga Dermatology Clinic, Fukuoka, Japan

Hisashi Kokuba
Sakurazaka Dermatology Clinic, Fukuoka, Japan

Kenji Tashiro
Tashiro Dermatology Clinic, Fukuoka, Japan

Ichiro Yano
Yano Dermatology and Urinary Clinic, Fukuoka, Japan

Shinichiro Yasumoto
Yasumoto Dermatology Clinic, Fukuoka, Japan

Philip M. Stephens, Brian Martin, Ghazal Ghafari, James Luong and Linda Pham
DeBusk College of Osteopathic Medicine, Lincoln Memorial University, Harrogate, TN, USA

Vinayak K. Nahar
Center for Animal andHuman Health in Appalachia, College of Veterinary Medicine, DeBusk College of Osteopathic Medicine and School of Mathematics and Sciences, Lincoln Memorial University, Harrogate, TN, USA

Jiangxia Luo
Department of English, Gannan Medical University, Ganzhou, Jiangxi, China
Carter and Moyers School of Education, Lincoln Memorial University, Harrogate, TN, USA

Marcelle Savoy
Lon and Elizabeth Parr Reed Health Sciences Library, DeBusk College of Osteopathic Medicine, Lincoln Memorial University, Harrogate, TN, USA

Manoj Sharma
Department of Behavioral & EnvironmentalHealth, School of Public Health, Jackson State University, Jackson, MS,USA

Abbas Darjani, Sareh Shafaei, Hojat Eftekhari, Narges Alizade and Kaveh Gharaei nejad
Skin Research Center, Dermatology Department, Guilan University of Medical Sciences, Razi Hospital, Sardare Jangal Street, Rasht, Iran

Rana Rafiei
Fellowship of Dermatopathology, Skin Research Center, Dermatology Department, Guilan University of Medical Sciences, Razi Hospital, Sardare Jangal Street, Rasht, Iran

Elahe Rafiei
Razi Clinical Research Development Center, Guilan University of Medical Sciences, Rasht, Iran

Behnam Rafiee
Department of Pathology, NYUWinthrop Hospital, 222 Station Plaza, No. 620, Mineola, NY 11501, USA

Sara Najirad
Department of Internal Medicine, Nassau University Medical Center, 2201 Hempstead Turnpike, East Meadow, NY 11554, USA

Arash Mostaghimi
Department of Dermatology, Brigham &Women's Hospital, Harvard Medical School, Boston, MA, USA

David G. Li
Department of Dermatology, Brigham &Women's Hospital, Harvard Medical School, Boston, MA, USA
Tufts University School of Medicine, Boston, MA, USA

Fan Di Xia and Forootan Alizadeh
Brigham &Women's Hospital, Harvard Medical School, Boston, MA, USA

Jasmine Rana
Santa Clara Valley Medical Center, San Jose, CA, USA

Grace J. Young
Harvard Medical School, Boston, MA, USA

Cara Joyce
Loyola University, Chicago, IL, USA

Shinjita Das
Department of Dermatology, Massachusetts General Hospital, Harvard Medical School, Boston, MA, USA

Mar-lia Bueno Savacini, Débora Tazinaffo Bueno, Ana Carolina Souza Molina and Ana Caroline Almeida Lopes
Ibramed Center for Education and Advanced Training (CEFAI), Amparo, Brazil

Renata Gomes Moreira, Stephani Almeida and Estela Sant'Ana
Clinical Laboratory of the Ibramed Center for Education and Advanced Training (CEFAI), Amparo, Brazil
Research, Development & Innovation Department IBRAMED, Ibramed Research Group (IRG), Amparo, Brazil

Caroline Nogueira Silva
Clinical Laboratory of the Ibramed Center for Education and Advanced Training (CEFAI), Amparo, Brazil
Research, Development & Innovation Department IBRAMED, Ibramed Research Group (IRG), Amparo, Brazil
Human Development and Technologies. Universidade Estadual Paulista (UNESP), Brazil

Renata Michelini Guidi
Clinical Laboratory of the Ibramed Center for Education and Advanced Training (CEFAI), Amparo, Brazil
Research, Development & Innovation Department IBRAMED, Ibramed Research Group (IRG), Amparo, Brazil
Electrical Engineering Department, Faculty of Medical Sciences, University of Campinas (Unicamp), Brazil

Richard Eloin Liebano
Department of Physiotherapy, Federal University of São Carlos, São Carlos, Brazil

Gia-Buu Tran, Nghia-Thu Tram Le and Sao-Mai Dam
Institute of Biotechnology and Food Technology, Industrial University of Ho Chi Minh City, 12 Nguyen Van Bao Street, Go Vap District, Ho Chi Minh City, Vietnam

Giuggioli Dilia, Colaci Michele, Cocchiara Emanuele, Spinella Amelia, Lumetti Federica and Ferri Clodoveo
Scleroderma Unit, Chair of Rheumatology, University of Modena and Reggio Emilia, Modena, Italy

Debajit Debbarma, Varinder Uppal, Neelam Bansal and Anuradha Gupta
Department of Veterinary Anatomy, College of Veterinary Science, Guru Angad Dev Veterinary and Animal Sciences University, Ludhiana 141004, Punjab, India

Susheera Chatproedprai, Vanvara Wutticharoenwong, Therdpong Tempark and Siriwan Wananukul
Department of Pediatrics, Faculty of Medicine, Chulalongkorn University and King Chulalongkorn Memorial Hospital,Bangkok 10330,Thailand

Moonyza Akmal Ahmad Kamil and Azura Mohd Affandi
Department of Dermatology, Kuala Lumpur Hospital, Kuala Lumpur, Malaysia

Azura Mohd Affandi, Iman Khan and Nooraishah Ngah Saaya
Department of Dermatology, Hospital Kuala Lumpur, Kuala Lumpur, Malaysia

Atena Barat, Michael J. Goldacre and Trevor W. Lambert
UK Medical Careers Research Group, Unit of Health-Care Epidemiology, Nuffield Department of Population Health, University ofOxford, Old Road Campus, Oxford OX3 7LF, UK

Mehdi Gheisari, Nilofar Nobari and Behzad Iranmanesh
Skin Research Center, Shahid Beheshti University of Medical Sciences, Tehran, Iran

Nikoo Mozafari
Skin Research Center, Shahid Beheshti University of Medical Sciences, Tehran, Iran
Department of Dermatology, Loghmen-e-Hakim Hospital, Shahid Beheshti University of Medical Sciences, Tehran, Iran

Arman Ahmadzadeh
Department of Rheumatology, Shahid Beheshti University of Medical Sciences, Tehran, Iran

Mehdi Ghahartars
Department of Dermatology, School of Medicine, Shiraz University of Medical Sciences, Shiraz, Iran

Shiva Najafzadeh, Shabnam Abtahi, Mohammad Javad Fattahi and Abbas Ghaderi
Shiraz Institute for Cancer Research, School of medicine, Shiraz University of Medical Sciences, Shiraz, Iran

Mina Mirnezami
Department of Dermatology, Faculty of Medicine, Arak University of Medical Sciences, Arak, Iran

Hoda Rahimi
Skin Research Center, Shahid Beheshti University of Medical Sciences, Tehran, Iran

Priyatam Khadka
Department of Microbiology, Tribhuvan University Teaching Hospital, Kathmandu, Nepal
M.Sc. Medical Microbiology, Tri-Chandra Multiple Campus, TribhuvanUniversity, Nepal

Januka Thapaliya
M.Sc. Medical Microbiology, Tri-Chandra Multiple Campus, Tribhuvan University, Nepal

Soniya Koirala
Department of Dermatology and Venerology, Tribhuvan University Teaching Hospital, Kathmandu, Nepal
M.D. Dermatology, Maharajgunj Medical Campus, Tribhuvan University, Nepal

Adane Bitew
Department of Medical Laboratory Sciences, College of Health Sciences, Addis Ababa University, Addis Ababa, Ethiopia

Giuseppe Giudice, Giorgio Favia and Michelangelo Vestita
Section of Plastic and Reconstructive Surgery, Department of Emergency and Organ Transplantation, University of Bari, 11, Piazza Giulio Cesare, Bari, 70124, Italy

Angela Tempesta and Luisa Limongelli
Department of Interdisciplinary Medicine, Complex Operating Unit of Odontostomatology, "AldoMoro" University, Piazza G. Cesare 11, 70124 Bari, Italy

Zohreh Tehranchinia, Bita Saghi and Hoda Rahimi
Skin Research Center, Shahid Beheshti University of Medical Sciences, Tehran, Iran

Jarso Sara
Affiliate of School of Public and Environmental Health, College of Medicine and Health Sciences Hawassa University, Ethiopia

Yusuf Haji and Achamyelesh Gebretsadik
School of Public and Environmental Health, College of Medicine and Health Sciences, Hawassa University, Hawassa, Ethiopia

Mohammad   Shahidi-Dadras,   Fahimeh Abdollahimajd , Razieh Jahangard and Parviz Toossi
Skin Research Center, Shahid Beheshti University of Medical Sciences, Tehran, Iran

Ali Javinani and Amir Ashraf-Ganjouei
Rheumatology Research Center, Tehran University of Medical Sciences, Tehran, Iran

Reem Dina Matzen and Steen Matzen
Department of Plastic Surgery and Breast Surgery, Zealand University Hospital, Roskilde, Denmark

Julie Zinck Leth-Espensen, Therese Jansson and Dennis Sandris Nielsen
Department of Food Science, Faculty of Science, University of Copenhagen, Denmark

Marianne N. Lund
Department of Food Science, Faculty of Science, University of Copenhagen, Denmark

Department of Biomedical Sciences, Faculty of Health and Medical Sciences, University of Copenhagen, Denmark

Ricardo Cardona
Group of Clinical and Experimental Allergy, IPS Universitaria, University of Antioquia, Medellin, Colombia

Jorge Sánchez
Group of Clinical and Experimental Allergy, IPS Universitaria, University of Antioquia, Medellin, Colombia
Foundation for the Development of Medical and Biological Sciences (FUNDEMEB), Cartagena, Colombia

Andres Sánchez
Group of Clinical and Experimental Allergy, IPS Universitaria, University of Antioquia, Medellin, Colombia
Foundation for the Development of Medical and Biological Sciences (FUNDEMEB), Cartagena, Colombia
Faculty of Medicine, Corporation University Rafael Nunez, Cartagena, Colombia

Sukhontha Hasatsri, Anuphap Pitiratanaworanat, Suwit Swangwit, Chadaporn Boochakul and Chamaipond Tragoonsupachai
Department of Pharmacy Practice, Faculty of Pharmacy, Rangsit University, PathumThani,Thailand

Dirk Höfer
Hohenstein Institute for Textile Innovation, Schlosssteige 1, 74357 Bönnigheim, Germany

Index